Global Impacts on Childhood Social Development

This important book combines insights from disciplines as diverse as developmental psychopathology, pediatrics, and public policy to offer a detailed description of the impact of global crises, such as armed conflict, climate change, and environmental degradation, on the developing child.

This book explores both the direct harms of these crises and those caused indirectly, including family separation, strained caregiving relationships, loss of cultural resources, and damage to children's self-efficacy and emotion regulation abilities. Using case studies from the last few decades, the authors demonstrate the interconnectedness of seemingly disparate systems, such as soil health, family cohesion, individual coping skills, nutrition availability, and economic policy, all with an eye to the urgent developmental processes unfolding within and around the child.

This text is core reading for upper-level undergraduates and graduate students in child psychology, social work, public health, healthcare, public policy, and public affairs. Also, by offering several roadmaps by which individuals, organizations, communities, and nations may leverage resources at each level of a child's ecology to support healthy development, this book will be of interest to professionals working in humanitarian sectors as well as leaders in global pediatrics.

Charles N. Oberg is Pediatrician and Professor Emeritus in Public Health at the University of Minnesota, United States. He is an outspoken advocate for children's rights and has an extensive teaching and research background in child development, pediatrics, and public health. Clinically, he has provided care to refugee and immigrant children both at home and abroad in low- and middle-income countries (LMIC).

Hopewell R. Hodges is an advanced doctoral student and PhD candidate in clinical and developmental psychology at the University of Minnesota's Institute of Child Development. In addition to providing therapy to children and families exposed to multisystem stressors and traumas, she conducts community-based research and trainings on strategies to promote resilient development.

International Texts in Developmental Psychology
Series editor: Peter K. Smith, Goldsmiths College, University of London, UK.

This volume is one of a rapidly developing series in *International Texts in Developmental Psychology*, published by Routledge. The books in this series are selected to be state-of-the-art, high level introductions to major topic areas in developmental psychology. The series conceives of developmental psychology in broad terms and covers such areas as social development, cognitive development, developmental neuropsychology and neuroscience, language development, learning difficulties, developmental psychopathology and applied issues. Each volume is written by a specialist (or specialists), combining empirical data and a synthesis of recent global research to deliver cutting-edge science in a format accessible to students and researchers alike. The books may be used as textbooks that match on to upper level developmental psychology modules, but many will also have cross-disciplinary appeal.

Each volume in the series is published in hardback, paperback and eBook formats. More information about the series is available on the official website at: https://www.routledge.com/International-Texts-in-Developmental-Psychology/book-series/DEVP, including details of all the titles published to date.

Published Titles

Visual and Motor Cognition in Infants and Children: What Develops and What Stays the Same
By Christiane Lange-Küttner

Children's Literacy Development: A Cross-Cultural Perspective on Learning to Read and Write, 3rd edition
By Catherine McBride

Global Impacts on Childhood Social Development: Building Resilience Amid Conflict, Environmental Degradation, and Climate Change
By Charles N. Oberg and Hopewell R. Hodges

'This compelling and readable book brings hope and guidance to the crucial task of building brighter futures for children in these turbulent times. Grounded in developmental theory and research on trauma, risk, and resilience, this volume highlights growing evidence on multisystem threats to child development and the multisystem strategies needed to counteract them. Drawing on research spanning multiple disciples, the authors identify practical ways to reduce risk and promote positive development in a world of increasing uncertainty and existential hazards for children everywhere. An illuminating resource for scholars, students, practitioners, and policymakers.'

Ann S. Masten, PhD, *Regents Professor Emerita of Child Development, University of Minnesota, and author of* Ordinary Magic: Resilience in Development *(2nd ed., 2025)*

'The threats posed by climate change, conflict, and social inequity to the physical and psychological well-being of children are the scourge of our times. Dr. Charles Oberg and Hopewell R. Hodges provide a comprehensive map of how children are impacted by these global threats and what we can do to prevent harm and help heal children in our communities. This is a must-read for researchers, practitioners, policymakers, and students who work on issues related to the well-being of refugee and immigrant children and families.'

Saida M. Abdi, PhD, LICSW, *Assistant Professor, School of Social Work, University of Minnesota*

'Charles Oberg and Hopewell Hodges have thoughtfully and painfully woven together descriptions of three existential threats to the health and development of children throughout the world. Their ability to engage the reader in considering the impact that human behavior and policy decisions have on future generations is both sobering and hopeful. I urge students, activists, policy makers and educators to read this textbook and make a commitment to engage in meaningful action to transform our collective behaviors in order to achieve a more hopeful and dynamic tomorrow. It is our individual and united responsibility to learn and think and act!'

Ellen Benavides, MHA, *Independent Health Policy Consultant*

'In a world increasingly defined by existential challenges to the rights of children to optimal survival and development, *Global Impacts on Childhood Social Development* provides a uniquely comprehensive and cogent discourse to understand and respond to the converging polycrises of our time. Grounded in science, policy, and the principles of human rights, the authors illuminate the devastating effects of inaction, and—most importantly—chart a powerful course forward framed in the context of resilience, justice, and hope. This book is essential reading for anyone committed to building a sustainable and equitable future for all children.'

Jeffrey Goldhagen, MD, MPH, *Professor and Chief of the Division of Community and Social Pediatrics, University of Florida College of Medicine-Jacksonville; President, International Society for Social Pediatrics and Community Health*

'*Global Impacts on Childhood Social Development* is a valuable resource for advocates, educators, practitioners, and researchers who are working with and for children to thrive. The scope and scale of this book creatively intertwines human and climate challenges impacting children's livelihood with innovative responses to collectively engage communities to champion children's rights and resilience. Through collaboration and reciprocity, the authors provide multiple possibilities for facing traumatic events, loss, and displacements head on by centering children as our heart and soul.'

Kristi Rudelius-Palmer, PhD, *Human Rights Educators USA, Strategy Advisor* and *Director*

Global Impacts on Childhood Social Development

Building Resilience Amid Conflict, Environmental Degradation, and Climate Change

Charles N. Oberg and Hopewell R. Hodges

Routledge
Taylor & Francis Group
LONDON AND NEW YORK

Designed cover image: Getty Images

First published 2026
by Routledge
4 Park Square, Milton Park, Abingdon, Oxon OX14 4RN

and by Routledge
605 Third Avenue, New York, NY 10158

Routledge is an imprint of the Taylor & Francis Group, an informa business

British Library Cataloguing-in-Publication Data
A catalogue record for this book is available from the British Library

ISBN: 9781032785325 (hbk)
ISBN: 9781032774879 (pbk)
ISBN: 9781003488385 (ebk)

DOI: 10.4324/9781003488385

Typeset in Galliard
by codeMantra

Contents

Figures and Tables

Figures

Tables

Case Studies

About the Authors

Charles N. Oberg is an outspoken advocate for children's rights. He is a Professor Emeritus in Public Health and Pediatrics at the University of Minnesota, USA. Dr. Oberg has an extensive background in teaching in child development, pediatrics, and public health. His primary clinical focus has been on providing access to primary care to refugee and immigrant families and their children. He has worked internationally in a number of refugee camps and low-income countries.

Dr. Oberg was a SRCD/AAAS Congressional Science Fellow in Washington, DC which broadened his expertise beyond medicine to include government, policy, and advocacy. Dr. Oberg is a founder of Global Child Health Consulting LLC, providing consultation for strategic planning, needs assessments, and program evaluations both in the United States and internationally. He has published over 100 scientific papers in peer-reviewed journals and written and/or edited several books, including *America's Children: Triumph or Tragedy* and *Children on the Move: The Health of Refugee, Immigrant and Displaced Children.*

Hopewell R. Hodges is a PhD candidate in the University of Minnesota's (UMN) joint-track doctoral program in developmental psychology and clinical psychology. In collaboration with clinical, academic, and community networks, she conducts community-engaged research on children's wellbeing. Her particular focus is on positive development in young people exposed to multisystem adversities like forced displacement and housing loss. Because children's health depends to such a large extent on the functioning of surrounding systems, Hopewell focuses much of her attention on building the capacity of the adult world to respond sensitively and creatively to children's needs using locally effective resilience mechanisms. Her clinical work with children and families exposed to trauma often relies on a similar lens of multisystem resilience.

Hopewell holds a bachelor's degree and a master's degree in literature from Yale University, both of which focused on communities' responses to collective trauma like war, genocide, and colonization. In recent years, she has received the P.E.O. Scholars Award, as well as UMN's Doctoral Dissertation Fellowship, the Norman and Edith Garmezy Fellowship, and the President's Student Leadership and Service Award.

Acknowledgments

Charles N. Oberg

I want to express gratitude to Dr. Jeffrey Goldhagen from the University of Florida College of Medicine and Pediatrics–Jacksonville, who has been a friend and colleague for close to 50 years. Dr. Goldhagen's dedication as a child rights advocate of the UN Convention on the Rights of Child has been an inspiration. I would like to extend my gratitude to Dr. Diane Cutts, Head of Pediatrics at Hennepin Healthcare and Co-PI at Children's Healthwatch for her vision of dedication for equitable healthcare and food security for all children. I also thank Jerry Cutts who provided the space and time for the exploration of new ideas. To Dr. Cindy Howard, the former Director of the Global Pediatric Program at the University of Minnesota, for her dedication to medical education and training in global pediatrics. I would also like to thank the International Society of Social Pediatrics (ISSOP) for its perspective that "what's right for all the world's children is children's rights." Many thanks to Kathryn Oberg and Ellen Benavides for their assistance in editorial support. I also thank my friend and co-author Hopewell Hodges for her insight, expertise, and passion for the well-being of marginalized communities. She was an essential necessity for bringing this project to completion. Finally, I am thankful to my family (Linda, Elizabeth, and Kathryn) for their support throughout the writing of this book and to my grandsons, Evan and Owen, wishing them a future in which they can thrive and grow.

Hopewell R. Hodges

I would like to first extend gratitude to my incredible mentors from the University of Minnesota. The guidance and opportunities that Dr. Ann Masten offered to me have ignited a lifelong curiosity about the diversity of resources and processes that can promote each child's positive development, even amid uncertainty and risk. Dr. Saida Abdi helped me grow more ambitious in designing systems that support families, while never losing sight of the children at the center of these processes. Working alongside Dr. Mimi Choy-Brown was a case study in methodological excellence and responsive leadership, and she also taught me how to work sustainably. Meanwhile, I was fortunate to build clinical skills with supervisors and educators like Drs. Danielle Vrieze, Katie

Lingras, Colleen Doyle, Kristina Reigstad, Bonnie Klimes-Dougan, and Linda Deters, and to learn more about systems of intervention delivery with staff, providers, and evaluators involved in Trauma Systems Therapy for Refugees. Continued support from members of Yale University's Clinical Affective Neuroscience and Development Lab (CANDLab)—especially Drs. Dylan Gee and Emily Cohodes—not only helped me find my place in the field, but also taught me how science can be a part of justice for developing individuals. Friends across the country (perhaps especially Marilyn Murray) have helped build my confidence as an advocate for children. I have always hoped for my work to be grounded in joy and relationships. I cannot imagine a better network of mentors and friends to have at my side as I build my identity as an emerging scholar in child development and learn to build lasting bridges between academic, clinical, and community circles.

I am beyond grateful to my husband, John, for continually reminding me of the most important work in the world: to love and be loved. Finally, I wish to thank my friend, Dr. Chuck Oberg, for inviting me to partner with him in building a better world for children. I hope to spend my career helping his lifelong vision—nothing less than thriving, for every child in the world—come nearer to reality.

We are both grateful to the editing and publishing teams at Routledge, including Shivranjani Singh, Shraddha Saikia, and Kathrin Immanuel, and most especially to Molly Selby, whose responsiveness and guidance made this book possible. We also offer grateful remembrance to Dr. Peter K. Smith, the editor of Routledge's series on *International Texts in Developmental Psychology*, who recently passed away. His work and dedication touched the lives of many children throughout the world.

Prologue

Global Risk, Global Opportunity

Most readers will be able to name several reasons that the 21st century is a challenging time in which to be a developing child. These reasons include well-documented damage to both global climate and local environments; widespread displacement; and armed conflict that appears to grow, unchecked, in pernicity. These humanitarian crises generate outrage, often in proportion to our access to accurate information and our commitment to fundamental human rights. The century's crimes against child development mobilize the century's adaptive systems.

This observation reveals a fundamental irony that has lain underneath child development for all of human history: Many of the structures that safeguard development also place it at risk. A drinking well dug in a 17th-century town offers a constant source of freshwater and reduces the amount of time parents must spend searching for water, to the benefit of caregiving availability. Yet if the well is infected with a pathogen, it may become a dangerous vector for diseases.

It is possible that much of what distinguishes the developmental landscape of the 21st century is a matter of scale. The very same internet platforms that enable prosocial civic engagement, facilitate post-disaster crowdfunding, and nurture remote communities are also the platforms that may host disinformation and promote political violence. The infrastructures of energy and trade that have preserved and improved lives worldwide are the same that exacerbate excess, inequity, and climate degradation. The human mind and heart carry the same irony, for it is these organs that both invent and dismantle systems of apartheid, that dreamt up sarin and penicillin. As our human population grows by close to 1% every year, we quantitatively compound our collective capacity for both harm and healing.

At the time of this writing, there are an estimated two billion children on the planet, with more arriving each day in the home we build for them. While current risks to child development are unevenly distributed across regions, nations, and social groups, all two billion face an uncertain future. Uncertainty, we are reminded, is a terrifying state. But it is also the state that makes *hope* possible, as no outcome is prescribed, and no fate is fully sealed (Bauer-Wu, 2022). And so we proceed with our eyes on the hope that presides, latent, over our 21st century. Two billion lives walking into an uncertain future may well face developmental failure on a catastrophic scale. At the same time, if the adults who host them in this world are truly hospitable, these children may grow into two billion people who are healthier, more connected, more creative, and more free than any generations the world has seen before. We hope we have the chance to meet them.

Thoughts from the Authors

This is a book about children. If you are still reading, you are probably aware that this implicates you as well. Whether you interact with them daily (as a caregiver, teacher, social worker, healthcare professional, etc.) or have gone a year without seeing one up close, your livelihood, leisure, beliefs, and the way you navigate the world are relevant to the development of children in your community and around the world. For children enter the world as we are building it.

I (Hopewell) began teaching a recent developmental psychology class by asking undergraduate students if they had ever met a human infant in real life. They all raised their hands, of course, and some laughed. I then asked if they had ever *held* a human infant. The room grew quieter; most still had their hands up. I asked how it felt to hold a baby. They answered: Honored. Scared of dropping it. Excited. Unqualified—"Why did someone trust me with this job?"

This reaction, we concluded together, is a microcosm of the task faced by each generation of adults since humanity emerged. Feeling barely grown ourselves, we are suddenly handed The Children, bundled up and often incomprehensible to us, and yet undoubtedly our responsibilities.

Children move into this world, into our home, as we are building it. And what is the home that we have built for our honored guests? We try to host them in accordance with our love for them—ensure they are given care, food, warmth. Perhaps we think about the invisible furniture in our house as well: economies with room to grow into; a stable jet stream to keep the weather liveable; a *zeitgeist* marked by hope, agency, belonging. How have we done? Is the baby still safely in our arms where it started?

To adults reading this book, we are grateful for the people, systems, and resources—visible and invisible to you—that have made your development possible. We encourage you to call them to mind as you begin reading and, with courage, to consider the ways you are equipped to support the development of children of today. (To precocious children who read this: We hope that you feel represented well—that we have been honest in describing the hurdles that we in the adult world have laid across your developmental journeys, but also that we have been honest about your potential as thrivers, creators, leaders, and so much more. We have tried to keep you in mind in our writing, as we always do.)

Hopewell R. Hodges

This book proceeded from my (Charles') past experiences as a pediatrician and child rights advocate providing care and support to children and families facing the stress of multisystem crisis.

I had the opportunity to travel as a pediatrician to provide care for refugee children in multiple locations including northern Jordan and on the island of Lesvos, Greece. In Jordan I served families at the Al Zaatari camp, at the time the second largest refugee camp in the world with over 80,000 inhabitants. On Lesvos, I worked at Moria, the camp surrounded by cement walls and fences. It was during the winter months, snow had fallen followed by freezing rain. Despite best efforts, resources were woefully inadequate. Referrals for specialty care were limited or non-existent. Quality shelter and nutrition were hard to provide in such settings. Children spent days, weeks, and months with little opportunity to play in a safe and nurturing environment. There were multiple NGOs providing assistance, including the United Nations High Commission on Refugees (UNHCR), Save the Children, Euro Relief, and the Red Cross/Red Crescent. These groups were dedicated to their mission and goals to assist families in need. However, there were limited resources such as playgrounds, toys, books, and learning spaces that help children be children. In addition, many of the children had experienced and/or witnessed trauma, both in their home country or on their exodus to safety and a new life (beatings, shootings, assaults, torture, family separation, etc.), and all had experienced the stress of living in unlivable conditions. Access to mental health services was woefully limited. The complaints we heard in the medical clinic were a blur of physical, emotional, interpersonal, and spiritual ailments.

Yet there was a palpable hope that one day things would be better. Families shared their aspirations for a better future. Daily, parents expressed gratitude that someone listened as they shared the story of their journey, affirmed their worth, acknowledged their struggle, and celebrated their humanity. You could see in their eyes and their smiles that each was seeking a better life for themselves and their children. The children I saw were just a fraction of the million children and youth who have been displaced from their homes due to war, conflict, natural disasters, and climate change. We have an obligation to believe in these children's potential and their right to a full and joyful future.

Charles Oberg

Introduction

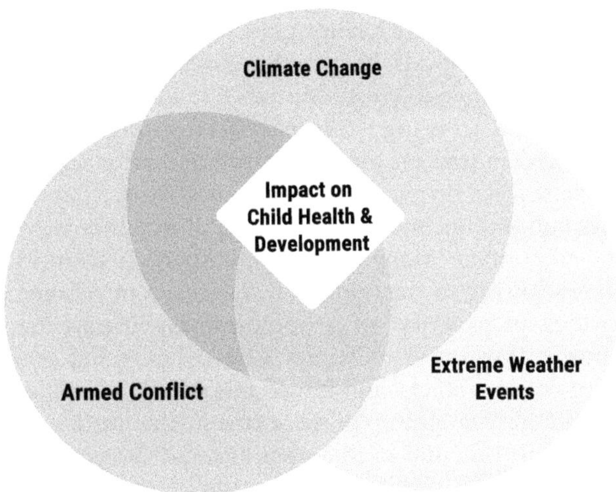

Figures 0.1 Impacts of geopolitical crises, environmental damage, and climate change on child health.

The 21st century is marked by converging and existential threats to the health and development of children, most especially geopolitical and inter-group tensions, environmental degradation, and climate change. These dangers converge to cause armed conflicts, natural disasters, poverty, and forced displacement, all of which disproportionately affect the lives of children. Conversations about large-scale global challenges must center on the vulnerability and needs of our planet's youngest members. As these crises accelerate, they not only impact greater numbers of children to greater extents, but they also deplete many of the resources and protective factors that can ensure a healthy future for developing people. If we do not acknowledge these risks that impact children's futures, we will fail to adequately protect them from these impending catastrophes. Our inaction may result in generations of children struggling to reach their potential, and, as a result, a global civilization with an uncertain future. Figure 0.1 provides a schematic of how geopolitical, environmental, and climate crises intersect to impact children's health and development.

Impact of Climate Change, Geopolitical Crises, and Extreme Weather Events

Geopolitical crises are growing more frequent and intense, impacting the development of an increasing number of children and families. These crises include international wars, intrastate conflict (civil wars), gang violence, growing wealth gaps, human trafficking, forced migration, closing of international borders to children on the move, and the rise in autocratic and dictatorial leaders. Armed conflict is increasingly urbanized and entails the targeting and damage of civilian targets. Unfortunately, as will be explored throughout this book, most people injured or killed in 21st-century armed conflicts are civilians like children.

Environmental crises are expected to continue accelerating, too, as the impact of human-caused climate change grows. These crises include food insecurity, droughts, famines, floods, hurricanes, and decreased availability of potable water. For example, in low-lying countries like Bangladesh, groundwater is becoming salinized due to rising sea levels. While armed conflict remains the main cause of forced migration globally, displacement is increasingly tied to climate-driven factors like drought-related resource scarcity and economic collapse due to agricultural decline. Indeed, these events themselves often cause or intensify armed conflict. Many nations now struggle to meet the needs of children who are growing in the middle of war zones or refugee camps.

Part I provides an overview of geopolitical, environmental, and climate change crises in the 21st century. Chapter 1 describes recent geopolitical (GP) events, including wars, conflicts, and forced migration, as well as the particular vulnerability of children caught up in these crises. Chapter 2 summarizes some of the extreme environmental events over the last 20 years, such as flooding, hurricanes/typhoons, wildfires, extreme temperatures, deforestation, and toxin exposure, again noting children's distinct vulnerability to these disasters. Chapter 3 concludes with an overview of climate change and its role as an exponential multiplier of geopolitical and environmental events.

Part II describes the mechanisms that influence child development during times of societal disruption, using Bronfenbrenner's socio-ecological framework as an organizational principle. Chapter 4 focuses on the *individual* child, with special emphasis on the pre- and perinatal periods, as well as infancy. This part of the text describes basic individual adaptive systems and the ways that these help children to meet their major developmental milestones, as well as the ways these systems may be threatened by crisis and upheaval. In Chapter 5, we discuss the *microsystem*, the environment closest to the developing child, with special attention to the quality of the caregiver-child relationship early in life and its impacts on subsequent development. This chapter also examines risks to the microsystem's functioning due to stress and trauma, as well as potential protective factors that help to mitigate the impacts of surrounding crises on these relationships. Chapter 6 discusses both the *mesosystem* and the *exosystem*. The mesosystem represents the connections between the different microsystems of the child's life (e.g., the home/family, caregivers, and schools) and with the exosystem, the larger community of extended family, neighborhood, and community, where children's exploration and activities help to further build their capacities for problem solving, self-esteem, mastery, competence, and identity. This chapter also describes the ways that conflict and disaster may impact the development of these age-expected competence skills. Chapter 7 focuses on the *macrosystem*, the cultural and broad societal structures that shape children's development (often via their impact on more proximal systems). We attend here especially to gender equality and its impact on social development through factors like access to primary education. The chapter shows how gender dynamics can be shaped by armed conflict, extreme environmental events, and climate change. Chapter 8 focuses on the *chronosystem*, a child's situation in time (e.g., in changing global landscapes and in their own lifecourse trajectories). It reviews how the prolonged exposure to adversity can impact development in the long term, and how resources like social capital can support resilient trajectories.

Part III explores in detail a few societal flashpoints accentuated by the three major themes of the textbook (armed conflict, environmental crises, and climate change). Chapter 9 examines forced displacement and the plight faced by children and youth who have had to leave their homes. Chapter 10 explores the convergences of conflict, famine, and climate degradation in the Sahel of Africa over the last several decades, showing how the structural adversities created in this area—and the developmental threats that accompany them—provide glimpses of the risks posed by climate change for current and future generations worldwide. Chapter 11 examines the difficult topic of genocide, war crimes, and crimes against humanity, encouraging readers to not only think of these as historical events from the past, but rather as persistent realities that continue in the 21st century. This chapter attends to the impacts of these atrocities on children's development, along with efforts by the international community to hold aggressors accountable. Chapter 12 describes multisystem processes that give rise to child labor exploitation, the impact of this practice on children's development, and global efforts to reduce child labor—efforts that, according to the International Labor Organization (ILO), have stalled after two decades of progress. Chapter 13 discusses the roles of technology in the lives of children, with focus on the intersections of social inequity with technological innovation. Chapter 14 is dedicated to a discussion of Indigenous populations and the disproportionate impacts of conflict and climate change on child development in these communities. Chapter 15 concludes this part with an overview of the challenges faced by "exceptional children," young people whose levels of need distinguish them from the rest of their age cohorts and who need special support to reach their full potential to thrive.

Part IV is dedicated to interventions that have potential to support development in light of the multisystem threats described throughout this book. Chapter 16 addresses the benefits of using a trauma-informed lens for care in medical systems, refugee resettlement practices, educational environments, and policies. Chapter 17 presents a child rights approach to advocacy and services, describing how practical approaches like UNICEF's Child Friendly Cities Initiatives can mobilize practical supports. Chapter 18 introduces the concepts of developmental resilience science (DRS) and resilience-informed systems, describing how systems, policies, and practices can be designed to promote resilient child development amid 21st-century risks. Chapter 19 describes ways that adults may be equipped to tell the truth about children's needs, children's rights, and children's potential in the world using ethical, effective research that responds to community needs and strengths.

Chapter 20 delves into advocacy, whether in the form of legislation and policy change or in the form of art. This part of the text posits that creative expression, one of the oldest and most resonant forms of communication, can bear witness to children's plight and potential, moving individuals and groups to create a better world for children. Chapter 21 discusses protest strategies that center and amplify youth's voices. Chapter 22 points to the growing fragility of our world's inter- and intranational unity, as well as promising strategies for promoting peace. We conclude with Chapter 23, which describes approaches to protecting children's global climate in the long term, with a special emphasis on sustainable systems of environmental protection and attention to young climate champions.

Conclusion

This text combines insights from the diverse disciplines of developmental psychology, pediatrics, public health, and public policy to describe the impacts of global crises on the developing child. The goal was to highlight the interconnectedness of seemingly disparate systems to promote the well-being of all future children. In the face of existential threats to children's survival and development, adults must prepare to show persistence, creativity, and collaboration. Of course, one cannot predict all the specific adversities that children will face in the coming decades. At the same time, a great deal is already known about the tools needed to protect, nurture, and restore children's wellbeing in the face of dynamic and diverse challenges. The text offers readers several roadmaps by which individuals, organizations, communities, and nations may leverage potent protective factors and resources to support healthy development. It ends with a call for hope, hospitality, and resilience, for the sake of our children's future.

Part I

Introduction

Convergence of Armed Conflict, Extreme Weather Events, and Climate Change

Adults in the 21st century are inundated with reminders of our world's instability in the form of natural disasters, economic crises, geopolitical conflicts, political extremism, and countless other reasons to turn on (or turn off) the news. Depending on readers' fields of study and awareness of global events, some of the content of the chapters that follow may already be familiar. What these chapters may offer, even to the seasoned climate scientists or avid reader of the news, is two-fold. First, they argue that most global and regional crises are more interconnected to one another than may initially meet the eye. In this sense, it is wise for, say, an expert in nutrition to become aware of the impacts of drought on long-term soil health and the impacts of conflict on food distribution infrastructure. Second, these chapters aim to bring discourse about armed conflict, environmental degradation, and climate change down to the level of the developing child. Natural and human-made crises alike disproportionately impact those who are already the most vulnerable, and so children's vulnerability must be centered in conversations about preventing and responding to future catastrophes.

The urgency of children's needs can serve as a beacon for the voyage through the remainder of the 21st century. Coordinated, intentional, and creative action for children in the coming decades can build resilient systems that support children's wellbeing and, in the process, support the health of entire communities. Such efforts can help communities apply a child-centered interpretive lens to global and local events alike—"How will this policy change impact family functioning?" "What must be prioritized in this disaster response effort?"—and equip communities of adults to ask these questions with skill and persistence.

DOI: 10.4324/9781003488385-1

1 Armed Conflict in the 21st Century

1.1 Introduction: Overview of Armed Conflict

The term "armed conflict" encompasses a wide range of crises, including those within and beyond national borders, conflicts involving only state actors, and conflicts involving non-state actors (Kadir et al., 2018). Armed conflict has always posed indirect threats to children, for reasons discussed throughout this book. It increasingly causes direct threats to them as well: It has been estimated that 90% of deaths in the first decades of the 21st century occurred among civilians (Garfield, 2008; Zwi et al., 2006). Figure 1.1 provides a visual depiction of the impact of geopolitical crises on children's health and development.

The darkened circles represent the type of conflicts that may arise, and the lighter circles represent the potential consequences of the conflicts. The causes of armed conflicts within and between nations include political differences, territory disputes, religious and ideological conflicts, and access to vital resources, to name just a few. This century, it has not been uncommon for

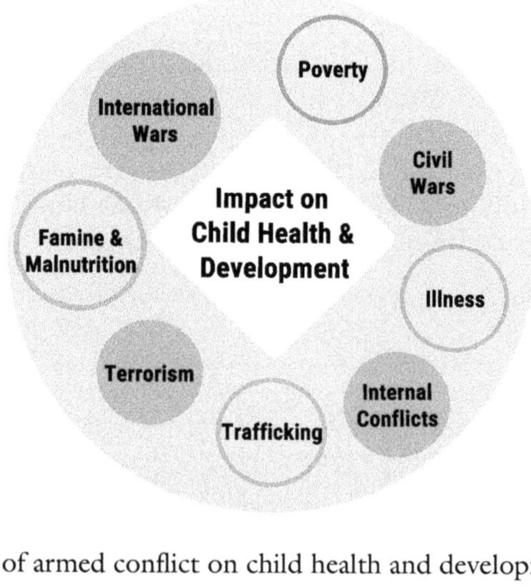

Figure 1.1 Impacts of armed conflict on child health and development.

DOI: 10.4324/9781003488385-2

outside countries to align with forces within a country attempting to sway the conflict toward their own interests. The threat of terrorism, both within and outside of nations, continues to play a large role in shaping global politics. Many of these trends will be discussed later in this chapter and throughout the textbook.

Conflict—both threatened and actual—has substantial impacts on children's health and development. Poverty very often co-occurs with conflict and is often severe enough to result in food macro-malnutrition (i.e., inadequate intake of calories, carbohydrates, proteins, and essential fatty acids) and micro-malnutrition (i.e., deficiencies of iron, zinc, electrolytes, or vitamins). As a result, children may suffer from growth delays, developmental disorders, and acute or chronic illnesses. War and conflict can also leave children more vulnerable to harm through maltreatment, exploitation, and trafficking. All these topics will be explored in more detail throughout the book, always with an emphasis on approaches to sustaining children's health, ameliorating trauma and harm, and promoting resilience.

Case Study: The Rohingya Crisis

The Rohingya are a minority group who have lived primarily for the last few centuries in Myanmar, formerly known as Burma. They are a Muslim minority in a largely Buddhist country. The Rohingya have been denied Myanmar citizenship since 1982 and are therefore a stateless population, often deprived of basic rights and protection. In 2017, renewed violence broke out against the Rohingya, spurred by social media postings (including some endorsed or posted by government officials). This conflict has resulted in widespread forced displacement, sexual exploitation, and gender-based violence. A number of international organizations have deemed that the Rohingya have suffered crimes against humanity and genocide. It is estimated that 2.6 million survivors were internally displaced in Myanmar, with 1 million refugees migrating to Bangladesh, more than 75% of whom are women and children.

Armed conflict and extreme weather events have interacted to amplify Rohingya people's vulnerability in recent years. Every June through October, Myanmar experiences monsoons, which bring torrential wind, rain, and landslides. Due to displacement and structural violence, many Rohingya people now live with contaminated water supplies, leaving them especially vulnerable to infectious diseases like hepatitis, malaria, dengue fever, and chikungunya that are accentuated by improper sanitation. In May of 2023, Cyclone Mocha caused particular damage in Myanmar and Bangladesh to Rohingya communities, which often lacked stable shelter and infrastructure. At present, many Rohingya people are dependent on organizations like the United Nations (UN) for daily living needs. In the meantime, local and international pressure has been mounting to ensure that Rohingya people can safely return to their homes in the long term, and that Myanmar's leadership is held accountable for ethnic cleansing, genocide, and crimes against humanity.

UNHCR (2024)

1.2 Major Recent Conflicts

Figure 1.2 shows a schematic of some of the major conflicts that have occurred or are still occurring during the first quarter of the 21st century. A number of these will be discussed in greater detail throughout this chapter.

Historically, the "archetypal war" was a governmentally sanctioned armed conflict between two or more countries' militaries. However, this type of engagement is the exception rather than the rule in the 21st century. For example, some of the major conflicts of the 21st century thus far are proxy wars, with international players that are not involved directly, but tangentially participate through, for example, sending money or weapons. Some conflicts reflect tensions between ethnic or religious groups, as with Boko Haram in Nigeria.

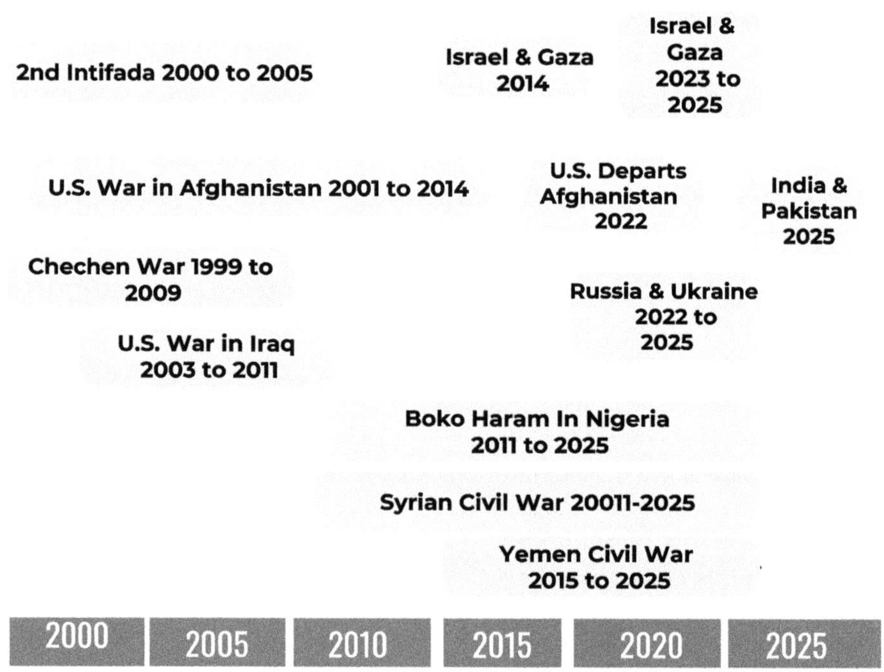

Figure 1.2 Timeline of selected armed conflicts in the 21st century.

The causes of armed conflict all originate in the adult world, yet too often the effects of armed conflict are felt most strongly by children. Through much of history, civilian status could be expected to protect a person from the worst of the direct effects of fighting, but the burden of war has increasingly shifted onto civilians (Rieder & Choonara, 2012). In addition to their limited mobility, their dependence on the systems around them, and the physical vulnerabilities that arise from their physiology and size (Meddings, 2001), children and the spaces they occupy are increasingly targeted by armed combatants. One notable example is the Russian bombing of the Maternity and Children's Hospital in Mariupol, Ukraine and of the Children's Hospital in Kiev (Reuters, 2022). The number of the world's children killed and injured by armed conflict in a given year can number in the tens of thousands, numbers which show no signs of slowing (UN, 2022; UN, 2024).

At the time of writing, one of the vivid examples of children's vulnerability in armed conflict is taking place in Palestine. After a Hamas terrorist raid into Israel killed 1,200 Israelis and took over 200 hostages in 2023, Israel began a military incursion into Gaza which quickly resulted in tens of thousands of deaths, with 70% of victims being women and children (PBS, 2024). Over 13,000 children had died by 2024, close to 800 of whom were under the age of one (UNICEF, 2024). In addition, in September of 2024, Israel opened another front in the Middle East by attacking southern Lebanon in an attempt to neutralize Hezbollah's capacity. In both Gaza and Lebanon, Israel has launched both ground and air assaults on housing units, hospitals, and schools, placing children in the crossfire. The rationale is that both Hamas and Hezbollah use such settings to hide in plain sight and to use civilians as human shields. As discussed later in the section on International Humanitarian Law, it is illegal to target such locations unless there is a documented use of civilians as protection there. However, even in these cases, the principle of "proportionality" states that the killing of civilians must be proportional to the value of the military target being attacked. There is significant debate in the international community as to the proportionality of these attacks by Israel. In 2023, the International Criminal Court (ICC) issued an arrest warrant for Prime Minister Benjamin Netanyahu and Yoav Ballant, Israel's Minister of Defense, alleging criminal responsibility for war crimes and crimes against humanity committed in Gaza (ICC, 2024).

As noted, armed conflicts frequently intensify existing adversities in affected communities. The invasion of Gaza followed a decade-long blockade of humanitarian aid, including food and water, that had already caused widespread hunger. In 2024, the UN Relief and Works Agency for Palestine Refugees estimated that 90% of the Gazans were faced with food insecurity without the influx of more humanitarian aid (UNRWA, 2024). By April 2025, with ongoing ballistic rocket attacks and the continual blockage of humanitarian food relief for 70 days, experts warned of a "critical risk of famine" for one in five Gazans (United Nations, 2025).

Finally, 2025 saw a reemergence of tension between the nuclear powers of India and Pakistan, focused on the territory of Kashmir, which has been a subject of dispute since the establishment of both countries. Presently, this region is divided between Pakistan in the west, India in the south, and China in the northeast. Conflict has usually centered on the Pakistan-India border. In May of 2025, militants entered the India-controlled territory and killed 26 civilians. Pakistan claimed it had no involvement in the terrorist attacks. India nevertheless responded with missile and drone attacks on presumed militant strongholds in the Pakistan region. Concern quickly mounted that this exchange, combined with ongoing and historic tensions, would escalate into a major regional war.

Many major 21st-century conflicts have involved the United States, including the wars in Afghanistan, Syria, Yemen, Somalia, and Mali, all conflicts with high rates of child casualties. It is important to note that these casualties are often underestimated due to the lack of systematic documentation (Adamkiewicz & Goldhagen, 2021).

1.3 Impact of Armed Conflict on Children

Armed conflicts increasingly invade children's backyards, neighborhoods, parks, and playgrounds. Children are often injured and killed by explosive devices, while they are playing, doing chores, or engaging in other daily activities (Frost et al., 2017). Compared to adults, children are more likely to experience severe injury or death during explosions, and such events are sadly among the most common civilian casualties of recent wars (Edwards et al., 2012; Creamer et al., 2009). The use of chemical weapons is prohibited under international law, including both the 1925 Geneva Protocol and the Chemical Weapons Convention (CWC) passed in 1993. However, there have been numerous examples of their use since these prohibitions. For example, authorities documented the use of chlorine gas and sarin during the Syrian Civil War (Brooks et al., 2018).

These weapons are also especially likely to harm children, since they are most damaging to those with small body size, faster breathing, and less mature cardiovascular regulation (Rotenberg & Newmark, 2003). Children also have more permeable blood-brain barriers, making them more vulnerable to nerve agents like sarin, and therefore to lasting neurodevelopmental damage (Rubin & Staddon, 1999).

Armed conflict also presents particular risk to young children due to their high dependence on surrounding infrastructures; indeed, people under the age of five have sometimes been those most likely to die from indirect effects of conflict (Guha-Sapir & Panhuis, 2004). Militant groups commonly take over hospitals or health clinics to use for hostage detention or firing locations, often killing or abducting healthcare workers in the process. One potent example occurred in South Sudan, where 170,000 people lost access to essential healthcare because a clinic was attacked. Sana'a, Yemen experienced an airstrike that cut off a hospital's electricity, which ended the lives of several infants who were on ventilators.

Armed conflict frequently results in an increase in preventable diseases by damaging multiple systems that usually help to keep children healthy. As children lose access to stable nutrition and preventative healthcare, their immune systems may weaken, leaving them more vulnerable to respiratory and gastrointestinal diseases. In Yemen, over 10,000 child deaths within the first few years of the most recent civil war were attributed to disrupted access to vaccines and routine healthcare (SHCC, 2016). Poliomyelitis has almost been eradicated from the globe in the past, but continues to emerge in war-torn areas. In Gaza, polio had been absent for over 25 years, but a case was identified in the fall of 2024. The case led to a temporary cease fire and a campaign to vaccinate 649,000 Palestinian children (WHO, 2024).

Access to prenatal care is often very hard during conflict, despite the fact that the risks of adverse outcomes are higher when pregnancies occur during armed conflict (Price & Bohara, 2013; Torche & Shwed, 2015). These harms occur through damage to maternal health, of course, and also through the cascading effects of parental trauma on children's development (Slone & Mann, 2016). Meanwhile, children often lose access to education during armed conflict, as their schools are inadvertently damaged, co-opted by military groups, or attacked intentionally—for example, by groups that seek to undermine girls' access to education (GCPEA, 2014).

As will be discussed in Chapter 5, one of the most pernicious dangers to the developing child is the loss of a stable caregiving relationship through death or separation. In addition to fostering children's healthy growth, a healthy caregiving relationship also helps to protect children from traumas like exploitation, abuse, and food insecurity. Children who have lost one or both parents are especially vulnerable to dangers during and after migration or conflict (Kibret, 2015).

1.4 Interconnectedness of Conflict, Environment, and Economy

Armed conflict has diverse and cascading impacts on a wide range of systems beyond the battlefield, often leading to environmental degradation, economic collapse, crop failure, and hunger, all of which present multisystem dangers to children. One of the major consequences of armed conflict is the widespread displacement of families, discussed further in Chapter 9.

Hunger and environmental crises relate to armed conflict both directly and indirectly, as discussed in Chapter 2. Political conflicts are increasingly among the primary causes of food insecurity globally (de Waal, 2018). Cases like the Ethiopian civil war of the 1980s show how commonly environment-related famine and armed conflict influence each other bidirectionally (Clay & Holcomb, 1986). Similarly, Bangladesh's economic and social resilience was drained following the devastating Bhola Cyclone in 1970, such that further flooding sent the nation into widespread food shortage (Fakir, 2019; Hossain,

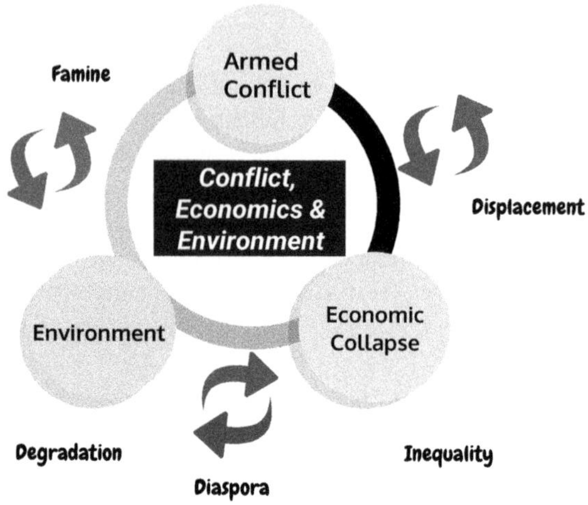

Figure 1.3 Interconnectedness of conflict, environment, and economy.

1999). In more recent years, Yemen has experienced a famine independent of environmental catastrophes. Since 2015, a civil war between internationally recognized government forces and Houthi resistance fighters has drawn shadow participation from many other nations. A resulting military stalemate has caused pervasive economic collapse, inflation, and a very high unemployment rate. Meanwhile, the country's food infrastructures have suffered serious damage. A coalition from the United Arab Emirates has blocked a major port, preventing nutritional aid from reaching the people of Yemen (Mohareb & Ivers, 2019). Elsewhere, combatants have intentionally destroyed crops. By 2018, more than 85,000 children had died, and UNICEF once estimated that over 12 million children needed life-saving humanitarian assistance (Graham 2021; UNICEF, 2020).

Most recently at the time of this writing, Russia's invasion of Ukraine has indirectly resulted in food insecurity for large parts of the world, as Russia blockaded several of the Black Sea ports involved in the international distribution of Ukraine's large grain reserves (Hussein & Knol, 2023). This blockade is a potent reminder of the interconnection of *all* nations, with conflict in one country cascading to impact the wellbeing of others around the world.

1.5 Conclusion

The first quarter of the 21st century has seen armed conflicts on an unprecedented scale that, tragically, shows no sign of abating. Conflicts increasingly harm children and the systems that usually help to keep young people alive and healthy. Economic, political, and environmental risks coalesce and lead to the initiation or intensification of conflict. In turn, conflict can exacerbate damage to economies, sociopolitical landscapes, and environments.

Those wishing to learn more about the impacts of armed conflict on child development are encouraged to read on. Part II applies a socio-ecological lens to children's health and wellbeing in light of surrounding insults to their development. Part III on Global Societal Flashpoints will examine the impact of specific conflict-related adversities on the wellbeing of children, such as forced displacement (Chapter 9) and conflict in the Sahel (Chapter 10). Finally, Part IV will provide a number of approaches to protect the lives of children facing armed conflict, including research, trauma-informed care, child rights, resilience-informed systems, advocacy, youth voices, and strategies for promoting peace.

Reflection Questions

At the end of each chapter, several questions are offered that reference some of the key content covered. Readers may benefit from these opportunities to reflect on the chapter and to assess their own responses. Such reflection may help with the consolidation of core arguments from the chapter and the integration of themes and ideas.

Question 1. Have any new wars or armed conflicts emerged in the world since this book came out? Have any of the ones described in the text been resolved? How did these conflicts begin and end?

Question 2. Can you describe three direct and three indirect ways in which armed conflict impacts children's development and wellbeing?

Question 3. Figure 1.3 attempts to capture the interconnectedness between conflict, economy, and environment. Can you think of examples from your lifetime?

Question 4. How can people in your own community work to protect children affected by armed conflict? What makes it easier or harder to do these things?

References

Adamkiewicz, T., & Goldhagen J. (2021). Mitigating Armed Conflict Casualties in Children. *Pediatrics*, 147 (2): e2020027847. 10.1542/peds.2020-027847

Brooks, J., Erickson, T. B., Kayden, S.Ruiz, R. Wilkinson, S. & Burkle, F.M. (2018). Responding to chemical weapons violations in Syria: Legal, health, and humanitarian recommendations. *Conflict and Health*, *12*, 12. https://doi.org/10.1186/s13031-018-0143-3

Clay, J. W., & Holcomb, B. K. (1986). *Politics and the Ethiopian Famine 1984–1985.* Transaction Books.

Creamer, K. M., Edwards, M. J., Shields, C. H., Thompson, M. W., Yu, C. E., & Adelman, W. (2009). Pediatric wartime admissions in U.S. military combat support hospitals in Afghanistan and Iraq: Learning from the first 2,000 admissions. *Journal of Trauma*, *67*(4), 762–768.

Declaration, S. S. (2015). Global Coalition to Protect Education from Attack. *N. d.) N. p.* URL: https://protectingeducation. org/wp-content/uploads/documents/documents_safe_schools_declaration-final. pdf. [in English].

de Waal, A. (2018). *Mass Starvation: The History and Future of Famine*. Polity Press.

Edwards, M. J., Lustik, M., Eichelberger, M. R., Elster, E., Azarow, K., & Coppola, C. (2012). Blast injury in children: An analysis from Afghanistan and Iraq, 2002–2010. *Journal of Trauma and Acute Care Surgery, 73*(5), 1278–1283. https://doi.org/10.1097/TA.0b013e318270d3ee

Fakir, A. (2019). Footprints of war and famine: Intrauterine and inter-generational effects of the 1971 Bangladesh Liberation War and the 1974 Bengal Famine. *Journal of Bangladesh Studies, 19*(1 & 2), 1–13.

Frost, A., Boyle, P., Autier, P., King, C., Zwijnenburg, W., Hewitson, D., & Sullivan, R. (2017). The effect of explosive remnants of war on global public health: A systematic mixed-studies review using narrative synthesis. *The Lancet Public Health, 2*(6), 286–296. https://doi.org/10.1016/S2468-2667(17)30099-3

Garfield, R. (2008). The epidemiology of war. In B. S. Levy, & V. W. Sidel (Eds.), *War and public health*. (2nd ed., pp. 23–36). Oxford University Press.

Graham, L. (2021). Pathways to accountability for starvation crimes in Yemen. *Case Western Reserve Journal of International Law, 55*, 401–440.

Guha-Sapir, D., & Panhuis, W. G. (2004). Conflict-related mortality: An analysis of 37 datasets. *Disasters, 28*(4), 418–428. https://doi.org/10.1111/j.0361-3666.2004.00267.x

Hossain A. (1999). Professor Amartya Sen and the 1974 Bangladesh Famine: Additional insights and policy implications. *Journal of Bangladesh Studies, 1*, 31–62.

Hussein, H., & Knol, M. (2023). The Ukraine war, food trade and the network of global crises. *The International Spectator*, *58*(3), 74–95. https://doi.org/10.1080/03932729.2023.2211894

International Criminal Court (2024). Statement of ICC Prosecutor Karim A.A, Khan, KC: Application for the arrest warrants in the situation in the State of Palestine. ICC Statement, May 20, 2024. https://www.icc-cpi.int/news/statement-icc-prosecutor-karim-aa-khan-kc-applications-arrest-warrants-situation-state

Kadir, A., Shenoda, S., Goldhagen, J., & Pitterman, S. (2018). Section on international child health. The effects of armed conflict on children. *Pediatrics, 142*(6), e20182586

Kibret, B. T. (2015). Armed conflict, violation of child rights and implications for change. *Journal of Psychology and Psychotherapy, 5*(4), 202.

Meddings, D. R. (2001). Civilians and war: A review and historical overview of the involvement of non-combatant populations in conflict situations. *Medicine, Conflict and Survival, 17*(1), 6–17. https://doi.org/10.1080/13623690108409551

Mohareb, A. M., & Ivers, L. C. (2019). Disease and famine as weapons of war in Yemen. *New England Journal of Medicine, 380*(2), 109–111.

PBS (2024). At least 43,000 Palestinians killed, more than half women and children in war in Gaza, Palestinian Health Ministry says. October 28. https://www.pbs.org/newshour/world/at-least-43000-palestinians-killed-more-than-half-women-and-children-in-war-in-gaza-palestinian-health-ministry-says

Price, J., & Bohara, A. K. (2013). Maternal health care amid political unrest: The effect of armed conflict on antenatal care utilization in Nepal. *Health Policy and Plan, 28*(3): 309–319. https://doi.org/10.1093/heapol/czs062

Reuters (2022). 287 Children Killed in Ukraine Since Russian Invasion Began, June 11. https://www.ndtv.com/world-news/287-children-killed-in-ukraine-since-the-russian-invasion-began-report-3057853

Rieder, M., & Choonara, I. (2012). Armed conflict and child health. *Archives of Diseases in Childhood, 97*(1), 59–62. https://doi.org/10.1136/adc.2009.178186

Rotenberg, J. S., & Newmark, J. (2003). Nerve agent attacks on children: Diagnosis and management. *Pediatrics, 112*(3), 648–658. https://doi.org/10.1542/peds.112.3.648

Rubin, L. L., & Staddon, J. M. (1999). The cell biology of the blood-brain barrier. *Annual Review of Neuroscience, 22*, 11–28. https://doi.org/10.1146/annurev.neuro.22.1.11

Safeguarding Health in Conflict Coalition (SHCC) (2016). No protection, no respect: Health workers and health facilities under attack. https://www.safeguardinghealth.org/sites/shcc/files/SHCC2016final.pdf

Sloan, M., & Mann, S. (2016). Effects of war, terrorism, and armed conflict on young children. *Child Psychiatry Human Development, 47*(6), 950–965. https://doi.org/10.1007/s10578-016-0626-7

Torche, F., & Shwed, U. (2015). The hidden costs of war: Exposure to armed conflict and birth outcomes. *Sociological Science, 2*(27), 558–581. https://sociologicalscience.com/download/volume-2/december/SocSci_v2_558to581.pdf

UNHCR (2024). The Rohingya refugee crisis explained. August 22. https://www.unrefugees.org/news/rohingya-refugee-crisis-explained/#Fires

UNICEF (2020). Millions of children's lives at high risk as Yemen inches closer to famine. https://www.unicef.org/press-releases/millions-childrens-lives-high-risk-yemen-inches-towards-famine

UNICEF (2024). More than 13,000 children reported dead in Gaza as famine nears. *UNICEF*, March 19. https://www.unicefusa.org/stories/more-13000-children-reported-dead-gaza-famine-nears

United Nations (2000). The impact of armed conflict on children: Filling knowledge gaps. A proposal by the Special Representative of the Secretary-General for Children and Armed Conflict. (UN 2000). Annex 2, December. https://www.mofa.go.jp/policy/human/child/survey/annex2.html#III_i

United Nations (2025). Gaza: Starvation looms for one in five people, say food security experts. *UN News*, May 12, 2025. https://news.un.org/en/story/2025/05/1163131

United Nations General Assembly Security Council (2022). Children and armed conflict: Report of the Secretary-General. A/74/845–S/2020/525. https://undocs.org/en/S/2020/525.

United Nations General Assembly Security Council (2024). *Secretary-General annual report on children and armed conflict.* United Nations. https://docs.un.org/en/S/2024/384

UNRWA, (2024). UNRWA situation report #149 on the humanitarian crisis in the Gaza strip and the West Bank, including East Jerusalem. November 27. https://www.unrwa.org/resources/reports/unrwa-situation-report-149-situation-gaza-strip-and-west-bank-including-east-jerusalem

WHO (2024). Humanitarian pauses vital for critical polio vaccination campaign in the Gaza Strip. *World Health Organization*, August 16. https://www.who.int/news/item/16-08-2024-humanitarian-pauses-vital-for-critical-polio-vaccination-campaign-in-the-gaza-strip

Zwi, A. B., Grove, N. J., Kelly, P., Gayer, M., Ramos-Jimenez, P., & Sommerfeld, J. (2006). Child health in armed conflict: Time to rethink. *Lancet, 367*(9526), 1886–1888.

2 The Environment

Extreme Weather Events and Human-Caused Pollution

2.1 Introduction

As discussed in the introduction, extreme weather events and environmental crises like droughts, floods, fires, and hurricanes can curtail a child's health and development and even cause death. Natural disasters can be categorized into two major types. The first are subsurface events like volcanoes, earthquakes, and tsunamis. The second are surface and atmospheric events like droughts, floods, hurricanes/cyclones, and fires; these have been increasing in

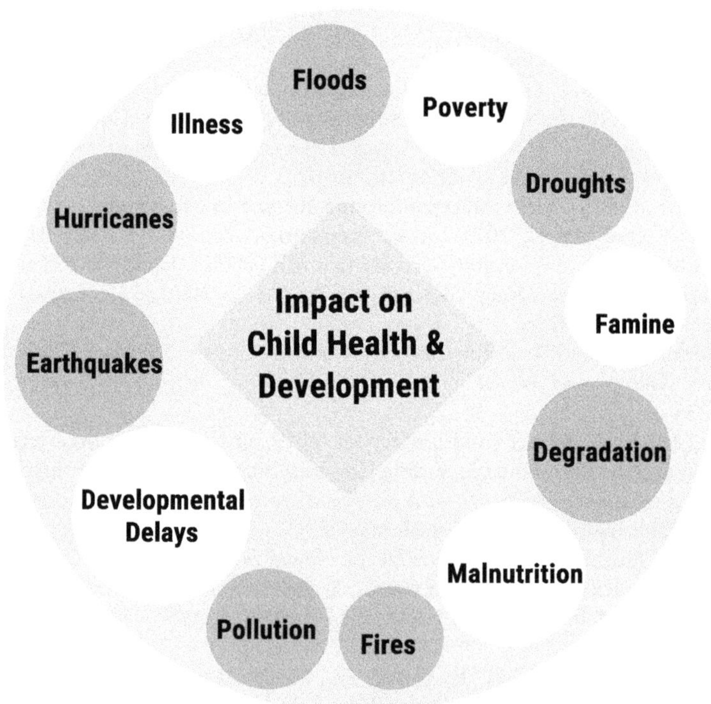

Figure 2.1 The impacts of weather and environmental events on child development.

DOI: 10.4324/9781003488385-3

frequency and intensity. Human-made environmental degradation and pollution also have lasting impacts on the lives of children. In addition to directly harming children (e.g., by exposing them to carcinogens), these patterns can both cause and exacerbate poverty, famine, malnutrition, and illness (Figure 2.1).

2.2 Subsurface Events: Earthquakes and Tsunamis

In 2004, an underwater earthquake of 9.1 magnitude occurred in the Indian Ocean, off the western coast of northern Sumatra. The resulting tsunami destroyed 800 km of coastal Aceh Province, with damage reaching 6 km inland. Approximately 230,000 people died, making this tsunami one of the deadliest disasters in modern history. Furthermore, 35,000 children were orphaned (UNICEF, 2004). Indirect harm accumulated in the following months, since the disaster disrupted sanitation, potable water supplies, and health care.

The 2010 Port-au-Prince earthquake in Haiti is estimated to have affected 1.2 million people and over half a million children in what is widely considered the poorest country in the Western hemisphere (UNICEF, 2011).

In 2011, the 9.0-magnitude Tohoku earthquake and tsunami struck Japan, causing widespread flooding and destruction of coastal towns, as well as the release of radioactive materials from the Fukushima Nuclear Power Plant. Like the Chernobyl nuclear disaster in 1986, much of this area will be uninhabitable for decades to come, with the human toll of injury and illness yet to be fully realized. The death toll was immense, with close to 20,000 people killed and thousands injured or missing. In addition, there was massive internal displacement of over 300,000 people with entire communities destroyed.

All of these calamities must be viewed from an equity lens. While an earthquake itself does not discriminate, it is common for damage to be unevenly distributed. Wealthy nations, of course, are often better positioned to invest in infrastructure to mitigate damage (e.g., levees and quake-resistant building practices), respond rapidly with critical aid to those affected, and rebuild. Within countries, people from marginalized communities often live, work, and play in areas more vulnerable to the impacts of natural disasters. They may also have fewer resources to rebuild or seek help in the aftermath of property loss and injury.

2.3 Surface and Atmospheric Events: Droughts, Flooding, Fires, and Hurricanes/Typhoons

According to the Intergovernmental Panel on Climate Change, Sixth Assessment Report (IPCC, 2021), the human-caused rise in greenhouse gases has increased the frequency and intensity of extreme weather events and surface and atmospheric natural disasters. In addition, human activity has increased the cost of destruction. For example, when coastal wetlands and marshes that ordinarily buffer inland areas from flooding are filled in to create more land for development (most commonly for more affluent populations), overall damage from flooding and rainfall is often more extensive.

Preparing for and responding to these events requires coordinated efforts within and across nations, and it has been all too common this century for children to suffer as a result of inadequate responses. An adaptive and functioning economy, societal peace, sustainable food production systems, resilient infrastructures, and international connections can help protect children and their communities before, during, and after these crises. When any of these protective resources are compromised, it is all too common for famine, conflict, and economic collapse to occur, disproportionately impacting those who are already most vulnerable. Similarly, damage to the environment reduces a community's resilience to future extreme weather events.

There have been 13 major hurricanes/cyclones in the 21st century that have caused over 1,000 deaths, including Hurricane Katrina, affecting the United States in 2005; Sidr, affecting Bangladesh in 2007; and Nargis, which caused over 138,000 fatalities around the North Indian Ocean in 2008.

Case Study: Cyclone Daniel

In September of 2023, Cyclone Daniel became the deadliest Mediterranean cyclone on record. Initially, it formed as a low-pressure system that impacted Greece, Bulgaria, and Turkey with extreme flooding. The low pressure then organized as a cyclone in the Mediterranean, causing catastrophic flooding in Libya that caused the collapse of major dams and the destruction of about a quarter of the city of Derna. By the time Cyclone Daniel weakened, it had affected multiple nations with tens of thousands of deaths, and 100,000 counted missing in Libya alone. This storm damaged critical infrastructure and left thousands homeless. Nearly 300,000 children were affected as floods and infrastructure loss caused the spread of waterborne diseases and, often, displacement.

Flooding is a part of many regions' annual environmental cycles, yet many communities are seeing increases in flood severity. The American Geophysical Union has documented that 100-year floods are anticipated to occur yearly by the end of 21st century due to rising sea levels (AGU, 2023). Severe flooding in India in 2020 and 2022 resulted in some of the costliest natural disasters in world history.

Droughts are prolonged precipitation deficiency that results in significant water shortage. An increasing number of droughts occurred around the globe in the 21st century across virtually every continent. These are often long-lasting; for example, Australia's Millennium Drought lasted from 2001 to 2009. Northern Africa and Somalia have experienced the most prevalent and persistent drought of the 21st century to date (NAPA, 2013). Meanwhile, environmental degradation, deforestation, desertification, and increasing soil dryness have diminished the land's resilience to extreme weather hazards (FAO, 2013).

Studies by the National Aeronautics and Space Administration (NASA) have found that extreme wildfires are becoming more frequent, more intense, and larger. Climate models project that the risk of very large wildfires will increase by up to six-fold in parts of the United States by the middle of the century (Cunningham et al., 2024). Increasing heat and drought fuel wildfires, secondary to the evaporation of moisture from the soil and the drying of underbrush. Recent examples of wildfires made worse by these phenomena include the Maui wildfires of 2023 and the fires in Australia's Victoria state in 2009.

2.4 Natural Disasters, Armed Conflict, and Famine

While famine has often been thought of as a natural phenomenon, scholars and activists increasingly describe it as a social one; after all, even a severe drought does not result in food availability decline (FAD) if a country's economy, supply chains, trading relationships, and transportation infrastructures are intact (Sen, 1981). In fact, natural disasters, famine, and armed conflict exist in strong bidirectional relationships with each other. A natural disaster can exacerbate inequality, inter-group tension, and poverty, leading to increased risk of armed conflict. Meanwhile, armed conflict frequently damages a region's agricultural, nutritional, and water infrastructures, while causing environmental degradation that increases the community's vulnerability to extreme weather in the future. Unfortunately, armed conflict and food insecurity frequently spread and escalate rapidly within regions.

In 2022, flooding across several African nations affected over 5.6 million people's access to food. For example, flooding along the Niger River caused food insecurity in Nigeria, South Sudan, and northwestern Malawi (Reed et al., 2022). Droughts have caused devastating famine in East Africa in recent years. Somalia in particular has seen droughts increasing in frequency and intensity over the past three decades, accompanied by declining food production, especially across central and southern Somalia (NAPA, 2013; Santur, 2019). A famine in 2010–2012 caused 260,000 deaths, half of which occurred in children under the age of five (Halakhe, A. 2022).

Famines in the 21st century have been especially likely to follow armed conflict (de Waal, 2018). For example, Sudan has seen conflict between the governmental army and several militia groups, causing an economic downturn, skyrocketing food prices, and a reduction in agricultural productivity. Affected areas have seen widespread FAD as a result, with two thirds of the population estimated to need food assistance, 18 million people experiencing acute hunger, and five million identified as facing a hunger emergency (WFP, 2024). The Democratic Republic of Congo (DRC) has also faced a severe famine tied to 25 years of armed conflict, with an estimated 25.4 million people living in households identified as food-insecure in the second half of 2023 (WFP, 2023). In addition, 4.4 million children, pregnant women, and breast-feeding women were acutely malnourished, with 900,000 children severely malnourished.

2.5 Exposure to Environmental Toxins

Despite national and international attempts at mitigation, the world remains dependent on plastic and other non-degradable products, toxic pesticides and herbicides, and other contaminants (lead, mercury, dioxin, arsenic, etc.) that impact fetal and child development (Sivakumar & Stefanski, 2007). Toxin exposure disproportionately affects vulnerable communities as industrial plants, waste facilities, strip mines, and other sources of pollution are frequently located in close proximity to economically marginalized families with children (Landrigan & Goldman, 2011). The environmental health burden from human-made pollution is also of immense importance. Pollution of air, water, and soil can cause disease in humans directly while also disrupting critical systems like sanitation and agriculture. The greatest risk of pollution is often felt by children (ALA, 2024).

Lead was one of the first pollutants and neurotoxins that was recognized as harmful to development, with awareness emerging early in the 20th century that lead exposure could cause encephalopathy, coma, and even death in children (Needleman, 1990). However, residual effects in children surviving lead poisoning went unrecognized for decades, and the toxin remained present in a range of commercial products, including paint, gasoline, plumbing pipes, and even toothpaste. In the 1960s, in response to research noting that high levels of lead exposure were related to impairments in intellect, behavior, and sensory-motor function, standards were established for the diagnosis and treatment of lead intoxication (WHO, 1995). However, it is now known that no level of lead exposure is healthy or acceptable, with even very small levels in the blood over a period of time proving detrimental to infant and child brain development (Roberts et al., 2022). Lead also binds to hemoglobin in the blood, displacing iron and leading to anemia. It can build up in children's bones, making it more difficult to remove the toxin through chelating agents.

Awareness and action around lead exposure has come slowly and in stages. In 1978, the U.S. Environmental Protection Agency (EPA) banned the use of lead in residential paints. It was outlawed as a fuel additive in 1973 and completely banned by the EPA in 1996. However, the legacy of lead poisoning remains a serious concern, especially in marginalized communities worldwide. In 2014, the predominantly Black U.S. community of Flint, Michigan, switched its water source from Lake Huron to the Flint River. The water supply from the Flint River contained corrosive agents that leached lead from the city's pipes. After this transition, communities complained about the look and smell of the water. Children's blood titers showed a doubling and tripling of lead levels (Hanna-Attisha et al., 2016). It is widely accepted that governmental responses to this crisis were insufficient due largely to systemic racism.

Global inequity shapes children's exposure to toxins like lead, with children in low- and middle-income countries (LMICs) often disproportionately likely to be exposed to pollutants (Erickson et al., 2021). Kabwe, a city 80 miles north of Zambia's capital (Lusaka), was home to one of the world's largest zinc and lead mines from 1906 to 1994. In 2022, the UN identified Kabwe as one of most lead-polluted places on the planet. Of 500 children under the age of 5 who were tested for lead, all had measurements that exceed safe levels (NPR, 2025). Children in this community also had an alarmingly high death rate.

There is also extensive data on the toxic developmental effects of mercury, polychlorinated biphenyls (PCBs), alcohol, and nicotine, as well as many pesticides and solvents (Stein et al., 2002). The effects of mercury on the developing brain were first recognized in Minamata Bay, Japan, in the 1950s, where people often consumed fish that swam in mercury-contaminated industrial runoff. Infants born to mothers who consumed the fish showed diverse challenges like cognitive impairment, gait disturbances, speech difficulties, and impairments in sucking, swallowing, and other reflexes (Harada, 1978). Often, their mothers showed no signs of mercury poisoning. Mercury poisoning, as with other types of poisoning, often occurs through bioconcentration, where a chemical builds up over time in an organism and reaches higher levels as one moves up the food chain; meanwhile, substances dispersed in water persist for long spans of time there, appearing in higher concentrations in fish that swim there. In this way, contaminants in water may be concentrated more than a million-fold in food consumed by people. The prenatal and infancy periods are times of rapid neurodevelopment, so transmission of concentrated mercury through the placenta or breastfeeding is particularly damaging. Many nations now issue guidelines on the safe consumption of fish (especially larger game fish) during pregnancy and breastfeeding (FDA, 2025). Critically, deficits in language, memory, and attention can result from even very low levels of prenatal mercury exposure (Weihe & Grandjean, 2012).

Dixons and other PCB compounds are a large group of 209 fat-soluble chemicals that were produced through the mid-20th century, used as lubricants and insulators in electrical equipment. Once released into the atmosphere, PCBs move with the winds and eventually settle on pastures and water bodies. Though PCB production has been banned or heavily restricted in most of the industrialized world for decades, it continues to bioaccumulate within the food chain, particularly in beef, dairy products, and fish that are relatively high in fat (Adamou et al., 2020; Lallas, 2001). Indigenous populations often face especially high risks of exposure to PCBs and dioxins. PCBs are thought to mimic estrogen, resulting in concerns about reduced fertility, abnormal menstrual cycles, and altered sex hormone levels (Eskenazi, et al., 1985). They appear to also be endocrine disruptors and to affect the functioning of the thyroid pathway in animal models, with human studies showing similar findings (Haddow et al., 1999). Specifically, even transient disruptions in the release of thyroid-stimulating hormone (TSH) from the hypothalamus, and subsequent production of Thyroxine T4, can alter neuronal branching and brain architecture. Newborns exposed to dioxins experience adverse developmental effects like reduced birth weight, and exposure may be associated with decreased cognitive ability, learning and memory challenges, and increased behavior problems in children (Mei-Lin et al., 1994).

Pesticides are biological or chemical compounds developed to kill animal and plant pests. The three major classes include insecticides (to kill insects), fungicides (to kill fungi and molds), and herbicides (to kill weeds). Scientific development of pesticides accelerated in the 1940s, and these compounds are still expansively used to promote crop production throughout the world. Many common pesticides have neurotoxic properties for humans. Several decades ago, the World Health Organization already reported three million acute, severe pesticide poisonings, with as many or more cases estimated to be unreported, and approximately 220,000 deaths annually (Ecobichon, 1996). Families living near agricultural operations are at an increased risk of exposure.

Visible plastic waste is everywhere in our world, including in our oceans and on our shorelines, wreaking havoc on flora and fauna. Furthermore, plastics do not biodegrade, but rather break down into smaller units, many of which are endocrine disruptor chemicals (EDCs) like bisphenol A (BPA), phthalates, per- and polyfluoroalkyl substances (PFAS) and brominated flame retardants (BFRs). This class of molecules is often referred to as "forever chemicals" (Ullah et al., 2023), circulated throughout our land, air, and water, and growing in bioconcentration as animals consume them.

Armed conflict, unsurprisingly, is a major source of toxin exposure for children. A recent article documented that chromium, uranium, tungsten, mercury, and other toxins appear in the hair of mothers and newborns in war zones, with the possibility of serious developmental consequences as infants grow (Punamäki et al., 2025). In fact, infants demonstrated problems in sensorimotor, cognitive, communication, and socioemotional skills like emotional regulation. A similar study found that exposure to old U.S. and U.K. munitions in Iraq was responsible for lead and mercury contamination, which was associated with increased risks of miscarriage, congenital defects, and infant heart malformations (Rubaii, 2020).

2.6 Deforestation

Deforestation entails cutting down forests for agriculture or development purposes, or to supply wood for fuel, industry, or construction. The results include loss of much-needed carbon sinks (systems that sequester or remove carbon from the atmosphere), ecological collapse, loss of flora and fauna, economic degradation, and displacement of communities. Unfortunately, wood is being harvested faster than it can regrow. The main agents in deforestation globally are large corporations that engage in activities like mining, dam construction, agriculture, ranching, and timbering (Bodo et al., 2021). Loss of trees can impact climate and rainfall even in geographically removed areas.

Deforestation also has disproportionate impacts on the most vulnerable people. One notable example comes from the case of fuelwood gathering. Historically, wood fuel has been used for cooking and heating by 70% of people in LMICs (Foley, 1985). The majority of wood in these regions is not commercially traded but is directly collected by the users, principally women and children. However, the wood supply has been vanishing in many nations due to the increasing demand for commercial fuels from wood and charcoal, and many individuals and families must travel further and further distances to find fuel (Waris & Antahal, 2014). When fuelwood is in short supply, families are forced to burn fuels such as cow dung, crop stems, and husks, which can sometimes rob the soil of needed nutrients. Eventually, fuel shortages can shorten the cooking time of meals and reduce the number of meals a family cooks, which increases malnourishment.

Conflict and deforestation are interrelated, with conflict-affected countries especially affected by the loss of forests, including Syria, Afghanistan, Ukraine, Angola, and Lebanon (CEOB 2021).

2.7 Conclusion

Environmental disasters, whether naturally caused, human-caused, or diversely caused, have a disproportionate impact on the most vulnerable, especially on children. These events and a community's collective response to them are closely related to armed conflict, inequality, and climate. Many types of environmental disasters are increasing in severity and frequency, such that they are likely to pose increasing risks to children in the coming years.

Reflection Questions

Question 1. Do you notice any trends in environmental events over the course of your lifetime?

Question 2. What has to happen for a community to fully recover from a major environmental event like a flood, hurricane, or tornado? How long do these events typically stay in the public's awareness?

Question 3. Do you think we are making progress in reducing or eliminating human-made environmental toxins? What needs to happen to make our efforts more effective?

Question 4. Are you aware of any social media advocacy initiatives that are addressing and making a meaningful contribution in awareness and response to environmental events? Give an example.

Question 5. How does public response differ to disasters that are perceived as natural versus human-caused?

References

Adamou, T. M., Riva, M., Muckle, G., Sidi, E. A. L., Lemire, M, & Ayotte, P. (2020). Blood mercury and plasma polychlorinated biphenyls concentrations in pregnant Inuit women from Nunavik: Temporal trends, 1992–2017. *Science of The Total Environment, 743*, 140495, ISSN 0048-9697, https://doi.org/10.1016/j.scitotenv.2020.140495.

ALA (2024). Who is most affected by outdoor air pollution. *American Lung Association*, September 18. https://www.lung.org/clean-air/outdoors/who-is-at-risk

American Geophysical Union (AGU) (2023). 100-year floods could occur yearly by the end of the 21st century, September 12. https://www.preventionweb.net/news/100-year-floods-could-occur-yearly-end-21st-century

Bodo, T., Gimah, B. G., & Seomoni, K. J. (2021). Deforestation and habitat loss: Human causes, consequences and possible solutions. *Journal of Geographical Research, 4*(2), 22–30.

CEOB(2021).Deforestationinconflictareasin2020.CouncilandEnvironmentObservatory.April21.https://ceobs.org/assessment-of-recent-forest-loss-in-conflict-areas/2

Cunningham, C. X., Williamson, G. J., & Bowman, D. M. J. S. (2024). Increasing frequency and intensity of the most extreme wildfires on earth. *Nature, Ecology & Evolution, 8*, 1420–1428. https://doi.org/10.1038/s41559-024-02452-2

de Waal, A. (2018). *Mass starvation: The history and future of famine*. Polity Press.

Erickson, B., Hu, H., Nash, E., Ferraro, G., Sinitsky, J., & Taylor, M. P. (2021). Blood lead levels in low-income and middle-income countries: a systematic review. *Lancet Planetary-health, 5*, e145–e153.

Ecobichon, D. (1996). Toxic effects of pesticides. In C. Klaassen (Ed.), *Casarett & Doull's toxicology: The basic science of poisons* (5th ed., p. 643). McGraw-Hill.

Foley, G. (1985). Wood fuel and conventional fuel demands in the developing world. *Ambio*, 14(5), 253–258

Halakhe, A. (2022). We Were Warned: Unlearned Lessons of Famine in the Horn of Africa. *Refugees International, https://www. refugeesinternational. org/reports/2022/12/7/we-were-warned-unlearned-lessons-of-famine-in-the-horn-of-africa.*

FDA (2025). Food and drug administration, advice about eating fish for those who might become pregnant or are pregnant or breastfeeding and children ages 1–11 years old. https://www.fda.gov/food/consumers/advice-about-eating-fish

Food and Agriculture Organization of the United Nations (FAO) (2013). *Resilient livelihoods-disaster risk reduction for food and nutrition security*, April.

Haddow, J. E., Palomaki, E., Allan, W. C., Allan, W.C.M., Williams, J.R., Knight,G.,J., Gagnon,J., O'Heir, C.E., Mitchell, M., L., Hermos, R.J., Waisbren, S.E., Faix, J.D., & Klein, R.,Z., 1999). Maternal thyroid deficiency during pregnancy and subsequent neuropsychological development of the child. *The New England Journal of Medicine, 341*(8), 549–55.

Hanna-Attisha, M., LaChance, J., Sadler, R. C., & Allison Champney Schnepp, A. C. (2016). Elevated blood lead levels in children associated with the Flint drinking water crisis. A spatial analysis of risk and public health response. *American Journal of Public Health, 106*, 283–290, https://doi.org/10.2105/AJPH.2015.303003

Harada, H. (1978). Congenital minamata disease: Intrauterine methylmercury poisoning. *Teratology, 18*, 285–288.

IPCC (2021). Summary for policymakers. In V. Masson-Delmotte, P. Zhai, A. Pirani, S. L. Connors, C. Péan, S. Berger, N. Caud, Y. Chen, L. Goldfarb, M. I. Gomis, M. Huang, K. Leitzell, E. Lonnoy, J. B. R. Matthews, T. K. Maycock, T. Waterfield,

O. Yelekçi, R. Yu, & B. Zhou (Eds.), *Climate change 2021: The physical science basis. Contribution of working group i to the sixth assessment report of the intergovernmental panel on climate change* (pp. 3–32). Cambridge University Press. https://doi.org/10.1017/9781009157896.001. https://www.ipcc.ch/report/ar6/wg1/downloads/report/IPCC_AR6_WGI_SPM.pdf

Lallas, P. L. (2001). The Stockholm convention on persistent organic pollutants. *American Journal of International Law*, *95*(3), 692–708. https://doi.org/10.2307/2668517

Landrigan, P. H., & Goldman, L. G. (2011). Children' vulnerability to toxic chemicals: A challenge and opportunity to strengthen health and environmental policy. *Health Affairs*, *30*(5), 842–850.

Mei-Lin, M.Y.,Hsu,C.,C., Guo, Y.L., Lai,T.J., Chen, S.J., Luo, J.M. (1994). Disordered behavior in the early-born Taiwan Yu-Cheng children. *Chemosphere*, *29*; 2413–2422.

National Adaptation Programme of Action on Climate Change (NAPA) (2013). Ministry of National Resources. Federal Republic of Somalia, April, p. 14.

Needleman, H. L. (1990). The future challenge of lead toxicity. *Environ Health Perspect*, *89*, 85–89.

NPR (2025). This may be the most lead polluted place on Earth. Is there any hope? March 30. https://www.npr.org/sections/goats-and-soda/2025/03/30/g-s1-51935/toxic-mines-zambia-polluted-lead-poisoning

Punamäki, R. L., Diab, S. Y., Vänskä, M., AlBarqouni, N., & Quota, S. R. (2025). Maternal and foetal exposure to potentially toxic metals of modern weaponry and infant cognitive, sensorimotor, and socioemotional development: The role of breastfeeding. *Infant Behavior and Development*, *79*, 102040.

Reed, C., Anderson, W., Kruczkiewicz, A. Nakamura, J., Gallo, D., Seager, R., & McDermid, SS. (2022). The impact of flooding on food security across Africa. *PNAS*, *119*(43), e2119339199. https://doi.org/10.1073/pnas.2119399119

Roberts, D., Bradberry, S. M., Butcher, F., & Busby, A. (2022). Lead exposure in children'. *BMJ*, *377*, e063950. https://doi.org/10.1136/bmj-2020-063950

Rubaii, K. (2020). Birth defects and the toxic legacy of war in Iraq. *Middle East Report*, *296*, 1. ISSN 0899–2851.

Santur, H. (2019). Weather and War: How Climate Shocks are compounding Somalia's problems. *The New Humanitarian*, *19*.

Sen, A. (1981). *Poverty and famines: An essay on entitlement and deprivation*. Clarendon Press.

Sivakumar, M. V. K., & Stefanski, R. (2007). Climate and land degradation—an overview. In M. Sivakumar, & N. Ndiang'ui (Eds.), *Climate and land degradation. Environmental science and engineering (environmental science)*. Springer. https://doi.org/10.1007/978-3-540-72438-4_6

Stein, J, Schettler, T., Reich, F., Wallinga, D., & Valenti, M. (2002). In harm's way: Toxic threats to child development. *Journal of Developmental and Behavioral Pediatrics*, S13–S22.

Ullah, U., Ahmad, S., Guo, S., Ullah, X., Ullah, S., Nabi, G., & Wanghe, K. (2023). A review of the endocrine disrupting effects of micro and nano plastic and their associated chemicals in mammals. *Frontiers in Endocrinology*, *13*, 1084236. https://doi.org/10.3389/fendo.2022.1084236

UNICEF (2011). How the earthquake in Haiti impacted the lives of children-Photo essay. August 17. https://www.unicef.org/lac/en/stories/how-earthquake-haiti-impacted-lives-children

UNICEF (2004). Indian Ocean earthquake and tsunami-UNICEF response at six months update. https://www.unisdr.org/files/2044_VL108103.pdf

Waris, V. S., & Antahal, P. C. (2014). Fuelwood scarcity, poverty and women: Some perspectives. *Journal of Humanities and Social Science* (IOSR-JHSS), *19*(8), 21–33. *e*-ISSN: 2279–0837, *p*-ISSN: 2279–0845.

Weihe, P., & Grandjean, P. (2012). Cohort studies of Faroese children concerning potential adverse health effects after the mothers' exposure to marine contaminants during pregnancy. *Acta Veterinaria Scandinavica*, *54*(Suppl 1), S7. https://doi.org/10.1186/1751-0147-54-S1-S7

WHO (1995). Inorganic lead. *Environmental Health Criteria*, *165*, 153.

World Food Program (WFP) (2023). https://www.wfp.org/countries/democratic-republic-congo

World Food Program (WFP) (2024). Emergency Sudan. February 19. https://www.wfp.org/emergencies/sudan-emergency#:~:text=Sudan%20is%20facing%20a%20rapidly,recorded%20during%20the%20harvest%20season.

3 Climate Change

The Existential Multiplier

3.1 Introduction

The United Nations Framework Convention on Climate Change (UNFCCC) conceptualizes climate change as alterations in climate patterns that are attributable, directly or indirectly, to human activity (IPCC, 2018). Importantly, the global climate has always been variable, and the planet has seen much colder and warmer periods than it has seen today. When climate change is referenced, the term typically refers to changes that are over and above the natural variability observed in global climate (e.g., over the course of seasons, decades, and centuries) and are human-caused. Much of the world's population already feels acute effects of climate change, and many readers will have likely reflected on changes in their regional climate over the course of their own lifetimes, such as decreases in precipitation or altered growing seasons.

Climate change presents the greatest existential risk to humanity in the 21st century and beyond, and its impending consequences demand a concerted international effort (Clark et al., 2020; UNICEF, 2025). These risks are thought to be especially high for children, who are likely to suffer to a greater extent from climate degradation. Half of the world's 2.2 billion children live in the 33 countries deemed at "extremely high risk" from the effects of climate change (UNICEF, 2021). Often, these are also countries facing increasing frequency and severity of armed conflict and weather-related disasters, which is not coincidental.

Adults have been aware of climate change for many decades, but ambivalence, denial, inaction, and conflicts of interest have dominated global responses through all these years of opportunity. The global scientific community identified that when annual average temperatures exceeded 1.5 degrees above preindustrial temperature, some of the most dangerous effects of climate change would occur with more speed and severity. Unfortunately, 2024 was the hottest year to date at the time of this writing, with an average temperature of 1.6 degrees Celsius above preindustrial temperatures (Scientific America, 2025).

This chapter defines climate change as a multiplier of life-threatening events, as shown in Figure 3.1, and describes some of the impacts that climate change is expected to have on the lives and development of children.

DOI: 10.4324/9781003488385-4

Preventing these risks would have been feasible through concerted international efforts. Instead, the danger has arrived. Adults can now work to develop mitigation strategies and attempt to reverse this damage where possible, all the while protecting children who are caught up in the effects of adult activity.

3.2 Climate Change and Natural Systems

Human activity alters global climate in several ways. First, industries and individuals engage in practices, from burning coal to flying planes to agriculture, that release gases like carbon dioxide and methane. These emissions alter the composition of the global atmosphere, resulting in more of the sun's heat becoming trapped close to the earth's surface. Meanwhile, deforestation and loss of marine plant life reduces the amount of carbon that is absorbed from the atmosphere each day. The result is that global temperatures rise over time.

Another important part of this equation is the existence of climate "feedback loops," where the early effects of climate change accelerate the damage. For example, ice coverage in the Arctic Circle has a powerful buffering effect to keep the planet's temperature habitable: This surface reflects much of the sun's radiation back out into the atmosphere. As rising temperatures begin to reduce the coverage of ice in the Arctic Circle, the world also loses access to this important buffering system, and temperatures rise faster (Bauer-Wu, 2024). Each time a forest fire reduces tree coverage, the world loses hectares' worth of carbon-absorbing power, also accelerating the rise of temperatures and, therefore, the risk of future fires. Many commonly referenced projections of climate change fail to account for these feedback loops.

The following sections discuss some of the common consequences of climate change.

3.2.1 Temperature and Ocean

At the time of this writing, the last two consecutive years have broken records for high global temperatures. Springs often start earlier, and fall lasts longer. In the summers, an increasing number of populated areas now experience long periods in which thermometers consistently reach above 37° or 38° Celsius (about 100°F), and even above 43°C (110°F). On average, the world now loses roughly 150 billion metric tons of ice per year in Antarctica and 270 billion tons in Greenland. The loss of ice from these two ice sheets is responsible for about a third of elevations in the global sea level to date (NASA, 2024). It estimated that global average sea level has risen 8–9 inches since 1880, and the rate is accelerating. Coastal lands and islands are increasingly threatened, compromising the health and economy of many nations. The subsequent loss of coastlines, reductions in arable and habitable land, and resource scarcity will cause increases in displacement and even armed conflict. UN Secretary-General António Guterres has stated that, "the world will witness a mass exodus of entire populations on a biblical scale" (United Nations, 2023), from small islands, coastal communities, and major population centers. In many places, the rising sea has already accelerated the salination of groundwater, such that people in some densely populated areas (e.g., large parts of Bangladesh) have lost access to safe water (Rakib et al., 2020).

Meanwhile, ocean currents appear to be weakening as global temperatures rise. Currents are created and maintained by a few factors, including the planet's rotation and surface winds, and also from the circulation of warmer and colder water. As water warms, it sinks more slowly, decelerating ocean currents (IPCC, 2021). Currents in polar regions are expected to continue weakening, as well as huge currents like the Atlantic Meridional Ocean Circulation (AMOC).

3.2.2 Global Weather

With changes in climate—that is, long-term patterns in the atmosphere—there are also changes in weather. Warming and rising waters have given rise to increases in the frequency and intensity of hurricanes and cyclones, as well as accompanying storm surges. Flooding and tornadoes are also growing more severe, and "hundred-year floods" occur nearly annually now in many regions. Rainfall often gets heavier, since warmer oceans result in more water evaporating into the atmosphere.

The fall of 2024 serves as its own case study in the scale and scope of the disasters exacerbated by climate change. Asheville, North Carolina was long considered one of the U.S.' "climate havens," sitting at over 2,000 feet of elevation and therefore held to be safe from many natural disasters. On September 28, 2024, the Asheville region experienced widespread and fatal destruction from Hurricane Helene. Just days later, Hurricane Milton caused 45 tornadoes to touch down in Florida. Meanwhile, torrential rainfall in North Africa brought flash floods to several cities, including Sousse, Tunisia. The same month, a slow-moving storm called Boris submerged entire neighborhoods across Europe, including Austria, Poland, Slovakia, and the Czech Republic. This storm's slow speed was attributed to the ineffectiveness of the jet stream, which ordinarily keeps winds moving through the region. Nepal, India, and Bangladesh also experienced unusually severe flooding at the end of September.

3.2.3 Water Cycles and Water Scarcity

The convergence of rising global temperatures, rising ocean levels, the weakening of air and water currents, water mismanagement, and disruptive land use has caused "unprecedented stress" on the global water cycle (Global Commission on the Economic of Water, 2024), which has historically distributed water atmospherically in predictable ways. As a result, some areas are commonly inundated with water surplus, while others face water scarcity. Four billion people experience severe water scarcity for at least one month each year and over two billion live in countries where water supply is consistently inadequate (Mekonnen & Hoekstra, 2016). Roughly a quarter of the world's children will be living in areas of extremely high water stress by 2040 (UNICEF, 2024), and the disruption of the water cycle threatens more than 50% of the world's food production (Global Commission on the Economics of Water, 2024).

3.3 Climate Crisis: An Exponential Multiplier to Risks for Children

In addition to increasing the impact of extreme weather events, climate change already appears to be intensifying social adversities like armed conflict, poverty, and food insecurity. As with climate feedback loops themselves, climate-related disruptions to human communities' protective resources can leave them more vulnerable to further adversity. As such, climate change can be thought of as exponentially multiplying individuals' and communities' risk of adversity.

3.3.1 Interpersonal Unrest and Armed Conflict

Extreme weather events, along with the loss of arable and habitable land due to rising sea levels, create contexts of resource scarcity as families struggle to access food, water, and livelihood opportunities. Globally, weather crises like floods are associated with onset and intensification of conflict and political tensions, and also with the economic downturns and food insecurity that often lead to revolts and widespread protests (Ide et al., 2021; Younes, 2015). Meanwhile, declines in agricultural productivity can exacerbate existing inequalities to increase the risk for conflict (UN, 2023). Climate change also causes widespread migration, which can increase tensions in transit communities and resettlement nations.

Hotter weather has long been associated with an increase in physically aggressive behaviors (O'Neal, 2016), with one study concluding that homicide rates would increase by 6% for every 1°C elevation in global temperatures (Perry & Simpson, 1987). Adverse climate events have been estimated to cause a 20–30% increase in human trafficking, along with a higher risk for domestic violence (UN Women, 2025). More children each decade will be raised by parents who themselves suffered early exposure to established risk factors for violent behavior, such as poor nutrition, witnessing conflict, and family disruption (Mares & Moffett, 2016).

3.3.2 Growing Inequities

As families face mounting resource scarcity amid natural disasters and loss of usable land, more children in lower- and middle-income countries (LMICs) will experience education disruptions. Environmental damage leads children to attend school less frequently (or cease formal education altogether) and enter the workforce to support their families (Putnick & Bornstein, 2015). The jobs given to children are often dangerous, and children are often injured

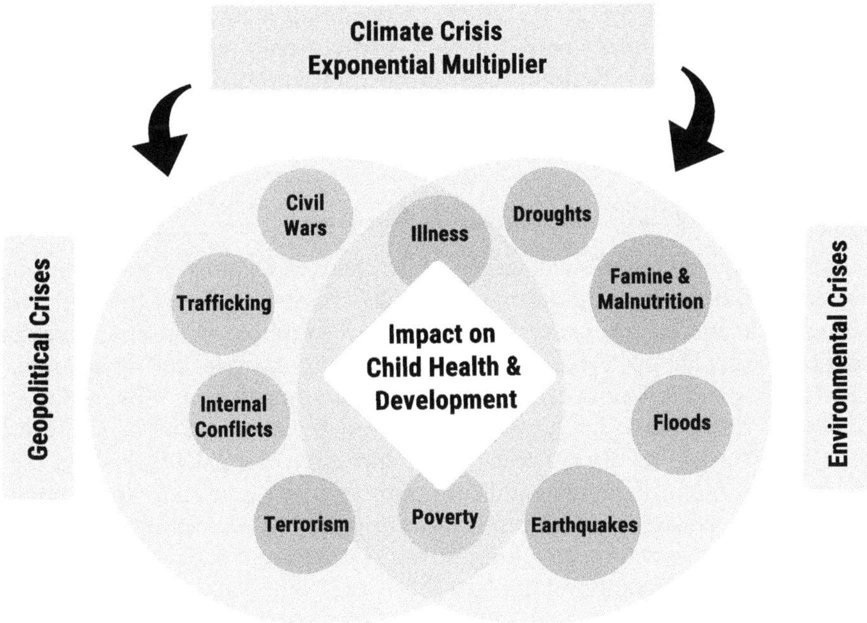

Figure 3.1 Climate change: The exponential multiplier.

or made ill through heat stroke or exposure to dust and heavy metals (Watts et al., 2019).

Needless to say, families and communities that are already economically marginalized are less able to rebound from environmental shocks and gradual climate degradation. After environmental disasters, children from lower-income families are less likely to receive nutritious meals, schooling, and medical attention (Fanzo et al., 2018). The cost of feeding a child is expected to rise in the coming years due to reductions in land productivity and infrastructure damage from conflict and natural disasters (Myers, 2017). Reliance on processed and high-preservative food will likely increase in nations of all income levels, with individual and population-level health suffering as a result (WHO, 2024).

3.3.3 Displacement

Acute weather events and prolonged climate-related crises alike can lead families to seek safety and livelihood elsewhere. Within-country climate migration alone is expected to affect 86 million people in sub-Saharan Africa and 40 million in South Asia by 2050 (Rigaud et al., 2018). As discussed in Chapter 9, displacement presents a multidimensional risk to children's development, with each stage of vulnerability posing particular risks for children, including trafficking, exploitation, disease, and loss of shelter

(Gerrard, 2017; Oberg et al., 2021). Coordinated international support during and after displacement can help protect children from these dangers. The UN's 1951 Refugee Convention, however, does not recognize climate-related displacement in its criteria for refugee status (Jayawardhan, 2017; Kar et al. 2007).

3.3.4 Harm to Family and Community Functioning

Climate change, as mentioned, can increase children's exposure to violence in their own communities and homes, but it also harms children's development through damage to the systems that ordinarily support children's development (Oberg et al., 2021; Sanson et al., 2019). For example, during droughts, adults may spend less time caring for children and more time walking longer and longer distances to fetch water (Mohamed & Ojwang, 2020). Children, too, may face risks of injury, heat stroke, and interpersonal adversity as they collect water. All in all, families and communities may spend more time acquiring resources, coaxing crops from unhealthy soil, and recovering from natural disasters, and less time engaging in the routines and activities that are so important for children's development.

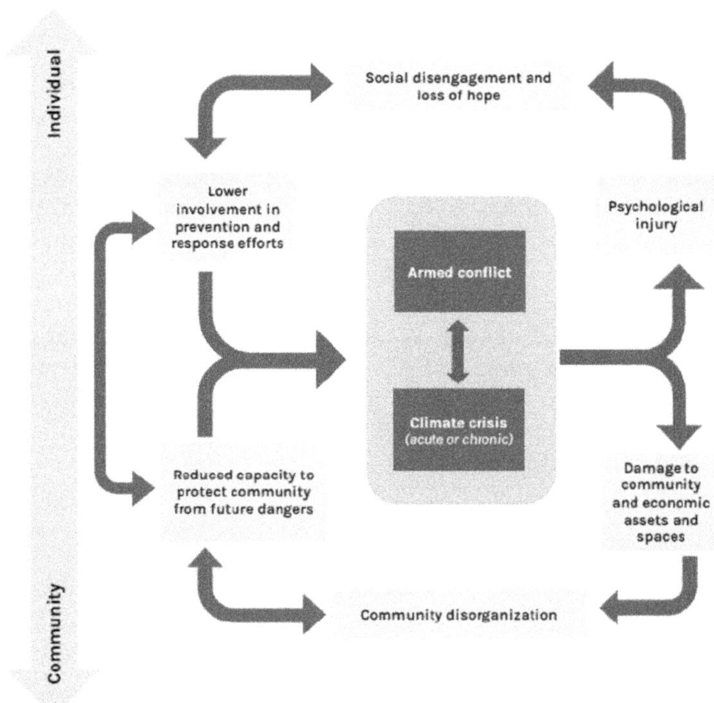

Figure 3.2 Convergence of armed conflict and the climate crisis.

There are countless adaptive systems at the community level that ordinarily buffer children from adversities, like effective responses to natural disasters, both preemptive and responsive. These depend on interpersonal engagement, individuals' adaptive capacity, and community organization. As shown in Figure 3.2, these are all assets that can be depleted when climate shocks are severe, prolonged, or particularly multisystem (e.g., when economic breakdown and famine accompany droughts).

Case Study: The Republic of Kiribati

The Republic of Kiribati is a collection of 32 low-lying islands in the Pacific Ocean and is the only country in the world that spans all four global hemispheres. Kiribati is also considered one of the most vulnerable countries in regard to climate change. Much of its population of 120,000 people is already impacted by rising sea levels, which have caused erosion, infrastructure damage, and salination of agricultural areas.

Kiribati's government has established formal plans to support community adaptation to climate change—for example, by building seawalls, planting mangroves in coastal areas, improving community climate education, increasing access to global financial assistance, and strengthening early warning systems (Government of Kiribati, 2023). Leaders have also begun to organize and implement the difficult process of helping portions of the population to strategically relocate. In the meantime, Kiribati increasingly calls on the international community to reverse the climate damage that has caused these dangers (WHO, 2024).

3.4 Conclusion

Climate change can justly be considered a form of violence against children, harming their bodies and damaging the systems that help them grow. Climate shocks increase the severity and frequency of extreme weather events, violence, famine, economic downturns, and other adversities, and they also degrade the systems that ordinarily help protect children's development when crises occur.

While individual behavior does matter for protecting the climate for children, a small number (i.e., less than 80) of corporate entities and state-affiliated producers have generated over 70% of all carbon emissions in history (Carbon Majors, 2024). Enforceable international legislation, combined with sustainable economic development, can help to slow down damage to the climate while ensuring that all communities around the world can enjoy prosperity without dependence on practices that harm the climate. In the meantime, as discussed in future chapters, adults can play a large role in protecting children from some of the acute impacts of climate change.

Reflection Questions

Question 1. How has climate change affected you personally in your life so far?

Question 2. What global events in your lifetime, both geopolitical and environmental, have likely been intensified by climate change?

Question 3. Consider your own household's daily rhythms. How might these be altered by instability in global climates?

Question 4. In what ways is climate change addressable through science? What about through social and political activities?

References

Bauer-Wu, S. (2024). A future we can love: Effective approaches to the climate crisis that begin with us. Shambhala Publications.

Carbon Majors. (2024). The Carbon Majors database: Launch report. Influence Map. https://carbonmajors.org/briefing/The-Carbon-Majors-Database-26913

Clark, H., Coll-Seck, A.M., Banerjee, A., Peterson, S., Dalglish, S.L., Ameratunga, S. (2020). A future for the world's children? A WHO-UNICEF-Lancet Commission. Lancet, 395, 605–658. https://doi.org/10.1016/S0140-6736(19)32540-1

Fanzo, J., Davis, C., McLaren, R., & Choufani, J. (2018). The effect of climate change across food systems: Implications for nutrition outcomes. Global Food Security, 18, 119. https://www.sciencedirect.com/science/article/pii/S2211912418300063

Gerrard, M. B. (2017). Climate change and human trafficking after the Paris agreement. The University of Miami Law Review, 72, 345.

Global Commission on the Economics of Water: Valuing the Hydrological cycle as a global common good. Executive Summary, October 17, 2024. https://watercommission.org

Government of Kiribati (2023). Kiribati development plan 2020–2023. A wealthy, healthy and peaceful nation. https://policy.asiapacificenergy.org/sites/default/files/Kiribati%20Development%20Plan%202020-2023.pdf

Ide, T., Kristensen, A., & Bartusevičius, H. (2021). First comes the river, then comes the conflict? A qualitative comparative analysis of flood-related political unrest. Journal of Peace Research, 58(1), 83–97.

IPCC (2018). Global Warming of 1.5°C: An IPCC Special Report on the Impacts of Global Warming of 1.5°C above Pre-industrial Levels and Related Global Greenhouse Gas Emission Pathways, in the Context of Strengthening the Global Response to the Threat of Climate Change, Sustainable Development, and Efforts to Eradicate Poverty. IPCC, Annex I, Glossary.

IPCC (2021). Climate change 2021. The physical science basis. Summary form policymakers. Intergovernmental Panel on Climate Change. Switzerland. ISBN 978–92–9169-158-6. https://www.ipcc.ch/report/ar6/wg1/downloads/report/IPCC_AR6_WGI_SPM_final.pdf

Jayawardhan, S. (2017). Vulnerability and climate change induced human displacement. Consilience, 17, 103–142. Retrieved February 21, 2021, at https://www.jstor.org/stable/26188784

Kar, N., Mohapatra, P. K., Nayak, K. C., Pattanaik, P., Swain, S. P., & Kar, H. C. (2007). Post-traumatic disorder in children and adolescents one year after a super-cyclone in Orissa, India: Exploring cross-cultural validity and vulnerability factors. BMC Psychiatry, 7(8), 1–9. https://doi.org/10.1186/1471-244X-7-8

Mares, D. M., & Moffett, K. W. (2016). Climate change and interpersonal violence: A "global" estimate and regional inequities. Climate Change, 135(2), 297–310.

Mekonnen, M., & Hoekstra, A. J. (2016). Four billion people severe water scarcity. Science Advances, 2. https://doi.org/10.1126/sciadv.1500323. https://www.science.org/doi/10.1126/sciadv.1500323#:~:text=The%20number%20of%20people%20facing%20severe%20water%20scarcity%20for%20at,15%2C%2027%E2%80%9330).

Mohamed, A. A., & Ojwang, R. A. (2020). Impact of climate change and vulnerability assessment of pastoralists located in South Central Somalia based on income and marital status. International Journal of Environment and Climate Change, 10, 101–112.

Myers L. (2017). The neglected link – effects of climate change and environmental degradation on child labour (Child labour report 2017). Terre des hommes. https://resourcecentre.savethechildren.net/node/13899/pdf/cl-report-2017-engl.pdf

NASA (2024). Ice Sheets Fact Sheet. https://climate.nasa.gov/vital-signs/ice-sheets/?intent=121#:~:text=Key%20Takeaway%3A,adding%20to%20sea%20level%20rise.

Oberg, C. N., Nathawad, R., Raman, S., & Goldhagen, J. (2021). Violence against children: Recognition, rights, responses. Pediatric Clinics of North America. https://doi.org/10.1016/j.pcl.2020.12.008

O'Neal, L. (2016). The link between natural disasters and domestic abuse. The Atlantic, September 28. https://www.theatlantic.com/health/archive/2016/09/disaster-domestic-abuse/501299/

Perry, J. D., & Simpson, M. E. (1987). Violent crimes in a city: Environmental determinants. Environment and Behavior, 9(1), 77–90. https://doi.org/10.1177/0013916587191004

Putnick, D. L., & Bornstein, M. H. (2015). Is child labor a barrier to school enrollment in low-and middle-income countries? International Journal of Educational Development, 41, 112–120. https://doi.org/10.1016/j.ijedudev.2015.02.001

Rakib, M. A., Sasaki, J., Matsuda, H., Quraishi, S. B., Mahmud, M. J., Bodrud-Doza, M., Atique Ullah, A., Fatema, K.,J., Newaz, A., Bhuiyan, M.,H.,B. (2020). Groundwater salinization and associated co-contamination risk increase severe drinking water vulnerabilities in the southwestern coast of Bangladesh. Chemosphere, 246, 125646.

Rigaud, K. K., de Sherbinin, A., Jones, B., Bergmann, J., Clement, V., Ober, K., Schewe, J., Adamo, S., McCusker, B., Heuser, S., & Midgley, A. (2018). Groundswell: Preparing for internal climate migration. World Bank. https://doi.org/10.1596/29461

Sanson A. V., Hoorn, J. V., & Burke, S. E. L. (2019). Responding to the impact of the ciliate crisis on children and youth. Child Development Perspectives, 13(4), 201–207.

Scientific America (2025). Earth surpasses 1.5 degree celsius in hottest year on record. Scientific America, January 10. https://apple.news/Ap0ghJ178RfOi5msQY_eqDg

UN (2023). Climate insecurity impacts on children and armed conflict. A discussion paper. office of the special representative of the secretary-general for children and armed conflict United Nations secretariat. https://childrenandarmedconflict.un.org/wp-content/uploads/2023/11/Climate-Insecurity-and-CAAC-Discussion.pdf

UN Women (2025). How gender inequality and climate change are interconnected. April 21. https://www.unwomen.org/en/articles/explainer/how-gender-inequality-and-climate-change-are-interconnected

UNICEF (2025). Unless we act now: The impact of climate change on children, United Nations Children Fund, United States of America p. 6. on 12 Sep 2025. https://sdgs.un.org/publications/unless-we-act-now-impact-climate-change-children-17989.
UNICEF (2021). United Nations children's fund. The Climate Crisis is a Child Rights Crisis: Introducing the Children's Climate Risk Index. UNICEF. https://www.unicef.org/media/105376/file/UNICEF-climate-crisis-child-rights-crisis.pdf
UNICEF (2024). Water scarcity, addressing the growing lack of available water to meet children's needs. https://www.unicef.org/wash/water-scarcity
United Nations (2023). Climate change-induced sea-level rise is a direct threat to millions around the world, Secretary-General tells Security Council. United Nations Security Council Meeting. February 14. https://press.un.org/en/2023/sc15199.doc.htm
Watts, N., Amann, M., Arnell, N., Ayeb-Karlsson, S., Belesova, K., Boykoff, M., & Montgomery, H. (2019). The 2019 report of The Lancet Countdown on health and climate change: Ensuring that the health of a child born today is not defined by a changing climate. The Lancet, 394(10211), 1836–1878. https://doi.org/10.1016/S0140-6736(19)32596-6
World Health Organization (WHO). (2024). Countering the climate crisis in Kiribati. World Health Organization: Western Pacific. https://www.who.int/westernpacific/newsroom/feature-stories/item/countering-the-climate-crisis-in-kiribati
Youness, M. A. (2015). How climate change contributed to the conflicts in the Middle East and North Africa. World Bank Blogs, December 10. https://blogs.worldbank.org/arabvoices/climate-change-conflict-mena

Part II

Introduction

Impacts of Global Crises on Child Development

At any age, exposure to events like armed conflict, famine, and forced displacement is associated with risks to a child's wellbeing. These risks include physical and mental health challenges, along with disruptions in social relationships and community functioning. Children's limited autonomy and mobility, coupled with their complete dependence on surrounding systems, makes them more vulnerable to harm during and after crises. In addition, events that occur during periods of heightened sensitivity to the environment and rapid developmental change—characteristic of much of infancy, childhood, and adolescence—can have disproportionately large impacts that cascade into other domains of functioning.

Part II describes the developmental impacts of the accelerating threats of climate crises, environmental degradation, and armed conflict. It is structured according to a socio-ecological model of human development, which holds that individual change occurs within social and structural "spheres" of varying proximity. The model begins with the child and expands to include families, communities, nations, and global systems. Each chapter in this part follows a common format, first describing some of the major developmental competence goals for children in a given socio-ecological sphere, referencing pediatric medicine and developmental science to discuss expectations around typical development. Much of each chapter is spent describing ways that adversities may impede children from meeting goals in a given domain. Throughout, the text mentions both direct and indirect processes, as political and environmental events often influence development through mediation or moderation models. Sensitive periods also receive special attention (i.e., the stages of life when environmental input can have particularly pronounced impacts on development).

Developmental psychopathology research contributes heavily to this discussion, as this field concerns itself with the cascading and interacting impacts of risks and resources on children over time. In particular, developmental psychopathology offers tools for describing multisystem interactions—for example, between environment and gene expression, or between childcare policies and parental stress. As such, Part II aims to help readers grasp the complex ways in which crises can influence children's development over time.

DOI: 10.4324/9781003488385-5

Research on the developing child exposed to adversity would be incomplete without a discussion on resilience, which will be explored throughout Part II. Because of the importance of resilience processes to children's development, each chapter includes discussions of factors and processes across levels of children's social ecologies that are associated with positive adaptation. The intention is that, amid discussion of mounting global and national risks to children's development, individuals, communities, and systems will be mobilized to invest in early life resilience factors, leveraging the sensitive developmental periods that characterize infancy, childhood, and adolescence to amplify the effects of positive resources.

This part of the book in particular aims to integrate perspectives from the fields of medicine, global health, developmental psychology, and clinical psychology, along with insights from educational studies and family social science. This combination of multidisciplinary perspectives may expand readers' imaginations for multi-sector collaboration and help them to grasp the interconnectedness of seemingly unrelated fields to their own.

4 The Child

Life's Journey Begins

Wonder of a Child

Wonder away like a child
She's shielded from the misty rain
Like a budding flower, wild
Knowledge flows like water
coursing through her brain...
Wonder is with this child
Quietly sits with her for a while

Philo Yan
Malaysia

4.1 Introduction

The individual child is at the center of the socio-ecological system around which each of the subsequent concentric circles emanates (Bronfenbrenner & Morris, 2006). Even in the earliest stages of life, a child interacts with the world through reciprocal relationships with each of the other spheres, such that it is impossible to completely separate children's attributes from their milieu. The activity level of a fetus shapes parental sleep and diet patterns, while prenatal exposure to the tones and prosody of spoken language shapes the auditory expectations of a newborn (Gervain, 2018).

This book rests on the assumption that children's interactions with the environment play a role in driving development, including through behaviors like eating, sleeping, cooing, laughing, or talking. To the keen and developmentally informed observer, it can be difficult to judge where a child ends and the environment begins, given how richly and mutually the individual and surrounding systems define one another. To what extent is an infant's fussiness a reflection of her temperament or physiology, as opposed to a mismatch between physiological needs and caregiving patterns? When one envisions the paths one has followed, personally and professionally, is it possible to parse the influence of one's own identity and nature from the influence of the surroundings? Yet for the purposes of narrative structure, it was necessary here to

DOI: 10.4324/9781003488385-6

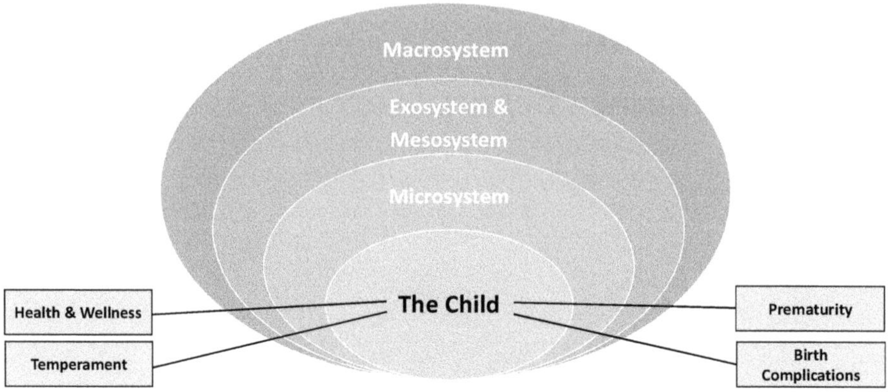

Figure 4.1 The socio-ecological model: The child.

draw a boundary around the attributes that are distinctly *of the child*, interfacing and interacting with its environment. The chapter will explore physical, physiological, sensorimotor, and emotional processes contributing to child development, attending with special focus to the developmentally dense period that spans the prenatal period and the first year of life. It will first describe markers of health and developmental competence relevant during this period, followed by some of the markers of individual competence that become relevant throughout early childhood and beyond (Figure 4.1).

4.2 Perinatal Period and Infant Morbidity

The perinatal period lasts from conception to a child's first birthday. This time is a sensitive developmental period during which even subtle disruption in the growth of the fetus and infant increases vulnerabilities to morbidity and mortality. In fact, one in four confirmed pregnancies in the United States ends in miscarriage or stillbirth—approximately the death rate of U.S. adults over age 85. Between 20 weeks of gestation and a baby's first birthday, rates of death are approximately equivalent to those expected of people in their sixties (Davis, 2016). To be sure, the causes of miscarriage and stillbirth are often difficult or impossible to discern, especially outside of extreme environmental adversity, such as famine. These statistics should serve as a reminder of the vulnerability of the perinatal period and encourage appreciation of just how many distinct systems within the developing individual must function in expected ways to ensure the survival and health of the young person.

Figure 4.2 provides a schematic of periods from preconception to the first year of life. The ***pre-pregnancy*** period is often neglected in discussions of perinatal health, but wellbeing and resource access of expectant parents before conception lay some of the foundations for the health of the subsequent pregnancy. It is common to hear public health experts, care providers, and acquaintances emphasize the health status of the gestational parent

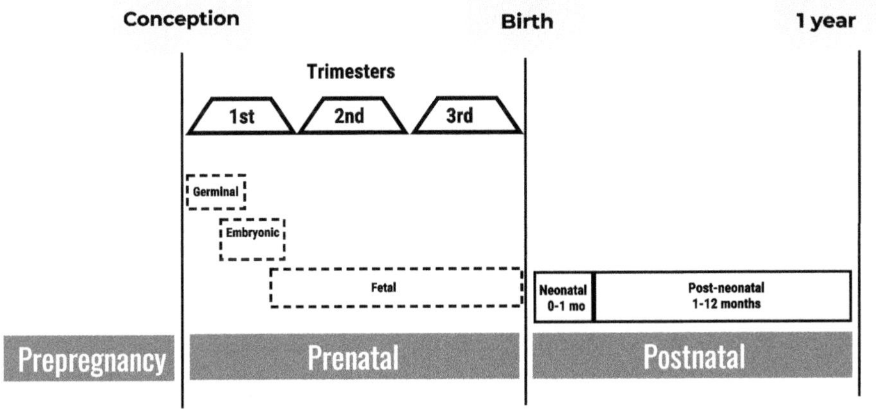

Figure 4.2 Critical periods from pre-pregnancy to postnatal.

leading up to pregnancy; indeed, most research on preconception health attends to maternal behaviors like alcohol consumption, tobacco use, and folic acid intake. Increasingly, there is a discussion of the impact of mothers' mental health in the preconception period on later infant health outcomes. Researchers are also beginning to focus on paternal health behaviors that impact spermatogenesis and may therefore influence fetal and infant development. For example, consumption of alcohol, meat, and plants; metabolic health; exercise; and stress may affect the likelihood of sperm leading to a viable pregnancy, as well as epigenetic expressions (Marcho et al., 2020; Tully et al., 2024).

Conception occurs when sperm and egg fuse into an embryo. Pregnancy begins when the embryo is implanted into the uterus after traveling down the fallopian tube or being implanted medically through a procedure like in-vitro fertilization (IVF). This second critical period is the ***prenatal period***, spanning the time between conception and birth. The prenatal period is often thought of as three evenly divided trimesters of around 13 weeks each, which together make up a 40-week ("full-term") pregnancy. However, in terms of development, a different set of periods may be more informative. These periods include:

- The *germinal period* lasts for the first two weeks after conception. It is marked by rapid increase of cell numbers of the dividing zygote and the implantation into the uterus.
- The *embryonic period* lasts around five weeks (weeks 3–8) and is a time of rapid organ development. It is in the first 7–8 weeks after conception when the fetus is most vulnerable to injury from certain metabolic or nutritional insults, such as folate deficiency, which may result in central nervous system abnormalities.
- Finally, the *fetal period* lasts from week eight to the time of delivery. A fetal period ideally lasts around 30–32 weeks, bringing the pregnancy to full term (38–40 weeks in total).

The ***postnatal period*** starts at birth and runs through the first year of life. For the purpose of this section, the first year of life is broken into two segments. The neonatal period consists of the first 28 days (or one month) after birth, and the post-neonatal period spans from 1 month to one year of age.

Presently, the earliest an infant can survive after delivery is roughly 22–24 weeks of gestation, if specialized neonatal intensive care services are available. Infants who are able to grow and mature in the womb have greater chances of survival (that is, lower infant mortality rates) and lower chances of major medical complications that disrupt infant growth and development (that is, lower infant morbidity rates). Infant mortality and morbidity prevention strategies focus on each of these critical time periods and are discussed below.

4.2.1 *Prematurity and Low Birthweight*

Infants with low birthweight (LBW) are those weighing less than 5 pounds 8 ounces (2500 grams) at birth. LBW can result from preterm birth and/or inadequate growth in utero. Contributing factors include maternal hypertension, tobacco exposure, inadequate weight gain during pregnancy, and multiple-birth pregnancy (e.g., twins). Babies born with LBW are at higher risk for both infant mortality and morbidity. Specifically, there is an incremental increase in mortality and morbidity for infants born at LBW compared to healthy-weight infants, another increase for those infants who are born at very low birth weight (VLBW, weighing less than 1,500 grams), and yet another increase for extremely low birthweight (ELBW) infants, weighing less than 1,000 grams.

Prenatal care is very important for achieving optimal maternal and infant health outcomes. Prenatal care providers work to support the health of parents, assess exposure to events or environmental insults that might influence the growth of the fetus, and provide additional resources to help the family raise a healthy baby. For example, providers may assess a family's nutrition access, stress levels, intentions to engage in substance use cessation plans, and pregnancy-related conditions, such as preeclampsia and gestational diabetes.

4.2.2 *Birth Complications and Neonatal Infections*

Birth complications may occur during the delivery process and the minutes and hours that follow. The complication that most commonly contributes to later child health concerns is birth asphyxia, or oxygen deprivation. During the pregnancy, the fetus receives all nutrition and oxygen through the umbilical cord. After delivery when the umbilical cord is cut, the infant needs to immediately start breathing, as oxygen allows the brain and the body to function adequately. One cause of oxygen deprivation is meconium aspiration. Meconium is the first stool from the infant's gastrointestinal tract and is usually passed in the first 24–72 hours after birth. Infants stressed during delivery—frequently due to a difficult delivery or birthing process—may pass the meconium while in the womb or birth canal. After delivery, when they take their first breaths, they can inhale the toxic meconium. This event may lead to chemical pneumonia, with a risk of death or long-term disability from lack of oxygen (i.e., hypoxia). Another leading cause of hypoxia is from the umbilical cord being wrapped around the neck during the birthing process, cutting off oxygen to the brain. Limited access to care providers, birth attendants, safe delivery facilities, and clean delivery supplies presents a potent risk factor for birth complications.

Neonatal infections are a major area of concern globally. These include maternal infections (such as HIV) that may be vertically transmitted to the infant during birth, as well as infections acquired soon after birth from the delivery space or other early environments. Possible serious bacterial infection (PSBI) is the most important clinical syndrome in this developmental period in low- and middle-income countries (LMICs). An estimated 6.9 million episodes of PSBI occur in young infants aged 0–59 days in LMICs every year (WHO, 2015). In 2023 alone, nearly 110,000 people globally died from measles, most of whom were children in the first few years of life (World Health Organization, 2024). Most infection-related infant deaths can be averted by preventive measures, early diagnosis, timely care-seeking, treatment with appropriate antibiotics, and follow-up.

4.2.3 Congenital Anomalies

Congenital anomalies occur when critical structures show abnormal growth or lack of development during the prenatal period. Frequently, the causes are unknown. Some are now understood to be related to maternal nutritional intake before the pregnancy, during the germinal and embryonic periods, and through organogenesis, particularly in the first 8 weeks after conception. For example, neural tube defects (NTDs) are a set of conditions that include spina bifida, encephaloceles, and anencephaly (the lack of development of the forebrain and cerebral cortex).

Folic acid is a water-soluble vitamin also known as pteroyl-glutamic acid, folacin, vitamin B9, and, historically, Lactobacillus casei factor. Folic acid is essential for the formation of new cells and the metabolism of deoxyribonucleic acid (DNA) and ribonucleic acid (RNA). The formation of tissues, bone marrow, and the entire nervous system depend on this B-vitamin; in fact, folic acid facilitates the closure of the neural tube around 4–5 weeks of gestation and the subsequent formation of the spinal cord and brain. Insufficient folic acid in the gestational environment can result in fetal development proceeding with an improperly closed neural tube. This can result in diverse NTDs. When closure fails on the lower end, toward the buttocks, the developmental outcome is known as spina bifida; at the upper end, an encephalocele or meningocele. These NTDs form as the result of an outpouching of either cerebral spinal fluid, meninges, and brain itself. The more severe the NTD, the greater the likelihood of significant morbidity or of mortality. If the infant lives, then the malformation needs to be corrected surgically and may still result in significant morbidity as the infant grows. Critically, the recommended dietary allowance of folic acid needs to be absorbed and sustained before conception occurs to make sure that adequate levels are present in the germinal phase of the pregnancy. Proactive intake of the recommended amount of folic acid before conception occurs—400 micrograms a day—reduces the incidence of NTDs by 50–70%.

Knowing the importance of folic acid in infant development, what must be done to ensure that people who may carry children have adequate intake and stores of folic acid? One approach might be to make prenatal vitamins with the appropriate amount of folic acid free or significantly subsidized and work with communities to ensure their equitable distribution. However, weeks may pass after fertilization before a pregnancy is detected, at which point the formation and closure (or lack thereof) of the neural tube may have already occurred, and so the critical window may have passed. Many public health professionals therefore feel that folic acid intake is best treated as a pre-pregnancy nutrition issue, relevant at the population level. Put simply, all women who may bear children should consume adequate folic acid prior to conception as a regular part of their diets.

Another approach, now adopted in many middle- to higher-income countries, is to supplement or fortify grocery items with these essential nutrients. Folic acid naturally exists in a variety of fruits, vegetables, beans, whole grains, egg yolks and milk products, and to distribute this nutrient on a population-wide level, governments may require or incentivize the fortification of grains with folic acid. Other examples of this principle—also of relevance to fetal and infant development—include the addition of iodine to salt, fluoride to water, and vitamin D to milk.

4.3 Motor Development

An important aspect of physical development is the infant's motor development. We may think of this as the ability to use one's body to effect changes in one's experience of the environment. For a baby, motor development includes skills like picking up a food object to feed herself, turning her head to look in the direction of a parent's voice, and, eventually, using her body to seek out entirely new spaces as she crawls or walks into another setting.

Even at birth, when infants are completely dependent on adults for nurture and protection, babies show roughly nine innate newborn reflexes, which disappear within weeks or months after birth and are replaced by voluntary action. For example, the *rooting* instinct occurs when stroking the side of the infant's cheek causes the baby's head to turn toward the source of stimulation, and *involuntary sucking* occurs when a finger or nipple is placed in a baby's mouth. Both of these instincts are essential for permitting feeding early in life. The *palmar grasp* occurs when a finger pressed into the infant's palm causes the infant to spontaneously grasp the finger, and the *stepping* instinct occurs when the infant lifts his bare feet in sequence after being allowed to touch them to a surface.

The emergence of gross and fine motor skills is like the emergence of a well-rehearsed dance. The infant begins in a supine position with little to no control of their posture or the use of their hands and feet. Then over the course of the first year of life, something incredible happens. The infant first learns to roll over and lift their head up, allowing them to look forward. Gradually, they are able to maneuver onto their hands and feet. Sitting at 4–6 months allows them to eventually stand and take their first steps, commonly between 12–15 months of age, and the development of running. Fine motor skills follow a similar path. Babies go from demonstrating a very basic voluntary palmar grasp and, gradually, an exquisite finger-and-thumb grip that facilitates the expert movement of objects to their lips. As these fine and gross motor skills develop, babies show growing capacities for greater interaction with their environments.

4.4 Cognitive Development

It has long been known that cognitive development follows similar patterns across children in different environments and communities (Piaget, 1952). As children's brains and bodies develop, they increasingly use their capacities to make discoveries about their world, thinking about objects, movement, and people in increasingly complex ways.

For cognitive development to proceed as expected, babies benefit from stable nutrition access (Kirolos et al., 2022). Other facets of the environment, such as predictability, can also safeguard cognitive development, helping to build the neural pathways of cause-effect response that help children navigate their worlds in the long term (Doom et al., 2024).

4.5 Emotional Development

Infant temperament is conceptualized in a variety of ways. Commonly, researchers refer to dimensions like *extraversion/surgency*, *negative emotionality*, and *effortful control.* That is, babies vary in their tendencies, respectively, to be sensitive to the environment, feel pleasure, and approach novelty; to feel sadness and distress; and to manage their own reactions and behaviors (Casalin et al., 2012). Notably, the basic foundations of effortful control are not expected to emerge in the first year of life; this variable becomes more relevant in later temperament classifications. The Thomas and Chess model (1977) of temperament consists of nine dimensions that cluster into three different temperament types: the easy child, the difficult child, and the slow-to-warm-up child. However, approximately a third of children do not fit in any of these categories. Some stability is commonly found in temperament over time, likely due both to psychobiological factors and to children's complex social and physical environments. Unsurprisingly, temperamental differences interact bidirectionally with caregiving environments; for example, babies who are seen as "easy" may receive more spontaneous positive affection, and these interactions confer additional developmental benefits.

Regardless of babies' baseline temperaments, when emotional development is proceeding as expected, babies react in response to their environments, explore appropriately as their bodies allow, show synchrony in close relationships, express a full range of emotions, and rely on safe adults around them to co-regulate these feelings. These abilities are linked to children's basic cognitive skills and neurological development (Walle et al., 2022). Needless to say, emotional difficulties may make it harder for children to meet these milestones. For example, a child who shows serious fear in response to new situations may have trouble exploring his environment (Fox et al., 2021).

4.6 Impact of Armed Conflict, Famine, and Climate Change on Individual Development

It has long been known that exposure to famine during pregnancy can result in adverse birth outcomes (Lumey, 1992). Research from the last 25 years has also found that armed conflict is associated with increases in maternal, neonatal, and infant mortality (Jawad et al., 2021), as well as in miscarriage, stillbirth, prematurity, LBW infants, congenital abnormalities, and premature rupture of membranes (PROM; Keasley et al., 2017). Simply living within 30 miles of a combat zone—a common experience in our world today—is associated with increased risk of maternal and child sickness, injury, and mortality (Bendavid et al., 2021), through pathways that include malnutrition and increased stress (Hogue & Vasquez, 2002). In the most recent war in Gaza, at least 50,000 pregnant women have been placed at risk for adverse birth outcomes from maternal stress, physical harm, and malnutrition (UNPF, 2024).

The risks of adverse pre-, perinatal, and maternal health outcomes are distributed unevenly even in middle- to high-income countries, due to entrenched systemic inequities like racism. In the United States, women of color—Black women in particular—face structural barriers to accessing quality healthcare, as well as bias from providers. Adjusting for education, income, and other factors, Black women in the United States consistently experience higher rates of preterm labor, preeclampsia, transient and pregnancy-induced hypertension, diabetes, placenta previa, placental abruption, PROM, infection, and cesarean section, all of which can contribute to preterm births and infant mortality risks (Shen et al., 2005; Singh & Stella, 2019). Meanwhile, Black women in the United States are substantially more likely to die during and after pregnancy than are women of other races (Joseph et al., 2021).

The current global hunger crisis is pushing one child into severe malnutrition every minute in 15 crisis-hit countries (UNICEF, 2022). Malnutrition in early life can cause a child to experience damage to the development of height, immune function, and cognition (Cravioto & DeLicardie, 1970; Kirolos et al., 2022). One syndrome related to malnutrition, marasmus, is associated with long-term difficulties in cognition, language, and learning. Kwashiorkor, or severe protein deficiency, can result in permanent cognitive damage and poor overall health (Latham, 1974). Any of these developmental insults can, in turn, reduce a child's resilience to future threats; for example, children with muscle loss may be less able to evade physical danger. Similarly, a community's adaptive capacity is, in many ways, bound up in individuals' adaptive capacity, and widespread cognitive damage may limit communities' future response to changing needs. Another insult to children's cognitive development comes in the form of environmental unpredictability. Disruptions to temporal routines, physical environment, and interpersonal interactions (e.g., consistent caregiving responses from a parent) are common during and after armed conflict and natural disaster—not to mention, the displacement, upheaval, scarcity, and stress that can follow. Interruptions or changes in these environmental patterns can harm children's neurological and cognitive development (Doom et al., 2024).

Children exposed to armed conflict and natural disasters are at a greater risk of injury and death than their adult counterparts are (Oberg et al., 2022). Psychological trauma can have diverse impacts on children's development as well, which can be difficult to assess and measure, but are potent nonetheless. Stress activates multiple physiological systems, including the hypothalamic-pituitary-adrenal (HPA) axis, causing cascades of cortisol and other hormones (Gunnar and Quevedo, 2007; Lupien et al., 2009). These cascades cause changes in the muscles, heart, lungs, and thyroid to prepare a person to mount a stress response (Van Der Kolk, 2014). This axis also functions with feedback mechanisms that prevent damage from prolonged cortisol exposure (Sapolsky et al., 2000). When cortisol levels remain elevated due to persistent stress, the HPA axis may adapt by changing its function (e.g., over- or under-responding to threatening cues) in ways that may eventually become maladaptive for youth's behavior. Cortisol itself can also contribute to differences in neural structures that are associated with emotional and cognitive health (Arnsten, 2009; Gee, 2021). Meanwhile, dysregulated cortisol patterns might contribute to persistent infections and atopic disease (e.g., asthma and allergies).

The next chapter will describe ways in which children's development may be impacted indirectly by stressors that impact caregiving relationships. It is important to note here, amid discussion of the individual child, that caregivers' traumatic stress resulting from natural disasters and other crises can have independent impacts on a child's long-term cognitive development, language acquisition, and socioemotional health (Laplante et al., 2004; Moss et al., 2017).

4.7 Safeguarding Individual Children's Health amid 21st-Century Crises

As future chapters will discuss in more detail, young children's health and development are closely tied to the resilience of the systems that surround them. Many of the most promising ways to impact child development involve investments in these surrounding systems. For example, improving families' long-term access to stable, affordable housing can help them to provide predictable environments for their infants and young children, to the benefit of cognitive and emotional development (Doom et al., 2024; Foster et al., 2024). Redesigning healthcare programs with equity in mind can improve maternal and child birth outcomes (Majebi et al., 2024). Ensuring that caregivers and children are kept together during and after crises and armed conflict can leverage the powerful buffering effects of this dyadic relationship for the benefit of young children's overall development (Qouta et al., 2021). The importance of the dyadic bond will be explored in more detail in Chapter 5.

Many approaches, of course, serve children directly. Sustainable nutrition support systems for children and families facing poverty or other adversities can be their own source of predictability, reduce parental stress, and, of course, provide children with the nutrients they need to grow and develop. Culturally tailored early childhood education programming can support emotional and cognitive development in humanitarian settings (Kohn et al., 2020). Culturally and developmentally sensitive therapies can help children and their caregivers to improve regulation and overall wellbeing in light of past trauma exposures. One of the highest priorities in safeguarding children's development is the prevention of further trauma, as each additional adverse event is associated with greater challenges to a young person's development (Evans et al., 2013).

To be sure, delivering these interventions for children—even when they are assets as conceptually simple as nutrition packs in humanitarian aid parcels—often requires coordinated efforts across dozens of systems in the adult world. International and local communities alike can work to ensure that the most basic interventions for children are simple to deliver, unimpeded by political or ideological disputes (Boukari et al., 2024).

4.8 Conclusion

The cumulative impacts of trauma and stress from armed conflict, natural disasters, and other crises can have lasting impacts on multiple generations simultaneously, making it more difficult for children to meet their developmental milestones and enjoy their environments. This harm can take place directly through illness or injury, and also indirectly, through damage to the systems that ordinarily help to keep children safe. Prioritizing the safety of children's bodies and minds can result in policies and practices that safeguard their development and improve the resilience of the broader community.

Reflection Questions

Question 1. In regard to the pre-pregnancy and pregnancy periods through the infant's first year of life, what strategies have shown success in reducing morbidity and mortality? What else is needed?

Question 2. In what ways is early-life development foundational for later development?

Question 3. What social and political actions have been effective for safeguarding the development of children exposed to serious adversity?

References

Arnsten AFT. (2009). Stress signaling pathways that impair prefrontal cortex structure and function. *Nature Reviews: Neuroscience, 10*, 410–422.

Bendavid, E., Boerma, T., Akseer, N., Langer, A., Malembaka, E. B., Okiro, E. A., Wise, P.H., Heft-Neal, S., Black, R.,E., Bhutta, Z.,A., and the BRANCH Consortium Steering Committee. (2021). The effects of armed conflict on the health of women and children. *The Lancet, 397*(10273), 522–532.

Boukari, Y., Kadir, A., Waterston, T., Jarrett, P., Harkensee, C., Dexter, E., Cinar, E. N., Blackett, K., Nacer, H., Stevens, A., & Devakumar, D. (2024). Gaza, armed conflict and child health. *BMJ Paediatrics Open, 8*(1), e002407. https://doi.org/10.1136/bmjpo-2023-002407. PMID: 38350977; PMCID: PMC10868171.

Brofenbrenner, U. (1994). Ecological models of human development. In *Husen T. & Postlethwaite, T., N., (Eds.) International Encyclopedia of Education* (2nd ed., Vol. 3, 1643–1647. Oxford: Pergamon/Elsevier Science.

Bronfenbrenner, U., & Morris, P. A. (2006). The bioecological model of human development. In *R. M. Lerner & W. Damon (Eds.), Handbook of child psychology* (6th ed., Vol. 1, pp. 793–828). Wiley.

Casalin, S., Luyten, P., Vliegen, N., & Meurs, P. (2012). The structure and stability of temperament from infancy to toddlerhood: A one-year prospective study. *Infant Behavior and Development, 35*(1), 94–108.

Cravioto, J., & DeLicardie, E. R. (1970). Environmental correlates of severe clinical malnutrition and language development in survivors from kwashiorkor or marasmus. *English Edition-Boletin De La OSP, 7*(2, 50–70.

Davis, D. L. (2016). Why is this so hard? In *Empty cradle, broken heart. 3rd Edition,* Fulcrum Publishing. ISBN: 1936218240, ISBN-13 : 978-1936218240

Doom, J. R., Han, D., Rivera, K. M., & Tseten, T. (2024). Childhood unpredictability research within the developmental psychopathology framework: Advances, implications, and future directions. *Development and Psychopathology, 36*(5), 2452-24631.

Evans, G. W., Li, D., & Whipple, S. S. (2013). Cumulative risk and child development. *Psychological Bulletin, 139*(6), 1342. https://doi.org/10.1037/a0031808

Fox, N. A., Buzzell, G. A., Morales, S., Valadez, E. A., Wilson, M., & Henderson, H. A. (2021). Understanding the emergence of social anxiety in children with behavioral inhibition. *Biological Psychiatry, 89*(7), 681–689.

Gee, D. G. (2021). Early adversity and development: Parsing heterogeneity and identifying pathways of risk and resilience. *American Journal of Psychiatry, 178*(11), 998–1013.

Gervain, J. (2018). The role of prenatal experience in language development. *Current Opinion In Behavioral Sciences, 21*, 62–67.

Gunnar, M., & Quevedo, K. (2007. The neurobiology of stress and development. *Annual Review of Psychology, 58*, 145–173.

Gunnar, M. R., & Vazquez, D. (2015). Stress neurobiology and developmental psychopathology. *Developmental Psychopathology: Volume Two: Developmental Neuroscience*, 2, 533–577.

Gunnar, M. R. (2014). The psychobiology of infnt temperament. In *Individual differences in infancy* (pp. 387–409). Psychology Press.

Hogue, C. J., & Vasquez, C. (2002). Toward a strategic approach for reducing disparities in infant mortality. *American Journal of Public Health, 92*, 552–556

Jawad, M., Hone, T., Vamos, E. P., Cetorelli, V., & Millett, C. (2021). Implication of armed conflict for maternal and child health: A regression analysis of data from 1881 countries for 2000-2019. *PLOS Medicine*, September 28. https://doi.org/10.1371/journal.pmed.1003810

Joseph, K. S., Boutin, A., Lisonkova, S., Muraca, G. M., Razaz, N., John, S., Mehrabadi, Azar, Sabr, Y., Ananth, C., & Schisterman, E. (2021). Maternal mortality in the United States: Recent trends, current status, and future considerations. *Obstetrics & Gynecology*, *137*(5), 763–771.

Keasley, J., Blickwedel, J., & Quenby, S. (2017). Adverse effects of exposure to armed conflict on pregnancy: A systematic review. *BMJ Global Health*, *2*(4), e000377. https://doi.org/10.1136/bmjgh-2017-000377. PMID: 29333283; PMCID: PMC5706483.

Kirolos, A., Goyheneix, M., Eliasz, M. K., Chisala, M., Lissauer, S., Gladstone, M., & Kerac, M. (2022). Neurodevelopmental, cognitive, behavioural and mental health impairments following childhood malnutrition: A systematic review. *BMJ Global Health*, *7*(7), e009330.

Kohn, S., Foulds, K., Murphy, K. M., & Cole, C. F. (2020). Creating a sesame street for the Syrian response region. *YC Young Children*, *75*(1), 32–41.

Laplante, D. P., Barr, R. G., Brunet, A., Galbaud, G., Du Fort, M., Meaney, L., Saucier, J. F., Zelazo, P., H., King, S. (2004). Stress during pregnancy affects general intellectual and language functioning in human toddlers. *Pediatric Research*, *56*(3), 400–410. https://doi.org/10.1203/01.PDR.0000136281.34035.44.

Latham, M. C. (1974). Protein-calorie malnutrition in children and its relation to psychological development and behavior. *Physiological Reviews*, *54*(3), 541–565. https://doi.org/10.1152/physrev.1974.54.3.541

Lumey L. H. (1992). Decreased birthweights in infants after maternal in utero exposure to the Dutch famine of 1944-1945. *Paediatr Perinat Epidemiol*, *6*(2), 240–53. https://doi.org/10.1111/j.1365-3016.1992.tb00764.x. PMID: 1584725.

Lupien, S. J., McEwen, B. S., Gunnar, M. R., & Heim, C. (2009). Effects of stress throughout the lifespan on the brain, behavior and cognition. *Nature Reviews Neuroscience*, *10*, 434–445.

Majebi, N. L., Adelodun, M. O., & Chinyere, E. (2024). Maternal mortality and healthcare disparities: Addressing systemic inequities in underserved communities. *International Journal of Engineering Inventions*, *13*(9), 375–385.

Marcho, C., Oluwayiose, O. A., & Pilsner, J. R. (2020). The preconception environment and sperm epigenetics. *Andrology*, *8*(4), 924–942.

Moss, K., Simcock, G., Cobham, V., Kildea, S., Elgbeili, G., Laplante, D., & King, S. (2017). A potential psychological mechanism linking disaster-related prenatal maternal stress with child cognitive and motor development at 16 months: The QF2011 Queensland flood study. *Developmental Psychology*, *53*(4), 629–641. https://doi.org/10.1037/dev0000272.

Oberg, C. N., Hodges, H. R., & Masten, A. (2022). Cascading consequences of armed conflict and famine on child health: A time for peace. *BMJ Paediatrics Open*. 6e001608. https://doi.org/10.1136/bmjpo-2022-001608

Piaget, J. (1952). *The origins of intelligence in children*. International Universities Press. (Original work published in 1932).

Qouta, S. R., Vanska, M., Ddiab, S. Y., & Punamaki, T. (2021). War trauma and infant motor, cognitive and socioemotional development: Maternal mental health and dyadic interaction as explanatory processes. *Infant Behavior*, *63*, 101532.

Sapolsky, R. M., Romero, M., Munck, A. U. (2000). How do glucocorticoids influence stress responses? Integrating permissive, suppressive, stimulatory, and preparative actions. *Endocrine Reviews*, *21*(1), 55–89.

Shen, J. J., Tymkow, C., & MacMullen, N. (2005). Disparities in maternal outcomes among four ethnic populations. *Ethnicity & Disease, 15*, 492–497.

Singh, G. K., & Stella, M. Y. (2019). Infant mortality in the United States, 1915-2017: Large social inequalities have persisted for over a century. *International Journal of Maternal and Child Health and AIDS, 8*(1), 19.

Thomas, A., & Chess, S. (1977). *Temperament and development.* Brunner/Mazel.

Tully, C. A., Alesi, S., McPherson, N. O., Sharkey, D. J., Teong, X. T., Tay, C. T., Silva, T., R., Puglisi, C., Barsby, J., P., & Mousa, A. (2024). Assessing the influence of preconception diet on male fertility: A systematic scoping review. *Human Reproduction Update, 30*(3), 243–261.

UNICEF (22022). Global hunger crisis pushing one child into severe malnutrition every minute in 15 crisis-hit countries. UNICEF Press Release, 22 June. https://www.unicef.org/press-releases/global-hunger-crisis-pushing-one-child-severe-malnutrition-every-minute-15-crisis

United Nations Population Fund. Crisis in Gaza. Retrieved August 21, 2024, at https://www.unfpa.org/crisis-gaza.

Van Der Kolk, B. (2014). *The body keeps the score. Brain, mind, and body in the healing of trauma.* Viking Press.

Walle, E. A., Lopez, L. D., & Castillo, A. (2022). Emotional development, p.61. In *The Oxford handbook of emotional development*, (Eds) Daniel, D., Samson, A.C., & Walle, E.A., Oxford University Press, United Kingdom. https://doi.org/10.1093/oxfordhb/9780198855903.001.0001

WHO (2015). Guideline-Managing possible serious bacterial infection in young infants when referral is not feasible. ISBN 978 92 4 150926 B

World Health Organization (2024). Measles cases surge worldwide, infecting 10.3 million people in 2023. *World Health Organization.* https://www.who.int/news/item/14-11-2024-measles-cases-surge-worldwide--infecting-10.3-million-people-in-2023

5 The Microsystem and Attachment

5.1 Introduction

Individual change occurs within social and structural "spheres" of varying proximity to a child (Bronfenbrenner, 1977) with the most proximal spheres exerting the most direct influence on children's development. The *microsystem* is the sphere closest to the developing child. Unsurprisingly, the most important features of this proximal environment are human; that is, children are shaped powerfully by the relationships that surround them as they grow. These influences are not unidirectional. Rather, processes in children (such as sleep patterns, emotion regulation, and bids for independence) respond to their proximal environments and simultaneously elicit responses from these environments (Gottlieb, 1991). In early life in particular, individual competence frequently reflects competence embedded in the microsystem. For example, a toddler's developmentally typical drive toward curiosity is made possible by caregivers' appropriate vigilance and allowance of independence. Meanwhile, consistent responses from adults organize a child's emerging understanding of communication as an infant learns, say, that a smile elicits a smile or that a cry results in comfort (Sroufe & Waters, 1977). In other words, it is nearly impossible to evaluate the

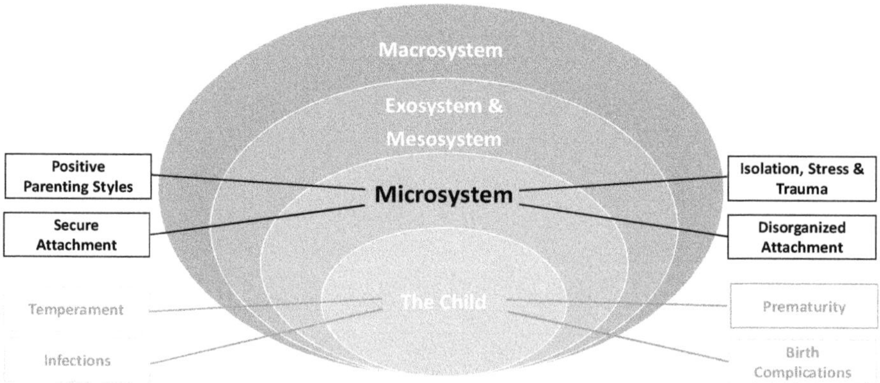

Figure 5.1 The socio-ecological model: The microsystem.

DOI: 10.4324/9781003488385-7

competence of infants and young children without attending to the functioning and health of their close relationships. Figure 5.1 depicts the microsystem and some of the assets and risks that may impact its health. Importantly, owing to its proximity to the developing child, the microsystem has the potential to be a locus of both potent developmental resources and also damage. When caregiving relationships are functioning well, they protect a child from many risks and also promote the development of positive outcomes like confidence, communication, and regulation skills (Masten & Palmer, 2019). Conversely, when these relationships are damaged or strained, the negative impacts on the developing child may be particularly strong.

5.2 The Developmental Tasks of Attachment

The smallest "unit" of a child's microsystem is the dyadic relationship they share with a caregiver. A major early marker of this dyad's functioning is the development of attachment. The earliest formulations of attachment reflected a few streams of observation. Scientists observed infants' and toddlers' responses to novel situations and temporary separations from caregivers and noted how often children seemed to inherently seek to restore the caregiver's proximity. John Bowlby (1969) observed, for example, that children had a wide range of responses to stressors, but that these behaviors often served to keep caregivers close, such as crying, bids for attention, or expression of affection. From their work, a theory emerged: These behaviors were important for a child's safety in the world and had emerged through evolutionary processes — in other words, children had survival advantages if their caregivers stayed nearby to guard them from threats and provide for their needs (e.g., nutrition). Another factor that inspired early attachment research was the observation that disruption to a caregiving relationship through maternal deprivation, separation, or other factors could have profound impacts on children's long-term behavior and development (Ainsworth, 1962). As Ainsworth and her team would come to show through their research studies, it was not merely physical separation from a caregiver that generated these "attachment injuries," but also "severely depriving relations with parents in the absence of separation" (p. 107). The quality of parent-child relationships, and not merely their existence, shaped a child's formation of attachment.

Case Study: Attachment-Friendly Healthcare

John Bowlby was a psychiatrist, psychoanalyst, and researcher who is credited with helping to establish attachment theory. Influenced by Dr. Konrad Lorenz's observations of young ducklings' bonds with their mothers, Bowlby took an ethological approach to identify parallels with human infants. With his colleagues, he noted ways that babies' behaviors helped keep caregivers close, which, in turn, gave them the emotional security they needed to explore their surroundings.

In addition to his research, Bowlby worked to help make healthcare spaces more conducive to children's emotional and attachment needs. For example, he helped support the redesign of labor and delivery practices to minimize the separation of infants and parents. He also collaborated with filmmaker James Robertson on a piece called *A Two Year Old Goes to the Hospital*, which depicts the experiences of hospitalization, surgery, and recovery from a toddler's perspective, showing how young Laura is hurt, afraid, and confused by separation from her mother and many other elements of the hospital environment. Projects like these spurred health systems to design and deliver care with children's developmental needs in mind.

Attachment research has identified several themes in infants' and young children's relational patterns toward their caregivers. These studies often introduce minor stressors like novelty or brief separations to see how the baby and the caregiving system respond (Ainsworth et al., 1978). Most infants show distress during separation from caregivers, seek caregivers' comfort and reassurance during and after the events, and show happiness when reunited. Often referred to as *securely attached* infants, these children are also better able to use the caregiver as a secure base in play and exploration: In essence, trusting that the caregiver will be there supportively no matter what happens, these children frequently show more confidence and independence in their own exploration. Other young children appear to self-soothe in the face of stress, including parental separation, and appear to be drawing on internal resources or distraction tactics to stay calm. These babies, frequently described as *insecurely-avoidantly* attached, may not immediately seek the caregiver upon reunion. Some, described as *insecurely-resistantly* attached, show persistent distress both during and after separation, and resist the comfort that their caregivers offer. A more recently formulated attachment style, *insecure-disorganized*, is marked by confusion or incoherence in a baby's response to the caregiver. For example, these children may appear apprehensive when approaching the caregiver for comfort or change strategies repeatedly. This pattern is thought to emerge sometimes in children who have experienced their caregiver as unpredictable or frightening. Broadly, all of these attachment behaviors are held to reveal what a child's internal working model may be of the caregiver—in other words, how predictable, present, sensitive, warm, and invested the child's mental representation of the caregiver is.

A few brief caveats are useful here. First, many attachment studies (including the original research) used dimensional measurements of children's reactions and behaviors but collapsed these into categorical groupings to support replicability and simplicity. Debate continues over the merit of categorical versus dimensional measurements of attachment behaviors (Raby et al., 2021).

Second, attachment research has not always accounted for cultural and contextual factors that impact the caregiving system. For example, in many communities, it is expected that multiple adults will care for children ("alloparenting"), and in some contexts, it is common practice for caregivers to keep infants and toddlers by their sides at all times. In such communities, children may exhibit some attachment behaviors toward non-parental adults, or may be expected to explore their environment only visually but not move through it on their own (Mesman et al., 2016). It is still common, though, for children to form a unique attachment relationship with primary caregivers even as other adults are important sources of comfort and support (e.g., to rely primarily on one adult for emotion regulation needs but to accept physical help from a large number of adults). Providers and researchers assessing attachment are wise to learn about caregiving practices common in a given community, as well as the types of child behaviors expected within stable dyadic relationships, before attempting to use established observational coding systems to categorize attachment behaviors.

As time passed, researchers began to describe the trajectories associated with various attachment styles across a child's development. For example, two-year-old children previously assessed as securely attached were found to show greater cooperation, persistence at tasks, and enthusiasm during problem-solving activities when compared to insecurely attached children (Matas et al., 1973). Four-year-olds who, as toddlers, were judged to be securely attached (as opposed to insecurely) were found to show greater ego resiliency (Sroufe, 1983). Attachment styles in infancy and toddlerhood have even been found to predict emotion regulation strategies used in adulthood, with clear implications for adult relational health (Girme et al., 2021). The benefits of a secure attachment relationship are long-lasting and diverse, seen in domains like problem-solving abilities, confidence, and overall emotional resilience. Secure attachments not only help to keep a child protected from danger and isolation, but also allow the child to thoroughly and efficiently access all of the adaptive resources available through the caregiving relationship, such as co-regulation of emotions, scaffolding of emerging mastery, a sense of self-efficacy (e.g., through the encouragement of appropriate independence), and positive identity development (Masten, 2025, p. 169).

Given its relevance to outcomes across the lifespan, the development of attachment has continued to generate substantial interest. Ainsworth's team demonstrated (1978) that early patterns of caregiving are related to subsequent patterns of attachment, including attachment to friends or romantic partners. In summary, a child raised in a caring, consistent, and sensitive manner is more likely to develop a secure attachment with the caregiver and to utilize the caregiver as a base from which to investigate and explore the environment. Conversely, children cared for in a more inconsistent or insensitive manner are more likely to develop an attachment pattern characterized as insecure or disorganized (Main & Solomon, 1990).

5.3 Risks in the Microsystem

Caregivers who show insensitivity toward their children's needs in infancy are at a higher risk of mistreating their children in the toddler and childhood periods, and their children are at greater risk of showing insecure attachment styles (Egeland & Sroufe, 1981; Yarrow et al., 1975). When caregivers are unable to access positive parenting practices, the risk to their children's development can be greater than the risk levied by exposure to four or more adverse events (Yamaoka & Bard, 2019). Infants and young children who receive insufficient care may experience heightened or chronic activation of neural networks that help to process threats in the environment. Cortical development may accelerate; that is, the young child's brain may build neural networks to help them process fear and compensate for the lack of a protective caregiver (Gee et al., 2013). While adaptive for the child's survival, these developmental differences can come at a cost. For example, children may experience dysregulated hormonal responses to stress (Gunnar & Reid, 2019). These response patterns can make it more difficult for children to benefit from anxiety-reducing resources around them and increase their risk of developing mental health conditions in the future (Gunnar & Quevedo, 2007).

Many of the crises and challenges already discussed in this book have clear implications for attachment relationships and the health of the microsystem. Most obviously, armed conflict, famine, natural disaster, and forced displacement may result in the death of the caring adults around a child. With over two thirds of children globally living in areas affected by conflict, and scores of others living in areas at risk of climate shocks and famine, orphanhood is a conceivable risk for many of the world's children (Mohamed & Homeida, 2024; Rigaud et al., 2018). Any of these crises may also separate a child from an attachment figure, of course. Any interruptions to the presence of a safe caregiver, especially in the context of other environmental risks, can have significant adverse consequences for neurological, cognitive, and emotional development (Cohodes et al., 2021; Waddoups et al., 2019).

Even when caregivers are able to stay physically present with their children, environmental stress can negatively impact the health of these relationships. It is very difficult to research attachment and caregiving practices during or immediately after armed conflict or natural disaster, of course, but a critical endeavor nonetheless (Masten & Osofsky, 2018; Okello et al., 2014). Unsurprisingly, exposure to armed conflict and other forms of violence has negative impacts on children's mental health and development in the long term, with factors in the microsystem often mediating and moderating these processes (Dimitry, 2012; Morina et al., 2018; Slone & Mann, 2016). For example, refugee mothers' PTSD symptoms appear to be associated with a weaker infant-parent bond and poorer attachment outcomes (Catalá et al., 2025). Meanwhile, chronic stressors like isolation, lack of social support, and economic strain can increase caregivers' emotional stress, making it harder to respond consistently and sensitively to children, to the detriment of parenting quality and child outcomes (Masarik & Conger, 2017; Vaughn et al., 1979). For expectant Palestinian mothers exposed to war, social support and maternal mental health mediated the relationship between trauma exposure and prenatal attachment, as well as parent-child interactions when babies were one year old (Punamäki et al., 2017).

5.4 Opportunities to Nurture Microsystem Resilience

From the earliest days of resilience research, scholars have noted that a healthy attachment relationship with just one caregiver is among the most fundamental predictors of positive development during and after adversity (Masten & Barnes, 2018; Masten & Palmer, 2019; Rutter, 1985). This relationship appears to be protective and promotive of children's social, emotional, and cognitive development even amid severe adversity (Yamaoka & Bard, 2019). Needless to say, parents are best able to provide security, nurture, and responsiveness to their children when they are physically present. Climate-related disasters, displacement, and armed conflict sometimes separate children from their parents, whether this occurs due to floods, a challenging migration process, parental death, or through income-driven parental migration, leaving children behind. In Somali youth, significant PTSD risk emerged from the interaction between traumatic experience and multiple separations (Rousseau & Drapeau, 1998). Among children exposed to severe natural disasters, parental separations and other attachment injuries predicted more negative mental health prognoses (Bryant et al., 2017; Osofsky et al., 2015). It is essential for governments and NGOs to make every possible effort to keep children and parents together during and after disasters, reuniting separated families as soon as feasible. Having a secure relationship with *two* caregiving adults may provide additional protection against childhood PTSD following conflict exposure, so it is ideal for humanitarian and resettlement processes to maintain children's connections to as many safe adults in the family system as possible (Punamäki, 2021).

Interventionists and policy makers who are developmentally informed may find themselves taking unconventional steps to support young children's connectedness to caregivers. One fascinating study examined the development of children of mothers who were incarcerated when the child was between 0 and 18 months old. Some children in the sample were separated from their mothers during the duration of parental incarceration, while the others were raised by their mothers in nurseries housed within the walls of prisons. As preschoolers, children fared better on measures of anxiety, depression, and behavioral problems if they had lived in prison nurseries where they could benefit from frequent contact with their mothers (Goshin et al., 2014).

As noted, environmental stressors and deprivation can impact the responsiveness and sensitivity of caregiving systems. Providing families with nutritional support is beneficial for children's long-term mental health and cognitive development, unsurprisingly (Molcho et al., 2007), with parental mental illness implicated in these processes (Althoff et al., 2016). Addressing food insecurity can improve the health of attachment relationships, as well as parental mental health and children's cognitive development. Broadly, reducing environmental strains on parents—for example, through increasing the safety of their environments, alleviating economic strain, and promoting social supports—constitutes a promising strategy for protecting attachment relationships (Mesman et al., 2016).

Evidence across cultures indicates that maternal mental health is associated with mental and physical wellbeing in children (Betancourt et al., 2014). The moderating influence of family functioning on the mental health of children affected by war may take two forms, depending on the quality of parenting provided: Parents or family members can provide a "protective shield" during hardship, or parents can accentuate the impact of the stress of war when they manage stress poorly. Any interventions to support the mental health of caregivers are likely to cascade to benefit attachment relationships. Among families impacted by armed conflict, the emotional availability of caregivers and the supportiveness of the home environment as a whole can moderate the effects of trauma exposure on children's behavior problems and hostility (Bosqui et al., 2017). Interventions that increase household predictability and caregivers' emotional capacity may support cognitive, social, and emotional development both directly and also indirectly through attachment health (Doom et al., 2024).

Parents reporting high levels of parenting-related stress may be at risk of forming less adaptive attachment relationships with their babies and young children, so efforts to identify dyads affected by parenting stress may help providers to plan targeted interventions, ideally even before a baby is born (Nordahl et al., 2020). Additionally, several parent-focused interventions have been found to help to increase parents' sensitivity and responsiveness to their babies' and young children's needs, to the benefit of attachment relationships. For example, the Attachment and Biobehavioral Catch-up (ABC) program delivers parent coaching in families facing risks to healthy parent-child relationships, such as after separations, maltreatment, or other attachment injuries. This program and others like it have shown promising results for improving attachment relationships, including in contexts marked by complexities like immigration-related needs and child welfare concerns (Benito-Gomez et al., 2022; Dozier & Bernard, 2017). Training in parental sensitivity, combined with exercises to help caregivers empathize with their babies, can have powerful impacts on attachment relationships and parents' own mental health (MacBeth et al., 2015; Slade et al., 2020; Swain et al., 2017). Culturally and contextually tailored interventions are likely to be especially effective (Ullmann et al., 2018). Other strategies include delivering education in concrete childcare skills. For example, responsive feeding is included in the UN's guidelines for protecting development, both nutritionally and also psychologically, as it can both rely on and amplify a caregiver's sensitivity to a baby's cues and may even support caregivers' sense of self-efficacy (WHO & UNICEF, 2003).

Reflection Questions

Question 1. What policies, practices, and resources in your country and community help to directly or indirectly support the health of early attachment relationships?

Question 2. Can you think of three ways that secure attachments support children's positive development? What about during stressful times?

Question 3. What would be done differently in your community if attachment was treated as a public health issue?

References

Ainsworth, M. D. (1962). The effects of maternal deprivation: A review of findings and controversy in the context of research strategy. *Public Health Papers*, *14*, 97–165.

Ainsworth, M., Blechar, E., Waters, & Wall, S. (1978). *Patterns of attachment*. Erlbaum.

Althoff, R. R., Ametti, M., & Bertmann, F. (2016). The role of food insecurity in developmental psychopathology. *Preventive Medicine*, *92*, 106–109. https://doi.org/10.1016/j.ypmed.2016.08.012

Benito-Gomez, M., Carrera, P., Zablah, F., Roben, C., & Dozier, M. (2022). Enhancing parental sensitivity in families with an evidence-based early intervention. *Papeles del psicólogo*, *43*(2), 110–116.

Betancourt, T. S., Abdi, S., Ito, B. S., Lilienthal, G. M., Agalab, N., & Ellis, H. (2014). We left one war and came to another: Resource loss, acculturative stress, and caregiver-child relationships in somali refugee families. *Cultural Diversity and Ethnic Minority Psychology*. Advance online publication. https://doi.org/10.1037/a0037538

Bosqui, T. J., Marshoud, B., & Shannon, C. (2017). Attachment insecurity, posttraumatic stress, and hostility in adolescents exposed to armed conflict. *Journal of Peace Psychology*, *23*(4), 372–382. https://doi.org/10.1037/pac0000260

Bowlby, J. (1969). *Attachment*, Volume 1. Basic Books. ISBN-10 0-465-00543-8

Bronfenbrenner, U. (1977). Toward an experimental ecology of human development. *American Psychologist*, *32*(7), 513.

Bryant, R. A., Creamer, M., O'donnell, M., Forbes, D., Felmingham, K. L., Silove, D., Malhi, G., Van Hoof, M., McFarlane, A. C. & Nickerson, A. (2017). Separation from parents during childhood trauma predicts adult attachment security and post-traumatic stress disorder. *Psychological Medicine*, *47*(11), 2028–2035.

Catalá, P., Gutiérrez, L., Écija, C., & Peñacoba, C. (2025). Maternal attachment and perinatal health in refugee women: A systematic review. *Psychiatry International*, *6*(1), 20.

Cohodes, E. M., Kribakaran, S., Odriozola, P., Bakirci, S., McCauley, S., Hodges, H. R., Sisk, L. M., Zacharek, S. J., & Gee, D. G. (2021). Migration-related trauma and mental health among migrant children emigrating from Mexico and Central

America to the United States: Effects on developmental neurobiology and implications for policy. *Developmental Psychobiology, 63*(6), e22158. https://doi.org/10.1002/dev.22158
Dimitry, L. (2012). A systematic review on the mental health of children and adolescents in areas of armed conflict in the middle east. *Child: Care, Health and Development, 38*(2), 153–161.
Doom, J. R., Han, D., Rivera, K. M., & Tseten, T. (2024). Childhood unpredictability research within the developmental psychopathology framework: Advances, implications, and future directions. *Development and Psychopathology, 36*(5), 2452–2463.
Dozier, M., & Bernard, K. (2017). Attachment and biobehavioral catch-up: Addressing the needs of infants and toddlers exposed to inadequate or problematic caregiving. *Current Opinion in Psychology, 15*, 111–117.
Egeland, B., & Sroufe, L. A. (1981). Attachment and early maltreatment. *Child Development, 46*, 71–76.
Gee, D. G., Gabard-Durnam, L. J., Flannery, J., Goff, B., Humphreys, K. L., Telzer, E. H., Hare, T. A., Bookheimer, S. Y. & Tottenham, N. (2013). Early developmental emergence of human amygdala–prefrontal connectivity after maternal deprivation. *Proceedings of the National Academy of Sciences, 110*(39), 15638–15643.
Girme, Y., Yuthika, U., Jones, R. E., Fleck, C., Simpson, J. A., & Overall, N. C. (2021). Infants' attachment insecurity predicts attachment-relevant emotion regulation strategies in adulthood. *Emotion, 21*(2), 260–272.
Goshin, L. S., Byrne, M. W., & Blanchard-Lewis, B. (2014). Preschool outcomes of children who lived as infants in a prison nursery. *The Prison Journal, 94*(2), 139–158.
Gottlieb, G. (1991). Experiential canalization of behavioral development: Theory. *Developmental Psychology, 27*(1), 4–13. https://doi.org/10.1037/0012-1649.27.1.4
Gunnar, M. R., & Quevedo, K. M. (2007). Early care experiences and HPA axis regulation in children: A mechanism for later trauma vulnerability. *Progress in Brain Research, 167*, 137–149.
Gunnar, M. R., & Reid, B. M. (2019). Early deprivation revisited: Contemporary studies of the impact on young children of institutional care. *Annual Review of Developmental Psychology, 1*(1), 93–118.
MacBeth, A., Law, J., McGowan, I., Norrie, J., Thompson, L., & Wilson, P. (2015). Mellow parenting: Systematic review and meta-analysis of an intervention to promote sensitive parenting. *Developmental Medicine & Child Neurology, 57*(12), 1119–1128.
Main, M., & Solomon, J. (1990). Procedures for identifying infants as disorganized/disoriented during the Ainsworht strange situation. In M. T. Greenberg, D. Cicchetti, & E. M. Cummings (Eds.), *Attachment in the preschool year: Theory, research, and intervention* (pp. 121–60). University of Chicago Press.
Masarik, A. S., & Conger, R. D. (2017). Stress and child development: A review of the Family Stress Model. *Current Opinion in Psychology, 13*, 85–90.
Masten, A. S. (2025). *Ordinary magic* (2nd ed.). Guilford.
Masten, A. S., & Barnes, A. J. (2018). Resilience in children: Developmental perspectives. *Children, 5*(7), 98.
Masten, A. S., & Osofsky, J. D. (2018). Disasters and their impact on child development: Introduction to the special section. *Child Development, 81*(4), 1029–1039.
Masten, A. S., & Palmer, A. R. (2019). Parenting to promote resilience in children. In *Handbook of parenting: The practice of parenting* (Vol. 5, 3rd ed., pp. 156–188). Routledge/Taylor & Francis Group. https://doi.org/10.4324/9780429401695-6

Matas, L. Arend, R. A., & Sroufe, L. A. (1978). Continuity of adaptation in the second years: The relationship between quality of attachment and later competence. *Child Development, 49*, 547–556.

Mesman, J., Van Ijzendoorn, M. H., & Sagi-Schwartz, A. (2016). Cross-cultural patterns of attachment. *Handbook of Attachment: Theory, Research, and Clinical Applications, 3*, 852–877.

Mohamed, A., & Homeida, A. (2024). Hunger in the shadow of conflict: Analyzing malnutrition and humanitarian challenges in Sudan. *Conflict and Health, 18*(1), 50.

Molcho, M., Gabhainn, S. N., Kelly, C., Friel, S., & Kelleher, C. (2007). Food poverty and health among schoolchildren in Ireland: Findings from the Health Behaviour in School aged Children (HBSC) study. *Public Health Nutrition, 10*, 364–370.

Morina, N., Stam, K., Pollet, T. V., & Priebe, S. (2018). Prevalence of depression and posttraumatic stress disorder in adult civilian survivors of war who stay in war afflicted regions. A systematic review and meta-analysis of epidemiological studies. *Journal of Affective Disorders, 239*, 328–338.

Nordahl, D., Rognmo, K., Bohne, A., Landsem, I. P., Moe, V., Wang, C. E. A., & Høifødt, R. S. (2020). Adult attachment style and maternal-infant bonding: The indirect path of parenting stress. *BMC Psychology, 8*, 1–11.

Okello, J., Broekaert, E., & Derluyn, I. (2014). War-trauma, attachment, and risk behavior in war-affected adolescents in Northern Uganda. (find link)

Osofsky, J., Kronenberg, M., Bocknek, E. *et al.* Longitudinal Impact of Attachment-Related Risk and Exposure to Trauma Among Young Children After Hurricane Katrina. *Child Youth Care Forum* 44, 493–510 (2015). https://doi.org/10.1007/s10566-015-9300-7

Punamäki, R. L. (2001). Resiliency factors predicting psychological adjustment after political violence among Palestinian children. *International Journal of Behavioral Development, 25*(3), 256–267.

Punamäki, R. L., Isosävi, S., Qouta, S. R., Kuittinen, S., & Diab, S. Y. (2017). War trauma and maternal–fetal attachment predicting maternal mental health, infant development, and dyadic interaction in Palestinian families. *Attachment & Human Development, 19*(5), 463–486.

Raby, K. L., Fraley, R. C., & Roisman, G. I. (2021). Categorical or dimensional measures of attachment? Insights from factor-analytic and taxometric research. In R. A. Thompson, J. A. Simpson, & L. J. Berlin (Eds.), *Attachment: Fundamental questions.* ISBN 97814625-46022. The Guilford Press.

Rigaud, K. K., de Sherbinin, A., Jones, B., Bergmann, J., Clement, V., Ober, K., Schewe, J., Adamo, S., McCusker, B., Heuser, S., & Midgley, A. (2018). Groundswell: Preparing for internal climate migration. *World Bank*. https://doi.org/10.1596/29461.

Rousseau, C., & Drapeau, A. (1998). The impact of culture on the transmission of trauma. In Y. Danieli (Ed.), *International handbook of multigenerational legacies of trauma. The plenum series on stress and coping.* Springer. https://doi.org/10.1007/978-1-4757-5567-1_29

Rutter, M. (1985). Resilience in the face of adversity: Protective factors and resistance to psychiatric disorder. *British Journal of Psychiatry, 147*, 598–611. https://doi.org/10.1192/bjp.147.6.598

Slade, A., Holland, M. L., Ordway, M. R., Carlson, E. A., Jeon, S., Close, N., & Sadler, L. S. (2020). Minding the Baby®: Enhancing parental reflective functioning and infant attachment in an attachment-based, interdisciplinary home visiting program. *Development and Psychopathology, 32*(1), 123–137.

Slone, M., & Mann, S. (2016). Effects of war, terrorism, and armed conflict on young children: A systematic review. *Child Psychiatry & Human Development, 47*(6), 950–965.

Sroufe, L. A. (1983). Infant caregiver attachment and patters of attachment in preschool: The roots of maladaptation and competence. In *Development and policy concerning children with special needs. The Minnesota Symposium on Child Psychology* (vol. 16), edited by M. Perlmutter. Erllbaum.

Sroufe, L. A., & Waters, E. (1977). Attachment as an organizational construct. In *Interpersonal Development* (109–124), edited by Rita Zukauskiene. Routledge.

Swain, J. E., Ho, S. S., Rosenblum, K. L., Morelen, D., Dayton, C. J., & Muzik, M. (2017). Parent–child intervention decreases stress and increases maternal brain activity and connectivity during own baby-cry: An exploratory study. *Development and Psychopathology, 29*(2), 535–553.

Ullmann, E., Bornstein, S. R., Lanzman, R. S., Kirschbaum, C., Sierau, S., Doehnert, M., Zimmermann, P., Kindler, H., Schauer, M., Ruf-Leuschner, M., Fegert, J.M. (2018). Countering posttraumatic LHPA activation in refugee mothers and their infants. *Molecular Psychiatry, 23*(1), 2–5.

Vaughn, B. E., Egeland, B., & Sroufe, L. A. (1979). Individual differences in infant-mother attachment at 12 and 18 months: Stability and change in families under stress. *Child Development, 50*, 971–975.

Waddoups, A. B., Yoshikawa, H., & Strouf, K. (2019). Developmental effects of parent-child separation. *Annual Review of Developmental Psychology, 1*(1), 387–410. https://doi.org/10.1146/annurev-devpsych-121318-085142

WHO & UNICEF (2003). *Global strategy for infant and young child feeding*. WHO. https://www.who.int/publications/i/item/9241562218

Yamaoka, Y., & Bard, D. E. (2019). Positive parenting matters in the face of early adversity. *American Journal of Preventive Medicine, 56*(4), 530–539.

Yarrow, L., Rubenstein, J., & Pedersen, F. (1975). *Infant and environment-Early cognitive and motivational development.* Wiley.

6 The Meso- and Exosystems

Mastery, Competence, and Identity

6.1 Introduction—The Mesosystem and Exosystem

As described previously, children's most proximal environments are often referred to as the "microsystem." The previous chapter focuses on caregiving relationships, which are among the most important facets of the microsystem in early life. Other important features of the microsystem include sibling relationships, close friendships, neighbors, and, as children enter school, teachers.

It is not hard to intuit that children's development is shaped not only by each of these relationships discretely, but also by the interactions between these parties. For example, a child's academic progress often varies greatly with the degree to which a caregiver is in communication with teachers and school staff. An entire sphere of Bronfenbrenner's model, the *mesosystem*, is dedicated to conceptualizing these interactions (Bronfenbrenner & Morris, 2007).

Beyond the microsystem, according to Bronfenbrenner's social-ecological framework, lie the formal and informal social institutions that shape children from an additional degree of removal, such as friends of the family, health systems, neighborhood organizations, religious institutions, welfare services, and family members' workplaces. This sphere is known as the *exosystem*. Children need not interact with it directly to be shaped by it. Parental leave policies can have substantial impacts on infant and childhood development, for example, while a caregiver's work schedule affects both their availability and mood at home (Gaston et al., 2015). Local school board decisions about funding and programming impact the quality of education a child receives. Assets at the community level (e.g., gainful employment opportunities, access to healthy and affordable food, and functional healthcare facilities), as well as risks (e.g., proximity to polluting industrial sites) are all relevant to children's development (Acevedo-Garcia et al., 2014).

Figure 6.1 provides a schematic of these two systems and names some of the developmental tasks discussed in this chapter.

DOI: 10.4324/9781003488385-8

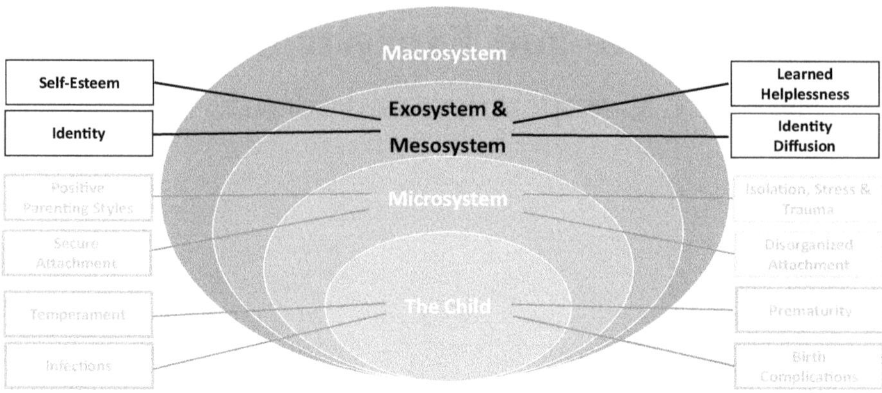

Figure 6.1 The socio-ecological model: The mesosystem and exosystem

6.2 Developmental Tasks in the Mesosystems and Exosystems

The foundations a child builds through stable, responsive caregiving relationships confer many of the skills they will need to navigate the environments outside of their homes (Sroufe & Waters, 2007). As they explore their neighborhoods, schools, and other environments, children have more and more opportunities to develop problem-solving skills, mastery motivation, self-esteem, and eventually a sense of identity.

A *mastery orientation* commonly develops during toddlerhood, preschool, and the early school years, as children approach the world with a desire to *achieve*, whether this achievement takes the form of stacking objects, helping with household chores, or showing off dances. In attempting these tasks, children also learn to measure themselves against standards (e.g., through earning praise from adults), incorporate feedback, and use reasoning skills to improve their performance—all the while, grasping that their success relates to their ability and effort (Eccles et al. 1998). Concurrently, children come to appreciate to a greater extent that they can learn and improve their abilities by attempting challenging tasks; that they can face and overcome new challenges; that failure is, at least in part, a result of factors that can be altered and changed; and that they are capable of persisting. Children who struggle to develop a mastery orientation may have low opinions of their own capacities, attributing their failure to a permanent lack of ability, but attributing success to luck or external events. Unlike those with a strong mastery orientation, children who view themselves from a lens of *learned helplessness* may have trouble applying themselves to tasks with persistence and hope (Cain & Dweck, 1995).

Self-esteem is another critical aspect of a child's emotional development, originating in early childhood and growing more elaborate in middle childhood. The construct is understood most broadly to reflect a global evaluation of oneself (Rosenberg, 1979). Another frequently used definition, by

Blascovich and Tomaka (1991), defines self-esteem as "the overall affective evaluation of one's own worth, value or importance." Other definitions reference specific domains of self-evaluation, such as one's academic aptitude, social skills, physical appearance, and athletic ability (Harter, 1982; Van den Bergh & DeRycke, 2003). A child's success at the most salient tasks at a given developmental stage (e.g., social competence in adolescence) are closely related to self-esteem, and this relationship is bidirectional. A child with high self-esteem is likely to be more proactive and adaptive when exploring their larger environment, learning new skills as a result that further benefit their sense of competence. Positive peer relations are also related bidirectionally to the development of self-esteem (Antonopoulou et al., 2019; Luijten, van de Bongardt, & Nieboer, 2023).

A youth's sense of ***identity*** emerges from their organized self-description and is therefore closely related to self-esteem. Closely tied to belonging, identity encapsulates a cohesive sense of one's self, one's values, one's expectations of the world, and one's frameworks for decision-making. It provides the foundation for an individual's interpersonal relations, choice of community, group membership, religious identification, political orientation, and more. A sense of identity is thought to emerge from engagement with the surrounding world over time, including family, peers, and cultural communities (Erickson, 1968). In particular, young people's identity development may benefit from sources of continuity (e.g., stable family relationships and positive engagement with religious or school communities) during periods of transition or novelty (Branje, 2022). With these supports, young people can feel safer exploring new dimensions of the self or frameworks for the world and consider whether to commit to them. Such positive exploration opportunities can beget youth's sense of competence and even help them to build patterns of positive civic engagement (Obradović & Masten, 2007). If these trajectories of identity exploration and commitment are threatened or disrupted, an individual's identity development may be compromised—for example, through failure to form a cohesive sense of self or long-term challenges with belonging. Wellbeing and competence in multiple domains may suffer as a result (Hatano et al., 2020).

In considering the influences of the mesosystem and exosystem on children's development, it is important to remember that the relationships and other resources of the microsystem are still implicated in developmental trajectories even as children engage in more activities outside of the home (de Souza Morais et al., 2021). Warm and affectionate parental relationships, for example, are closely related to young people's development of self-esteem, and coherent family identity can support the development of individual identity (Branje, 2022; Ojanen & Perry, 2007). In fact, the extent of a child's intuitive trust in the world and in relationships first shaped in infancy and toddlerhood continues to be implicated in the development of interpersonal interaction styles, mastery motivation, and positive identity (Erickson, 1968; Sroufe & Watters, 2007).

6.3 The Impact of Humanitarian Emergencies on Child Development

Complex humanitarian emergencies, whether from armed conflict, environmental crises, or other causes, can disrupt nurturing family and community relationships, and even the infrastructure of society. This is a particularly potent risk when disasters are multisystem and prolonged. Even when children are physically safe, these disasters can impede their ongoing development by interfering with opportunities to explore, solve problems, connect with safe others, and develop the essential attributes of mastery and self-esteem (Betancourt & Williams, 2008).

When adversity occurs at the family level (e.g., through parental loss or separation, or through toxic levels of stress introduced to caregiving relationships), children not only lose access to co-regulation support from the safe adults around them but also to the parental praise that forms the foundation of mastery; to the coherent narratives about family and community identity that can help them form a sense of self; and many other resources (Branje, 2022; Masten & Palmer, 2019). In fact, childhood adversity has been found to impact children's hormonal and stress regulation patterns through family processes and, specifically, diminished development of self-esteem (Zilioli et al., 2016).

Another domain of child development that is vulnerable to the impact of humanitarian emergencies is the development of positive exploration and play. Play is one of the first casualties of war. It is common for these basic developmental needs to be inadvertently neglected during emergencies as concrete needs take priority, to the detriment of children's mastery motivation, self-esteem, problem-solving skills, social development, and basic sense of competence (Wessells, 1998). Meanwhile, the risk of death or injury from the relics of war, such as chemical contaminants or unexploded ordnance, keeps many children from freely exploring their environments (Frost et al., 2017). Humanitarian settings like refugee camps are often unsafe places to play and are rarely designed with children's needs at the center (Hyder, 2005). Even after children and their families are physically safe, lingering levels of fear (their own and their caregivers') may result in lower levels of exploration and play. Even playful and exploratory cognitive processes (e.g., imagination) can be diminished in children who have experienced serious adversities (Rubinstein & Lahad, 2023).

In the broader community, prolonged collective stress may make it more difficult for children to treat one another with kindness. The resulting interpersonal adversities can diminish children's sense of social competence, and therefore their self-esteem (Hodges et al., 1999). Furthermore, damage to community gathering spaces, or loss of these spaces during and after displacement, can rob children of critical opportunities to build their developmental competence in the ways described above. When children develop in contexts that are hostile to their identity groups in some way—for example, when youth are displaced to resettlement societies marked by xenophobia, or when post-disaster resource scarcity in a nation results in heightened ethnic tensions—they may have difficulty safely exploring and committing to their own ethnic and cultural identities (Suárez-Orozco et al., 2018).

The prolonged sense of powerlessness and fear that so often accompanies exposure to armed conflict can make it hard for children to develop a sense of mastery motivation and self-efficacy. In fact, exposure to political violence is associated with lower self-esteem in children (Haj-Yahia et al., 2021). Climate change, as discussed, can significantly increase the likelihood of exposure to an array of adverse conditions known to affect health, wellbeing, and development (Oberg et al., 2021). There is an emerging field of scientific study documenting the risk that climate change poses to children, including through damage to caregivers' mental health and wellness, with negative impacts on children including increased anxiety and depression, a sense of powerlessness, and challenges with learning and emotion regulation (Burke et al., 2018; Olson & Metz. 2020).

Case Study: The Aftermath of the 2004 Tsunami

A major tsunami occurred in the Indian Ocean on December 26, 2004. It was the deadliest natural disaster to date in the 21st century and one of the worst tsunamis in recorded history, with over 250,000 people killed and thousands more injured. The tsunami's massive waves came in pairs or triads, with crests as high as 20 feet traveling at hundreds of miles per hour. The impact of the crashing waves and the flooding of surrounding areas left a desolate landscape in which survival was challenging.

In addition to this catastrophic loss of life, microsystems and exosystems were damaged across the region, with schools, religious communities, child-care facilities, markets, and other gathering spaces destroyed or damaged. Widespread trauma in the adult world doubtless shaped many people's interaction styles with one another. Unsurprisingly, children's trauma symptoms were worse when the usual supports around them were damaged, such as protective caregiving relationships or social and practical resources in the community (Agustini et al., 2011). At the same time, for people who survived this disaster, the ongoing impacts of trauma often coincided with positive developmental outcomes. In particular, children's development benefited from religious activities and involvement in spiritual communities, meaning-making, opportunities to fulfill meaningful social roles, and connection with others (Math et al., 2008; Taube Dayan, 2023).

6.4 Interventions

Children have the right to explore, discover, and play during times of war and displacement. As van Gils (2007) stated so clearly, "the right to play is the right to be a child"; in fact, this is captured in Article 31 of the UN Convention on the Rights of the Child. A child rights framing (discussed further in Chapter 17), especially when coupled with enforceable rules around the care of children in humanitarian settings, may help international parties to safeguard children's access to play areas, education spaces, and community gatherings even amid conflict and natural disasters (Bennet & Friel, 2014). There is growing interest in developing educational and life skills training opportunities for youth in humanitarian settings, which can benefit their sense of self-efficacy (Schlecht et al., 2017). When these programs are embedded in trusted community institutions (e.g., schools or religious organizations), children may additionally benefit from increases in belonging and social connection.

Ensuring that families' material needs are met can help caregiving systems to continue functioning as buffers from ongoing adversity, improve caregiver mental health, and help give children the freedom to engage in developmentally typical exploration, play, and socialization (Meyer et al., 2019). Meanwhile, children who have been through forced displacement may benefit from targeted mental health programs in schools and communities that can improve their self-esteem, motivation, and self-efficacy (Tyrer & Fazel, 2014), while therapies based in play and creativity may help to rebuild children's sense of imagination and play (Rubinstein & Lahad, 2023). Hodges and Abdi (2024) describe more approaches to support healthy adolescent development after displacement.

There is a paucity of research on the development of children facing complex emergencies (Jordans et al., 2009). Partnering with young people and the adults who support them through community-based research and needs assessment (discussed further in Chapter 19) can help teams gain insights about the specific needs of youth depending on their gender, social identities, and developmental stages (Chávez et al., 2018).

6.5 Conclusion

Armed conflict, natural disasters, and other crises can interfere with children's psychological and social development, including the sense that they belong and can make a difference in the world. Adults are responsible for creating environments that nurture children's development, including opportunities to explore, solve problems, develop mastery, build self-esteem, and explore positive identities. These opportunities are likely to have cascading effects on children's wellbeing, especially when they help children to connect with supports in their own communities.

Reflection Questions

Question 1. What are two ways that large disasters like the 2004 Indian Ocean tsunami can impact children's identity development?
Question 2. How does a sense of agency, mastery, and empowerment benefit children's future development? Can you name two ways that armed conflict exposure might damage this?
Question 3. Describe a program you have learned about or experienced that is likely to help children build mastery, self-esteem, belonging, and identity during or after trauma exposure. How do you think this program is helpful?

References

Acevedo-Garcia, D., McArdle, N., Hardy, E. F., Crisan, U. I., Romano, B., Norris, D., Baek, M., & Reece, J. (2014). The child opportunity index: Improving collaboration between community development and public health. *Health Affairs*, *33*(11), 1948–1957.

Agustini, E. N., Asniar, I., & Matsuo, H. (2011). The prevalence of long-term post-traumatic stress symptoms among adolescents after the tsunami in Aceh. *Journal of Psychiatric and Mental Health Nursing*, *18*(6), 543–549.

Antonopoulou, K., Chaidemenou, A., & Kouvava, S. (2019). Peer acceptance and friendships among primary school pupils: Associations with loneliness, self-esteem and school engagement. *Educational Psychology in Practice*, *35*(3), 339–351.

Bennett, C. M., & Friel, S. (2014). Impact of climate change on inequities in child health. *Children*, *1*(3), 461–473.

Betancourt, T. S., & Williams, T. (2008). Building and evidence base on mental health interventions for children affected by armed conflict. *Intervention*, *6*(1), 39–56. https://doi.org/10.1097/WTF.0b013e3282f761ff

Blascovich, J., & Tomaka, J. (1991). Measures of self-esteem. In J. P. Robinson, P. R. Shaver, & L. S. Wrightsman (Eds.), *Measures of personality and social psychological attitudes* (pp. 115–160). Academic Press.

Branje, S. (2022). Adolescent identity development in context. *Current Opinion in Psychology*, *45*, 101286.

Bronfenbrenner, U., & Morris, P. A. (2007). The bioecological model of human development. *Handbook of Child Psychology*, *1*.

Burke, S. E. L., Sanson, A. V., & Van Hoorn, J. (2018). The psychological effects of climate change on children. *Current Psychiatry Reports*, *20*, 35. https://doi.org/10.1007/s11920-018-0896-9

Cain, K. M., & Dweck, C. S. (1995). The relation between motivational patterns and achievement cognition through the elementary school years. *Merrill-Palmer Quarterly*, *41*, 25–52.

Chávez, C., Cuesta, J., Godwin, M., & Shusterman, J. (2018). The long-term effect of humanitarian emergencies on adolescents: Existing evidence, gaps and considerations for research and practitioners.

de Souza Morais, R. L., de Castro Magalhães, L., Nobre, J. N. P., Pinto, P. F. A., da Rocha Neves, K., & Carvalho, A. M. (2021). Quality of the home, daycare and neighborhood environment and the cognitive development of economically disadvantaged children in early childhood: A mediation analysis. *Infant Behavior and Development*, *64*, 101619.

Eccles, J. S., Wigfield, A., & Schiefele, U. (1998). Motivation to succeed. In W. Damon, & N. Eisenberg (Eds.), *Handbook of child psychology: Social, emotional, and personality development* (pp. 1017–1095). John Wiley.

Erickson, E. H. (1968). *Identity, youth, and crisis.* Norton.

Frost, A., Boyle, P., Autier, P., King, C., Zwijeneburg, W., Hewitson, D., & Sullivan, R. (2017). The effect of explosive remnants of war on global public health: A systematic mixed- studies review using narrative synthesis. *Lancet Public Health*, *2*(6), 286–296.

Gaston, A., Edwards, S. A., & Tober, J. A. (2015). Parental leave and child care arrangements during the first 12 months of life are associated with children's development five years later. *International Journal of Child, Youth and Family Studies*, *6*(2), 230–251.

Haj-Yahia, M., Greenbaum, C. W., & Lahoud-Shoufany, L. (2021), Palestinian Adolescents' prolonged exposure to political violence, self-esteem, and post-traumatic stress symptoms. *Journal of Interpersonal Violence*, *36*(9–10), 4137–4164.

Harter, S. (1982). The perceived competence scale for children. *Child Development*, *53*, 87–97.

Hatano, K., Sugimura, K., Crocetti, E., & Meeus, W. H. (2020). Diverse-and-dynamic pathways in educational and interpersonal identity formation during adolescence: Longitudinal links with psychosocial functioning. *Child Development*, *91*(4), 1203–1218.

Hodges, E. V. E., Boivin, M., Vitaro, F., & Bukowski, W. M. (1999). The power of friendship: Protection against an escalating cycle of peer victimization. *Developmental Psychology*, *35*(1). 94–101.

Hodges, H. R., & Abdi, S. M. (2024). Forced displacement. In *Encyclopedia of Adolescence* (Vol. 2). Elsevier.

Hyder, T. (2005). *War, conflict, and play* (p. 24). Open University Press.

Jordans, M., J., D., Wietse, A. T., Komproe, I. H., J., V., T., M., de Jong. (2009). Systematic review of evidence and treatment approaches: Psychosocial mental health care for children in war. *Child and Adolescent Mental Health*, *2009*, 2–14.

Luijten, C. C., van de Bongardt, D., & Nieboer, A. P. (2023). Adolescents' friendship quality and over-time development of well-being: The explanatory role of self-esteem. *Journal of adolescence*, *95*(5), 1057–1069.

Math, S. B., Tandon, S., Girimaji, S. C., Benegal, V., Kumar, U., Hamza, A., Jangam, K., & Nagaraja, D. (2008). Psychological impact of the tsunami on children and adolescents from the Andaman and Nicobar Islands. *Primary Care Companion to the Journal of Clinical Psychiatry*, *10*(1), 31.

Meyer, S. R., Meyer, E., Bangirana, C., Mangen, P. O., & Stark, L. (2019). Protection and well-being of adolescent refugees in the context of a humanitarian crisis: Perceptions from South Sudanese refugees in Uganda. *Social Science & Medicine*, *221*, 79–86.

Oberg, C. N., Hodges, H. R., & Masten, A. S. (2021). Risk and resilience of Somali children in the context of climate change, famine and conflict. *Journal of Applied Research on Children: Informing Policy for Children at Risk*, *12*, 1–26.

Obradović, J., & Masten, A. S. (2007). Developmental Antecedents of Young Adult Civic Engagement. *Applied Developmental Science, 11*(1), 2–19. https://doi.org/10.1080/10888690709336720

Ojanen, T., & Perry, D. G. (2007). Relational schemas and the developing self: Perceptions of mother and of self as joint predictors of early adolescents' self-esteem. *Developmental Psychology, 43*(6), 1474–1483.

Olson, D. M., & Metz, G. A. S. (2020). Climate change is a major stressor causing poor pregnancy outcomes and child development. *F1000Res, 9*, F1000 Faculty Rev-1222. https://doi.org/10.12688/f1000research.27157.1. PMID: 33093942; PMCID: PMC7549179.

Schlecht, J., Lee, C., Kerner, B., Greeley, M., & Robinson, C. (2017). Prioritizing programming to address the needs and risks of very young adolescents: A summary of findings across three humanitarian settings. *Conflict and Health, 11*, 1–8.

Sroufe, L. A., & Waters, E. (2017). Attachment as an organizational construct. *Interpersonal Development*, 109–124.

Suárez-Orozco, C., Motti-Stefanidi, F., Marks, A., & Katsiaficas, D. (2018). An integrative risk and resilience model for understanding the adaptation of immigrant-origin children and youth. *American Psychologist, 73*(6), 781.

Rosenberg, M. (1979). *Conceiving the self*. Basic Books.

Rubinstein, D., & Lahad, M. (2023). Fantastic reality: The role of imagination, playfulness, and creativity in healing trauma. *Traumatology, 29*(2), 102.

Taube Dayan, S. (2023). Trauma is not the whole story: Trajectories of responses to childhood disasters intertwining with Life following the Indian Ocean tsunami. *Infant and Child Development, 32*(4), e2437.

Tyrer, R.A, & Fazel, M. (2014). School and community-based interventions for refugee and asylum seeking children: A systematic review. *PLoS One, 9*(2), e89359.

Van Gils, J. (2007). The child's right to play: The right to be a child. *The UN children's rights convention: Theory meets practice: Proceedings of the International Interdisciplinary Conference on Children's Rights* (pp. 18–19). Intersentia.

Vanden Bergh, B. R. H., & De Rycke, L. (2003). Measuring the multidimensional self-concept and global self-worth of 6–8 year olds. *Journal of Genetic Psychology, 164*, 2010–225.

Wessells, M. G. (1998). Children, armed conflict, and peace. *Journal of Peace Research, 35*(5), 635–646.

Zilioli, S., Slatcher, R. B., Chi, P., Li, X., Zhao, J., & Zhao, G. (2016). Childhood adversity, self-esteem, and diurnal cortisol profiles across the life span. *Psychological Science, 27*(9), 1249–1265.

7 The Macrosystem and Gender Equity

7.1 Introduction—The Macrosystem

Bronfenbrenner (1994) described the macrosystem as the overarching patterns of the micro-, meso-, and exosystems of a given culture or subculture. This sphere includes belief systems, bodies of knowledge, material resources, customs, lifestyles, opportunities, and life course options that are embedded in societal standards. From a bioecological perspective, competence in the macrosystem can be thought of as attainment of life paths and roles that are available to them by virtue of their communities' laws (e.g., legal conduct), customs, and cultures (e.g., particular educational milestones, particular religious practices, respected roles in family or friend circles).

In an ideal world, the opportunities available by which a person can "succeed" at macrosystem goals are options that are compatible with their own and others' thriving. Section 7.3, and Chapter 17, both discuss in more detail how rights-based approaches have been used thus far to increase the likelihood

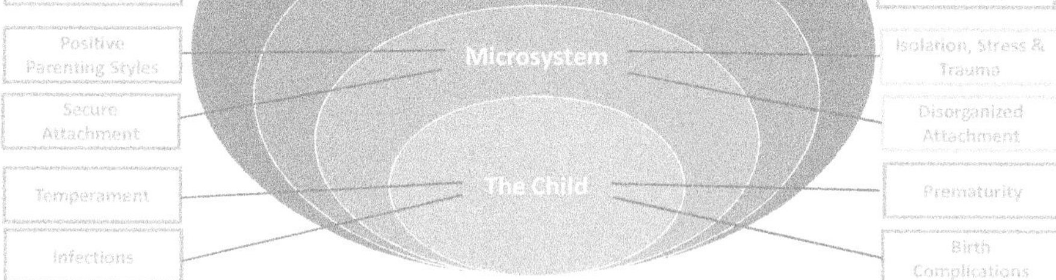

Figure 7.1 The socio-ecological model: The macrosystem.

DOI: 10.4324/9781003488385-9

that macrosystem forces converge to offer children healthy, safe, and fulfilling options for living. Figure 7.1 shows possible features of macrosystems.

7.2 Challenges in the Macrosystem to Healthy Development

Anyone who has read a news article about disparities in education quality; spent time in neighborhoods that have been deprived of economic opportunities for generations; or seen differential treatment in families, clinics, or classrooms based on a child's marginalized identity status can grasp easily that forces far larger than an individual human can interfere with the needs and rights of a child.

This chapter cannot, of course, evaluate all laws and customs in all societies in the world from a lens of child equity. Gender equity is presented as an example of a macrosystem pattern that cuts across many contexts worldwide. Some other identity markers subject to inequity (e.g., national origin, economic status, Indigeneity) are discussed further in Part III, and readers will doubtless be able to think of many more types of identity-based marginalization with the potential to interfere with children's wellbeing.

Gender inequity exists in most if not all countries on the globe to a greater or lesser degree, often interacting with other identity markers (e.g., race, ethnicity, parental status) to amplify people's risks of adverse experiences and discrimination (Baird et al., 2021). As one example affecting the adult world (and, by extension, the children that adults raise), the gender pay gap in the U.S. has doubled in recent years, from 2.9% to 6% in April 2024. The gap is especially large in STEM fields such as science and engineering, and those most affected by these inequities are women of color and women with children (Roussille, 2024). The following sections describe evidence of gender inequities in the domains of education, health, and safety, as well as ways that climate change, armed conflict, and environmental disasters can exacerbate risks.

7.2.1 Gender Inequity in Primary Education

Equity in primary education means that schools provide equal learning opportunities for all students independent of children's identity and backgrounds. Equitable education opportunities increase the chances that children will achieve their developmental milestones, perform well academically, and enjoy social and emotional wellbeing (OECD, 2018). Poverty is the single most important factor keeping children out of school worldwide, as many children are compelled to go to work to supplement their family's income (Roser, 2021). Children from the poorest households are more likely to be out of school compared to their wealthier counterparts. Here, too, it is clear that 21st-century crises escalate this risk to children, as half of the world's out-of-school children live in conflict zones.

Despite being enshrined in Article 28 of the UN Convention on the Rights of the Child, primary school-age girls throughout the world are still less likely to attend school than their male counterparts. Some factors behind this disparity relate to menstruation, including shame girls may feel during their periods, inadequate hygiene facilities in schools, and the high cost of menstrual products (Jaafar et al., 2023). Critically, "period poverty" occurs even in wealthy nations, and menstrual products have historically been taxed as luxury goods in some countries.

Other times, gender disparities are intentional, reflecting targeted threats to girls' education or policies forbidding them from attending school. Recently, it was estimated that 130 million girls around the world are denied an education (UNHR, 2023). Table 7.1 names some of the countries with some of the greatest educational disparities by gender and gives select examples of the barriers families may face to bringing their daughters to school (Theirworld, 2017).

Case Study: Malala Yousafzai

Malala Yousafzai was an adolescent from Pakistan who nearly gave her life to fight for girls' rights to education. Her advocacy stems from lived experiences. Her father was a teacher who ran a girls' school in the Swat Valley of Pakistan that, like many others, was closed when the Taliban took over the area and implemented an interpretation of Islamic law that forbade female education.

In 2009, Ms. Yousafzai began writing a blog opposing Taliban restrictions on female primary education, both in her village and also across Pakistan. On October 9, 2012, while returning from school, a masked gunman boarded her bus, attacked her, and shot her in the head. Many thought she would not survive, but after multiple surgeries and extensive rehabilitation she literally and figuratively regained her voice to speak out. Her stories and advocacy resulted in worldwide protests. Over two million people soon signed a petition for the right to female education, and Pakistan's National Assembly ratified the Right to a Free and Compulsory Education in response. In 2017, the United Nations Secretary General, António Guterres, designated Ms. Yousafzai as a Messenger of Peace to raise awareness of the need for primary education for all children regardless of gender. Ms. Yousafzai was awarded the Nobel Peace Prize in 2014 and four years later she entered Oxford University to continue her studies with a focus on philosophy, education, politics, and economics. The Malala Fund was established to promote the cause of universal primary education.

Beyond those listed below in the table, the United Nations reported that there were attacks on schools in at least 70 countries between 2009 and 2014 (OHCHR, 2015). There are huge benefits to the young girls and adolescents who are guaranteed a primary education, yet many girls are still denied this basic right. Education provides adolescent girls with the tools that help to generate economic opportunities for themselves and their families. It also reduces the prevalence of child marriage, early pregnancy and childbirth, and victimization (UNICEF, 2007).

Table 7.1 Examples of gender inequities in education

Afghanistan	More than 200 girls' schools were closed in 2016, denying over 50,000 girls access to education as policy of the Taliban and their restrictions on female education. The Taliban currently bans girls' education past primary school.
India	In July 2013, four girls 12–14 years of age were abducted from a Christian school and sexually assaulted.
Iraq	The Islamic State has persecuted Yazidi girls attending school and subjected many to sex trafficking.
Mali	Girls have been targeted violently for failure to adhere to the strict dress requirements imposed by armed groups.
Nigeria	Boko Haram has been responsible for the abduction of hundreds of girls in northeast Nigeria, along with attacks on teachers. Boko Haram has destroyed over 900 schools and closed more than 1500.
Pakistan	In 2009, Taliban attacks resulted in 120,000 female students in the Swat district losing access to education. In 2014, girls' schools were blown up in Bara and Bajaur.
Somalia	In 2010, girls were kidnapped from schools to become "wives" of Al-Shabaab fighters.
Syria	An Islamic State mortar attack on a Harabesh primary school for girls killed nine students and injured another 20 in northeast Syria.
Uganda	The Lord's Resistance Army has targeted girls' schools in northern Uganda, killing, kidnapping, and sexually assaulting students.
Yemen	In 2015, nearly half of primary school-aged girls did not go to school, due in large part to escalating conflict.

7.2.2 *Gender Inequity in Health*

One other consequence of structural gender inequity is the disinvestment in health issues affecting girls and women. In the United States, for example, research on diseases affecting primarily women and girls receives considerably less federal funding than research on male-dominant diseases, with the result that many providers and individuals lack the information they need to best promote girls' and women's health (White & Clayton, 2022). Mental health differs by gender as well: In many countries, girls are found to experience more distress, less positive emotion, and a lower sense of overall life satisfaction (Campbell et al., 2021). As with many of the themes discussed in this chapter, vulnerabilities compound intersectionally, with children facing higher risks of adverse outcomes when they experience marginalization based on other identity markers (Hoffman et al., 2022). In many countries, young people with transgender and nonbinary identities are disproportionately likely to attempt suicide and suffer from other serious mental health challenges, due in large part to discrimination, isolation, fear, and difficulty accessing supports (Kingsbury et al., 2022).

Features of a child's macrosystem clearly shape the opportunities available to them, and therefore their health. When clinicians and the systems they work in are insufficiently equipped to promote the wellbeing of youth with minoritized gender identities, it is much harder to access quality care. When girls are unable to attend school, they miss out on critical opportunities to interact with peers and build a sense of competence and self-esteem, to the detriment of their mental health (Baird et al., 2021). Climate change, environmental disasters, and armed conflict are thought to amplify gender disparities in health (van Daalen et al., 2020).

One domain of girls' and women's health that can be especially difficult to talk about and address is female genital mutilation (FGM), also known as female genital cutting, circumcision, or excision. The World Health Organization (WHO) defines FGM/cutting as all procedures that involve total or partial removal of or modification to the external female genitalia for non-medical reasons (WHO, 2024). These procedures range from partial excision of the clitoris and labia minora, to infibulation or narrowing of the vaginal opening. It is estimated that more than 230 million girls and women alive today have undergone these procedures in over 30 countries, across a wide range of ethnic, religious, and cultural communities (United Nations, 2023). Typically, FGM/cutting procedures are carried out on young girls between infancy and 15 years of age (WHO, 2024). There are no documented health benefits of these surgeries, and they are associated with a range of short- and long-term health difficulties for the girls and women who experience them, including increased risk of mortality and of future newborn deaths. Some research finds that these procedures are more common in families that face existing vulnerabilities, such as poverty (Ahinkorah et al., 2020). Additionally, armed conflict and related difficulties (e.g., forced displacement and education disruption) may increase the implementation of FGM/cutting procedures while widening gender inequities in general (Ayang, 2024; Esho et al., 2021).

The UN considers FGM/cutting a human rights violation, and the UN Sustainable Development Goal 5 (Gender Equality) also calls for intensified global efforts to end the use of these procedures by 2030. In many countries, a decline is already underway, driven largely by the advocacy of women, girls, and allies; legislation; grassroots education efforts; and, critically, by access to schooling, which is associated with a lower likelihood of intergenerational continuity of FGM/cutting (UNICEF, 2022). Of note, international discourse on these procedures has sometimes been marked by high levels of paternalism, racism, and essentializing. Cultural outsiders addressing FGM/cutting sometimes fail to attend to local contexts, needs, and strengths, as well as the complex multisystem causes and consequences of these practices (Khosla et al., 2017; Monahan, 2007). For example, there is often minimal consideration of how bans on FGM/cutting may impact the social wellbeing of women and girls in communities in which these practices have been the norm. Furthermore, international discourse and resourcing in this domain has attended primarily to *prevention* of these procedures rather than, say, addressing root causes of inequity, promoting wellbeing in those who have already undergone FGM/cutting, and training healthcare providers to offer excellent care to these individuals. As is the case with other public health and social movements, these conversations must center on the agency and insights of leaders within communities that are working to prevent FGM/cutting.

7.2.3 *Autonomy and Safety*

Globally, girls and women face a higher likelihood of experiencing many types of violence, with serious implications for physical and mental health (Potter et al., 2021). The rate of childhood sexual abuse is thought to be close to one in four (Pan et al., 2021), and further trauma and fear is sadly common among those who come forward to report these experiences (Kennedy & Prock, 2018). Critically, events like childhood sexual abuse, assault, and intimate partner violence affect young people of all genders.

One practice that can both reflect and perpetuate gender inequities is child marriage, which is most likely to affect girls in rural areas whose families are experiencing serious poverty. More than 650 million women worldwide who are alive today were married as children, with an additional 12 million girls married each year before they reach the age of 18 (OHCHR, 2023). Girls who are in this vulnerable position frequently stop attending school, to the detriment of their social mobility, employment opportunities, and mental health. They also face heightened risks of early pregnancy, maternal and infant mortality, and exposure to sexually transmitted infections. HIV/AIDS is the second leading cause of death in adolescent girls in large parts of sub-Saharan Africa and the third most common cause of death among adolescents globally.

Fortunately, child marriage rates are declining, though crises like the COVID-19 pandemic and armed conflict increase its prevalence, threatening global progress in girls' rights (Human Rights Watch, 2020; UNICEF, 2023). In many families, marriage may emerge as a way to protect a daughter from the dangers of armed conflict (DiGiuseppe & Haer, 2023). Natural disasters are also associated with increases in child marriage in some countries, likely due to the poverty that follows these crises and the need to ensure that a daughter is cared for materially (Corno et al., 2020; Kumala Dewi & Dartano, 2019). Culture and context (e.g., whether brides' or grooms' families typically cover the costs associated with marriage) shape these trends, of course.

When male children are seen as more desirable than female children, and when resources for raising children are scarce, families often make the difficult choice to invest in boys over girls. In 1990, the economist Amartya Sen noted something surprising: that there were 100 million fewer women in Asia than would be expected from overall population size. China saw several decades of family planning laws, like mandatory waiting periods between children, restrictions on the number of children allowed per family, and fines for families who have more children than allowed (Zhang, 2017). Though none of these policies are explicitly intended to reduce the ratio of girls to boys, it is speculated that gender biases have interacted with these policies to lead to increasing rates of sex-selective abortion (although this practice is illegal in China), reduced health and financial supports for baby girls, and, in very rare cases, infanticide (Mei & Jiang, 2025; Nie, 2009). China now sees a high ratio of males to females (Ding & Hesketh, 2006).

The UN's Department of Social Affairs studied 150 countries over 40 years and found that China and India were the only two countries where female infant mortality was higher than male infant mortality. One analysis found that one in 12 female infants born in India each year died in the first year of life, and girls aged 1–5 were 75% more likely to die than their male peers (UN, 2011). There, factors like dowry prices can interact with gender inequities to shape the perceived desirability of raising girls and, therefore, the high ratio of males to females in many regions, particularly in the north of the country.

7.3 Interventions

International dialogue around children's rights is one step to addressing the impacts of gender inequities and other inequities on children's health and development. The United Nations adopted the UN Convention of the Rights of the Child (CRC) in 1989, and when it was ratified in 1991, it was the fastest ratification of a treaty in the history of the United Nations (Jeria & Milman, 2020). Article 28 of the CRC states that countries must "recognize the right of the child to education." Chapter 16 provides a more in-depth discussion of the CRC and the history of children's rights. In tandem, the 2001 Millennium Development Goals (MDGs) established by the UN are an attempt to implement and monitor the CRC. The MDGs—and, later, the Sustainable Development Goals (SDGs)—established eight domains in which the adult world is encouraged to work toward higher standards of living and sustainable priorities for the climate (Fehling et al., 2013). These goals include gender equity and access to quality education (Hák et al., 2016; SDG Report, 2023). It is important that international efforts to improve gender equity and other developmental needs for children work to build the capacity of local communities to meet goals in ways that align with cultural and contextual values and needs; honor the diverse identities of communities and individuals; and amplify the voices and ideas of children and their advocates from their own communities (Baird et al., 2021; Khosla et al., 2017). When the sovereignty and insights of communities are honored, international goals for child rights are more likely to be pursued in ways that are effective, sustainable, culturally harmonious, and attentive to varying needs within communities.

Access to high-quality education—discussed further in Chapter 12—is a multifaceted protective factor worldwide. For girls, it can increase social connection, self-esteem, health literacy, civic engagement, and self-advocacy, while also increasing their earning potential and employment opportunities in the future. Investments in girls' human capital is likely to reduce rates of exploitation and premature marriage, especially as mounting pressures of armed conflict and climate change threaten to amplify gender inequities in many places (Corno et al., 2020; UNICEF, 2022).

7.4 Conclusion

Factors in the macrosystem constrain the opportunities available to children as they develop. As climate shocks, armed conflict, and poverty mount worldwide, the time is now to ensure that children's life opportunities expand rather than contract in the coming decades, and that children benefit equitably from global efforts to improve child rights. Education and social capital are pathways to such equity. The coming decades will, hopefully, see an increase in research and global advocacy related to the intersections of climate change, armed conflict, and various dimensions of inequality (van Daalen et al., 2020).

Reflection Questions

Question 1. Ms. Malala Yousafzai almost died while working to promote gender equity and education in Pakistan. Did the men who attempted to assassinate her for her efforts ever face consequences? How do factors like legal impunity influence gender inequities?

Question 2. Cultural humility is understood to involve self-reflection and critique toward one's own values and assumptions, as well as curiosity about those of others (Yeager & Bauer-Wu, 2013). How does the practice of cultural humility shape international discourse on children's rights? How might it shape the quality of the solutions that are implemented?

Question 3. What are two reasons that local community efforts (e.g., grassroots organizing) may be especially effective in promoting equity and justice for children? What are two ways that international communities may be ethically, effectively involved in these efforts?

References

Ahinkorah, B. O., Hagan, J. E., Ameyaw, E. K., Seidu, A. A., Budu, E., Sambah, F., Yaya, S., Torgbenu, E. and Schack, T. (2020). Socio-economic and demographic determinants of female genital mutilation in sub-Saharan Africa: Analysis of data from demographic and health surveys. *Reprod Health*, *17*, 162. https://doi.org/10.1186/s12978-020-01015-5

Ayang, P. (2024). Female genital mutilation continues amid Sudan's conflict and forced displacement. *OCHA*. Published February 27, 2024. https://reliefweb.int/report/sudan/female-genital-mutilation-continues-amid-sudans-conflict-and-forced-displacement

Baird, S., Camfield, L., Ghimire, A., Hamad, B. A., Jones, N., Pincock, K., & Woldehanna, T. (2021). Intersectionality as a framework for understanding adolescent vulnerabilities in low and middle income countries: Expanding our commitment to leave no one behind. *The European Journal of Development Research*, *33*(5), 1143–1162.

Bronfenbrenner U. (1994). Ecological models of human development. In T. Husen, & T. N., Postlethwaite (Eds.), *International Encyclopedia of Education* (2nd ed. Vol. 3, 1643–1647. Pergamon/Elsevier Science.

Campbell, O. L., Bann, D., & Patalay, P. (2021). The gender gap in adolescent mental health: A cross-national investigation of 566,829 adolescents across 73 countries. *SSM-Population Health*, *13*, 100742.

Corno, Lucia, Nicole Hildebrandt, & Alessandra Voena (2020). Age of marriage, weather shocks, and the direction of marriage. *Econometrica*, *88*(3), 879–915.

DiGiuseppe, M., & Haer, R. (2023). The wedding bells of war: The influence of armed conflict on child marriage in West Africa. *Journal of Peace Research*, *60*(3), 474–488.

Ding, Q. J., & Hesketh, T. (2006). Family size, fertility preferences, and sex ratio in China in the era of the one child family policy: Results from national family planning and reproductive health survey.

Esho, T., Komba, E., Richard, F., & Shell-Duncan, B. (2021). Intersections between climate change and female genital mutilation among the Maasai of Kajiado county, Kenya. *Journal of Global Health*, *11*, 1–10.

Fehling, M., Nelson, B. D., & Venkatapuram, S. (2013). Limitations of the millennium development goals: A literature review. *Global Public Health*, *8*(10), 1109–1122.

Hák, T., Janoušková, S., & Moldan, B. (2016). Sustainable development goals: A need for relevant indicators, *Ecological Indicators*, *60*, 2016; 565–573.

Hoffmann, J. A., Alegría, M., Alvarez, K., Anosike, A., Shah, P. P., Simon, K. M., & Lee, L. K. (2022). Disparities in pediatric mental and behavioral health conditions. *Pediatrics*, *150*(4), e2022058227.

Human Rights Watch (2020). Child marriage, pregnancies soar during pandemic. October, 12. https://www.hrw.org/news/2020/10/12/child-marriage-pregnancies-soar-during-pandemic

Jaafar, H., Ismail, S. Y., & Azzeri, A. (2023). Period poverty: A neglected public health issue. *Korean Journal of Family Medicine*, *44*(4), 183.

Jeria, M. B., & Milman, H. M. (2020). Celebrating the 30th anniversary of the un convention on the rights of the child. *Lancet/Child-Adolescent*. 4, 8–9.

Kennedy, A. C., & Prock, K. A. (2018). "I still feel like I am not normal": A review of the role of stigma and stigmatization among female survivors of child sexual abuse, sexual assault, and intimate partner violence. *Trauma, Violence, & Abuse*, *19*(5), 512–527.

Khosla, R., Banerjee, J., Chou, D., Say, L., & Fried, S. T. (2017). Gender equality and human rights approaches to female genital mutilation: A review of international human rights norms and standards. *Reproductive Health*, *14*, 1–9.

Kingsbury, M., Hammond, N. G., Johnstone, F., & Colman, I. (2022). Suicidality among sexual minority and transgender adolescents: A nationally representative population-based study of youth in Canada. *CMAJ*, *194*(22), E767–E774.

Kumala Dewi, L., P., R., & Dartano, T. (2019). Natural disasters and girls' vulnerability: Is child marriage a coping strategy of economic shocks in Indonesia? *Vulnerable Children and Youth Studies*, *14*(1), 24–35.

Mei, L., & Jiang, Q. (2025). Sex-selective abortions over the past four decades in China. *Population Health Metrics*, *23*(1), 6. https://doi.org/10.1186/s12963-025-00368-y

Monahan, K. (2007). Cultural beliefs, human rights violations, and female genital cutting: Complication at the crossroad of progress. *Journal of Immigrant & Refugee Studies*, *5*(3), 21–35.

Nie, J. B. (2009). Limits of state intervention in sex-selective abortion: the case of China. Culture, Health & Sexuality, 12(2), 205–219.

OECD (2018). *Equity in education: Breaking down barriers to social mobility, PISA*, OECD Publishing. https://www.oecd.org/en/publications/equity-in-education_9789264073234-en.html

Pan, Y., Lin, X., Liu, J., Zhang, S., Zeng, X., Chen, F., & Wu, J. (2021). Prevalence of childhood sexual abuse among women using the childhood trauma questionnaire: A worldwide meta-analysis. *Trauma, Violence, & Abuse*, *22*(5), 1181–1191.

Potter, L. C., Morris, R., Hegarty, K., García-Moreno, C., & Feder, G. (2021). Categories and health impacts of intimate partner violence in the World Health Organization multi-country study on women's health and domestic violence. *International journal of epidemiology*, *50*(2), 652–662.

Roser, M. (2021). Access to basic education-almost 60 million children of primary school age are not in school. Published online at WourWorldInData.org. https://ourworldindata.org/children-not-in-school

Roussille, N. (2004). The role of the ask gap in gender pay inequality. *The Quarterly Journal of Economics*, *139*(3), 1557–1610.

Sustainable Development Goals Report, Special Edition-2023. https://unstats.un.org/sdgs/report/2023/The-Sustainable-Development-Goals-Report-2023.pdf.

Theirworld (2017). 10 countries where girls' education has been under attack. https://theirworld.org/news/10-countries-where-girls-education-has-been-attacked/

UNICEF (2007). *The state of the world's children. Women and children: The double dividend of gender equality*. The United Nations Children's Fund (UNICEF), New York. ISBN-10: 92–806–3998-6

UNICEF (2022). *The power of education to end child marriage*. UNICEF. https://data.unicef.org/resources/child-marriage-and-education-data-brief/

UNICEF (2023). Child marriage is a violation of human rights but is all too common. June. https://data.unicef.org/topic/child-protection/child-marriage/

United Nations, Department of Economic and Social Affairs, Population Division (2011). *Sex differentials in childhood mortality (United Nations publication, ST/ESA/SER.A/314)*.

United Nations (2023) Human Rights Office of the High Commissioner. The world is failing 130 million girls denied education: UN experts. January 23. https://timor-leste.un.org/en/216447-world-failing-130-million-girls-denied-education-un-experts.

UNICEF (2022) United Nations International Children's Emergency Fund. *The power of education to end female genital mutilation*. https://data.unicef.org/resources/the-power-of-education-to-end-female-genital-mutilation/

OHCHR (2015) Background paper: On Attacks against girls seeking to access education. https://www.ohchr.org/sites/default/files/Documents/Issues/Women/WRGS/Report_attacks_on_girls_Feb2015.pdf

OHCHR (2024) Submission for the UN Secretary General report on progress towards ending child, early and forced marriage, responding to the OHCHR's Guiding Questions. https://www.ohchr.org/en/women/child-and-forced-marriage-including-humanitarian-settings#:~:text=Worldwide%2C%20more%20than%20650%20million,is%2028%20girls%20every%20minute.

van Daalen, K., Jung, L., Dhatt, R., & Phelan, A. L. (2020). Climate change and gender-based health disparities. *The Lancet Planetary Health*, *4*(2), e44–e45.

White, J., & Clayton, J. (2022). The gender health innovation gap: A perspective from the NIH Office of Research on Women's Health. *Med*, *3*(5), 298–301.

World Health Organization (WHO) (2024). Female genital mutilation, Fact Sheet, February 5. https://www.who.int/news-room/fact-sheets/detail/female-genital-mutilation

Yeager, K. A., & Bauer-Wu, S. (2013). Cultural humility: Essential foundation for clinical researchers. *Applied Nursing Research*, *26*(4), 251–256.

Zhang, J. (2017). The evolution of China's one-child policy and its effects on family outcomes. *Journal of Economic Perspectives*, *31*(1), 141–160.

8 The Chronosystem and Life Course Trajectories

8.1 Introduction

This chapter is intended to tie together the previous ones by providing overall developmental frameworks by which to understand the impacts of resources and risks on children's wellbeing. To this end, the present chapter attends to the *chronosystem*, the infusion of time into a socio-ecological model. Bronfenbrenner's original conceptualization of the ecological spheres surrounding children did not include the chronosystem, but he incorporated it after gradually seeing the ways in which the passing of time presented its own set of internal and external variables (1994). Social transitions and normative developmental trajectories find their way into the chronosystem. These include changes in family structure, trends in urbanization, the navigation of puberty, social mobility, and the acquisition of new developmental milestones. With the addition of the chronosystem, the bioecological model affirms explicitly that these spheres are not static, but change over time. Developmentalists are better equipped to capture trajectories, the continuous patterns in a person's physiological, psychological and social states (with the possibility of transitions and/or discontinuities).

Figure 8.1 provides a schematic of the chronosystem.

The pace and progress of a child's development change over time due to internal factors (e.g., development of new medical conditions, acquisition of new attitudes) and external factors (e.g., making a new friend, political shifts in a nation). Importantly, these phenomena are not independent from each other, but inform the impact of other internal and external factors on a child's development. The resources available around a child can constrain and support their neurological development and, following this, their patterns of response to other events and environments in the future. Even the expression of genes can be shaped by environmental factors and, in turn, influence a child's physiological, psychological, and behavioral responses to their world (Gottlieb, 1992). In other words, development is cumulative, and events at each level of a child's body, mind, relationships, and broader environments act on one another bidirectionally to shape the likelihood of future outcomes. Likelihood is a critical construct here, as internal and external events rarely cause an outcome directly, but rather shape its probability. In fact, developmentalists

DOI: 10.4324/9781003488385-10

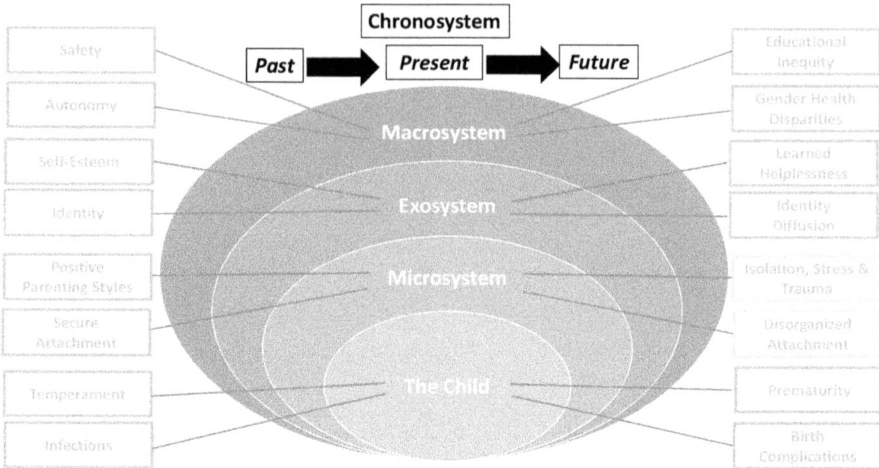

Figure 8.1 The socio-ecological model: The chronosystem.

often use the term ***probabilistic epigenesis*** to refer to the complex relationships between inputs and outcomes that occur during development.

Children differ significantly in how responsive they are to changes in their inner and outer ecologies. Summarized briefly, there is natural variation across individuals in how much or little input it takes, and for how long a time, to effect changes in a person's neurobiology (Ellis et al., 2011). The concept of ***differential susceptibility*** refers to the fact that environmental changes (whether helpful, unhelpful, or neutral to a person's positive adaptation) may have greater impacts on some individuals' long-term developmental trajectories than on others'.

Individual children also vary over time in their susceptibility to certain environmental inputs, just as the impact of alcohol on brain development is very different for a fetus at 12 weeks gestation than for a 25-year-old adult, or how language exposure, broadly speaking, is more likely to result in fluency when exposure occurs earlier in life (Newport et al., 2001). ***Sensitive periods*** are often understood to be times during which a developing individual's neurobiology and physiology are more plastic, unstable, and primed to receive input from the environment that will shape their future functioning (Zeanah et al., 2011). The emergence of these periods varies by domain; for example, infancy is often marked by greater sensitivity to environmental signals about the predictability and safety of one's environment, whereas adolescence may be marked by enhanced sensitivity to cues about one's social competence (Blakemore & Mills, 2014; Gee & Cohodes, 2021).

8.2 Risk Factors and Developmental Outcomes: Insights from Observations

A ***developmental risk*** is defined as an association between a factor and increased chances of a future negative outcome. Risks are often multisystem and highly complex. For example, it is well documented that exposure to poverty is a developmental risk factor (Jensen et al., 2017). Digging deeper, it becomes clear that poverty can include food insecurity, housing instability, exposure to environmental dangers, and family stress (Masarik & Conger, 2017). Together and individually, these factors increase the risk of adverse cognitive, neurological, emotional, physical, and social development. As described above, these impacts vary by developmental timing, the severity of exposure, chronicity, and other factors shaping the child's unique susceptibility.

Michael Rutter, a British psychiatrist and developmental researcher, quantified the associations of multiple risk factors (including poverty, residential overcrowding, parental mental health, and incarceration of family members) with children's outcomes (specifically, emotional and/or conduct difficulties at 10 years of age). He found that as the number of risk factors increased, the chance of an adverse outcome increased not linearly, but rather exponentially, as depicted in Figure 8.2 (Rutter, 1979). What was shown was that stressors "potentiate" each other, such that the effect on behavioral and emotional outcomes is more than the summation of the individual risk factors.

An important step in contemporary understanding of adversity's long-term impacts occurred with the initiation of the Adverse Childhood Experiences (ACE) Study, which began in California in 1995 and enrolled nearly 10,000 participants (Felitti et al., 1998). In this study, participants who received standardized physical examinations in the health system were invited to complete surveys regarding difficult experiences they had faced in their early lives, their current health behaviors, and current health status. They also completed multiple surveys regarding childhood maltreatment and family dysfunction. Researchers then computed adjusted odds ratios evaluating the relationship between childhood adversities and the incidence of known health risks.

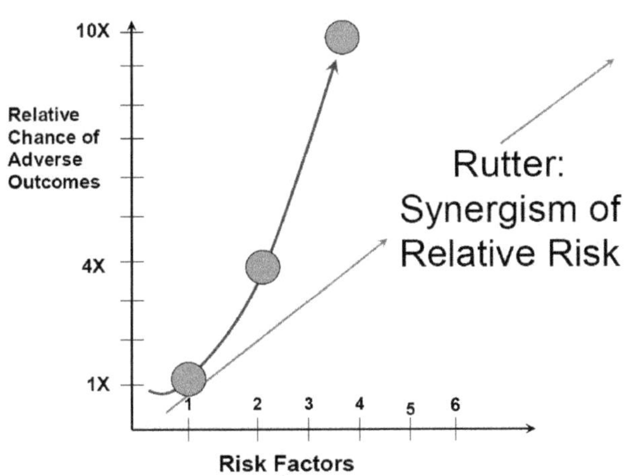

Figure 8.2 Relative risk and adverse outcomes

Table 8.1 Examples of Adverse Childhood Experiences in Felitti et al. (1998)

Household Dysfunction
- Problematic substance and alcohol use by people in the household
- Suicidality or other mental health challenges among household members
- Incarceration of household members
- Violence against female caregiver

Abuse
- Emotional/Verbal
- Physical
- Sexual

(Adapted from Felitti et al., 1998)

They found that each additional adversity to which a person was exposed in childhood was associated with increased risks of physical health problems in adulthood, including risks for some of the leading causes of death in the United States. Table 8.1 displays some of the categories of adverse experiences assessed in the original ACE Study.

This study was understood to have some limitations, such as dependence on retrospective measures of childhood adversity. It was also limited in racial, ethnic, and educational diversity. Additionally, the categories of adversities included in this original study were limited—for example, it did not include structural or systemic adversities or those that occurred outside of the context of the home. At the same time, its influence on public health has been profound, and preventing childhood adversity is increasingly understood to be a key strategy for population health and longevity (Hughes et al., 2017). In helping to establish that there is a "risk gradient" between childhood adversity and adult health (i.e., that an increase in the "dose" of exposure contributes to an increase in the likelihood of negative outcomes; Evans et al., 2013), this research has contributed powerfully to simple public health methods. Research on ACEs has also helped the world to grasp how common these experiences are. About 64% of adults in the United States reported that they had experienced at least one type of ACE before age 18. Three quarters of high school students reported experiencing one or more ACEs, and one in five experienced four or more ACEs (Swedo et al., 2024). Nearly one in six (17.3%) adults reported having experienced four or more types of ACEs (Swedo et al., 2023).

As use of ACE measures continues, there are efforts to expand their content to include adversities like exposure to armed conflict, bullying, foster care entry, lack of safety in the neighborhood, experiences of racism, or housing loss (Cronholm et al., 2015). A recent review of the research on ACEs also noted that these studies commonly attend to the impacts of adversity on long-term health, rather than the factors that cause these adversities, their unequal distribution across populations, or strategies for preventing them (Karatekin et al., 2022).

8.4 Developmental Perspectives on Adversity

Earlier-life adversities are clearly related to challenges later in life, including in the domain of physical health. Longitudinal life course research has added to this understanding, showing that adversity can function causally to increase the chances of health difficulties as individuals grow up (Dube et al., 2003; Larson et al., 2008; Lu & Halfon, 2003). The adversity implicated in these trajectories is varied and includes systemic difficulties (e.g., living with the stress of structural racism) as well as acute adversities (e.g., witnessing a natural disaster).

Developmental research on the mechanisms by which adversities confer greater risk for physical, mental and social problems has identified that stress can have deleterious effects on physiological functioning (Juster et al., 2010). For example, among children going through homelessness, those who have experienced more stressful life events have differences in cortisol function, an important homeostatic agent that interfaces with autonomic response systems, immune functioning, and inflammatory processes (Cutuli et al., 2010). Children exposed to poverty have been observed to show heightened cardiovascular reactivity and heightened inflammatory profiles, with associated risks for diseases like asthma (Miller et al., 2009). Such findings offer plausible mechanisms by which stress in childhood contributes to socioeconomic disparities in health and, perhaps, the increased rates of health problems among children who have been through housing instability and housing loss. Of particular concern to developmentalists is "toxic stress," often understood to occur when a child is subject to intense, frequent, and/or prolonged activation of physiological stress response systems, but without adequate external regulation from an adult (Shonkoff et al., 2009). Children's brain structures may undergo altered development as a result, with possible impacts including long-term dysregulation of emotional responses or other difficulties with age-expected functioning (NSCDC, 2005; Rosenzweig & Sundborg, 2022; Shonkoff & Garner, 2012).

A perspective of probabilistic epigenesis can also help to clarify how domains outside of biology can form a link between early-life adversity and later health difficulties. When children are exposed to stress, they may develop cognitive, behavioral, and emotional patterns that help them adapt. For example, children exposed to childhood maltreatment may develop a cognitive style of assuming hostile intent in others (Zhu et al., 2020), or a pattern of hyperreactivity to stress, both of which can increase the likelihood of responding quickly to new possible threats (Loman & Gunnar, 2010). With these internal patterns, though, a child may have trouble engaging kindly with peers or paying attention in classroom settings (Shonkoff, & Garner, 2012). As children begin to fall behind at key developmental tasks like social or academic competence, they face increased risks of internalizing difficulties (e.g., depression, anxiety) and externalizing difficulties (e.g., aggression, problematic substance use), all of which have known associations with morbidity and mortality (Obradović

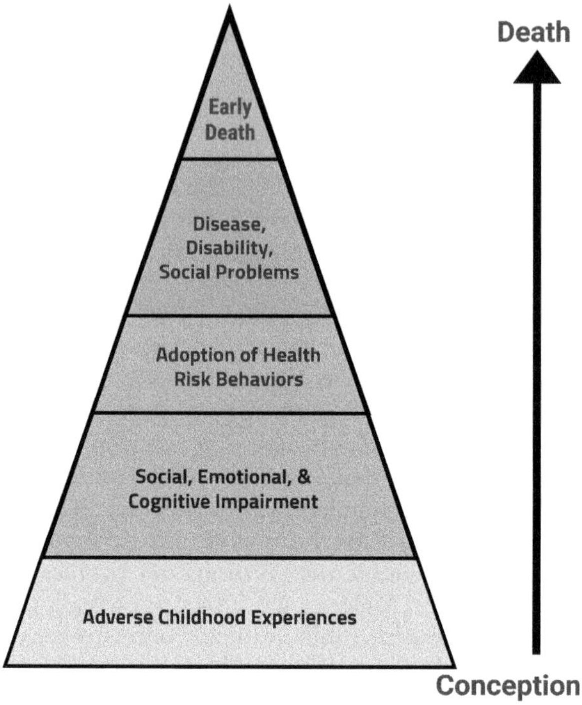

Figure 8.3 Example of impacts of ACEs through the life course.

et al., 2009). Figure 8.3 offers one example of how early adversity can impact health outcomes in the long term.

Expanding the temporal perspective beyond the individual's lifespan, it becomes clear that one person's adversity can be associated with intergenerational risk processes. ACEs are associated with increased risk for maternal and child health problems like pregnancy complications, preterm birth, and fetal death (Hillis et al., 2004). In addition, when individuals suffering from ACE-related health risks go on to become parents, their own physical and mental health struggles may interfere with their availability and wellness as they raise children. Communities and families that have suffered from oppression may sometimes show these lingering effects across generations. Chapter 14 discusses this in more detail.

Clearly, whether ACEs are defined narrowly (i.e., as a select set of difficulties in one's household) or more broadly, these all increase in the face of the multisystem risks discussed thus far in the text (Bhutta et al., 2023).

8.4 Positive Developmental Trajectories

Fortunately, positive resources and inputs from the environment work in much the same way as adverse ones, increasing the chances that children attain milestones, gain competence, and enjoy relationships, to the benefit of later development. Critically, children exposed to serious adversities often have access to key resources and "buffering" factors that can support positive developmental processes (Merrick et al., 2019). For example, effective caregiving amid adversity can mitigate the impact of stress on children's neurobiological development and scaffold the development of self-regulation and executive functioning skills (Blair & Raver, 2012; Loman & Gunnar, 2010). These skills buffer the effects of future risks. They also predict school success and positive social-emotional functioning, particularly when children are exposed to adversity, and are associated with better health during middle childhood and adolescence (Lengua et al., 2015; Zelazo & Carlson, 2012).

As threats to children's development escalate, so does the interest in identifying the factors that can support positive life trajectories. *Social capital* is one concept that has relevance for both individuals and communities responding to multisystem adversities (Carmen et al., 2022). Whether applied to individuals or collective groups, social capital refers to the tendency for relationships to be marked by stability, reciprocity, and trust; for social norms to be agreed upon; for social networks to interconnect well with one another; and for parties to participate in shared life activities. Individuals, families, or communities with higher social capital are often better able to adapt together to connect children with resources necessary for their developmental health, a key protection in the face of war, natural disasters, and other crises (Masten 2021).

Other innovations in the study of positive developmental trajectories come in the domain of measurement. For example, the Benevolent Childhood Experiences (BCEs) survey was created to parallel measures of ACEs. This list of 10 items assesses whether individuals had access to assets like a safe caregiver, enjoyable school experiences, and comforting beliefs in childhood (Merrick et al., 2019). While the science on the mechanisms of BCEs is nascent, emerging evidence suggests that BCEs are implicated in protecting caregivers' mental health and wellbeing amid difficult experiences (Narayan et al., 2018). More discussion of positive developmental trajectories is available in Chapter 18.

8.5 Conclusion

Robert Frost's well-known 1916 poem, "The Road Not Taken", feels a fitting end to discussion of the chronosystem.

The Road Not Taken

Two roads diverged in a yellow wood,
And sorry I could not travel both
And be one traveler, long I stood

And looked down one as far as I could
To where it bent in the undergrowth;

Then took the other, as just as fair,
And having perhaps the better claim,
Because it was grassy and wanted wear;
Though as for that the passing there
Had worn them really about the same,

And both that morning equally lay
In leaves no step had trodden black.
Oh, I kept the first for another day!
Yet knowing how way leads on to way,
I doubted if I should ever come back.

I shall be telling this with a sigh
Somewhere ages and ages hence:
Two roads diverged in a wood, and I—
I took the one less traveled by,
And that has made all the difference.

Attending to the chronosystem and the ways in which children's development unfolds over time opens up a set of tools for grasping the enduring and changing impacts of life experiences, with clear implications for health at the individual level, as well as for families, communities, nations and the global ecosystems. An understanding of the mechanisms by which children develop over time—including the biological embedding of adversity, the emergence of sensitive periods, and the independent impacts of protective and risk factors—can help to plan supports and interventions for children as global crises escalate. Safeguarding children from the neurobiological effects of stress requires preventing adversity, and also investing in the health and responsiveness of the adults who surround a child, improving their ability to buffer a child from the effects of stress (Garner & Yogman, 2021; Masten, 2025).

Reflection Questions

Question 1. How does normative stress (e.g., nervousness about exams, minor sibling conflict, etc.) differ in its developmental impacts from chronic, severe, or toxic stress?

Question 2. Consider a humanitarian crisis in the news today. How do you think these events may be damaging the emotional, cognitive, physical, and behavioral development of children? What protective factors are most important for children there?

Question 3. What are three ways that ACEs and BCEs research could help shape developmentally informed policies?

Question 4. Reflect on Robert Frost's poem and how it relates to Bronfenbrenner's socio-ecological framework, the chronosystem, life course trajectories, and resilience.

References

Bhutta, Z. A., Bhavnani, S., Betancourt, T. S., Tomlinson, M., & Patel, V. (2023). Adverse childhood experiences and lifelong health. *Nature Medicine*, *29*(7), 1639–1648.

Blair, C., & Raver, C. C. (2012). Child development in the context of adversity: Experiential canalization of brain and behavior. *American Psychologist*, *67*, 309–318.

Blakemore, S. J., & Mills, K. L. (2014). Is adolescence a sensitive period for sociocultural processing? *Annual Review of Psychology*, *65*(1), 187–207.

Bronfenbrenner, U. (1994). Ecological models of human development. In T. Husen, & T. N., Postlethwaite (Eds.), *International encyclopedia of education* (2nd ed. vol. 3, pp. 1643–1647). Pergamon/Elsevier Science.

Carmen, E., Fazey, I., Ross, H., Bedinger, M., Smith. F. N., Prager, K., McCymont, K., & Morrison, D., (2002) Building community resilience in a context of climate change: The role of social capital. Ambio 51, 1371–1387. https://doi.org/10.1007/s13280-021-01678-9

Cronholm, P. F., Forke, C. M., Wade, R., Bair-Merritt, M. H., Davis, M., Harkins-Schwarz, M., Pachter, L. M. & Fein, J. A. (2015). Adverse childhood experiences: Expanding the concept of adversity. *American Journal of Preventive Medicine*, *49*(3), 354–361.

Cutuli, J. J., Wiik, Kristen L., Herbers, Janette E., Gunnar, Megan R., & Masten, Ann S. (2010). Cortisol functions among early school-aged homeless children. *Psychoneuroendocrinology*, *35*, 833–845. https://doi.org/10.1016/j.psyneuen.2009.11.008

Dube, S. R., Felitti, Vincent J., Dong, M., & Anda, R.F. (2003). The impact of adverse childhood experiences on health problems: Evidence from four birth cohorts dating back to 1900. *Preventive Medicine*, *37*, 268–277.

Ellis, B. J., Boyce, W. T., Belsky, J., Bakermans-Kranenburg, M. J., & Van Ijzendoorn, M. H. (2011). Differential susceptibility to the environment: An evolutionary–neurodevelopmental theory. *Development and Psychopathology*, *23*(1), 7–28.

Evans, G. W., Li, D., & Whipple, S. S. (2013). Cumulative risk and child development. *Psychological Bulletin*, *139*(6), 1342.

Felitti, V. J., Anda, R. F., Nordenberg, D., Williamson, D. F., Spitz, A. M., Edwards, V., & Marks, J. S. (1998). Relationship of childhood abuse and household dysfunction to many of the leading causes of death in adults: The Adverse Childhood Experiences (ACE) study. *American Journal of Preventive Medicine*, *14*(4), 245–258.

Garner, A., & Yogman, M. (2021). Committee on psychosocial aspects of child and family health, section on developmental and behavioral pediatrics, council on early childhood, preventing childhood toxic stress: Partnering with families and communities to promote relational health. *Pediatrics, 148*(2), e2021052582. https://doi.org/10.1542/peds.2021-052582

Gee, D. G., & Cohodes, E. M. (2021). Influences of caregiving on development: A sensitive period for biological embedding of predictability and safety cues. *Current Directions in Psychological Science, 30*(5), 376–383.

Gottlieb, G. (1992). *Individual development and evolution: The genesis of novel behavior.* Oxford University Press.

Hillis, S. D., Anda, R. F., Dube, S. R., Felitti, V. J., Marchbank, P. A., & Marks, J. S. (2004). The association between adverse childhood experiences and adolescent pregnancy, long-term psychosocial consequences, and fetal death. *Pediatrics, 113*(2), v320–7.

Hughes, K., Bellis, M. A., Hardcastle, K. A., Sethi, D., Butchart, A., Mikton, C., Milton, C., Jones, L., & Dunne, M. P. (2017). The effect of multiple adverse childhood experiences on health: A systematic review and meta-analysis. *The Lancet Public Health, 2*(8), e356–e366.

Jensen, S. K., Berens, A. E., & Nelson, C. A. (2017). Effects of poverty on interacting biological systems underlying child development. *The Lancet Child & Adolescent Health, 1*(3), 225–239.

Juster, R-P, McEwen, Bruce S., & Lupien, S. J. (2010). Allostatic load biomarkers of chronic stress and impact on health and cognition. *Neuroscience and Biobehavioral Reviews, 35*, 2–16.

Karatekin, C., Mason, S. M., Riegelman, A., Bakker, C., Hunt, S., Gresham, B., Corcoran F., & Barnes, A. (2022). Adverse childhood experiences: A scoping review of measures and methods. *Children and Youth Services Review, 136*, 106425.

Larson, K., Russ, S. A., Crall, J. J., & Halfon, N. (2008). Influence of multiple social risks on children's health. *Pediatrics, 121*; 337–344.

Lengua, L. J., Moran, L., Zalewski, L. Ruberry, E., Kiff, C., & Thompson, S. (2015). Relations of growth in effortful control to family income, cumulative risk, and adjustment in preschool-age children. *Journal of Abnormal Child Psychology, 43*, 705–720.

Loman, M. M., & Gunnar, M. R. (2010). Early experience and the development of stress reactivity and regulation in children. *Neuroscience & Biobehavioral Reviews, 34*(6), 867–876.

Lu, M. C., & Halfon, N. (2003). Racial and ethnic disparities in birth outcomes: A life-course perspective. *Maternal and Child Health Journal, 7*(1), 13–30.

Masarik, A. S., & Conger, R. D. (2017). Stress and child development: A review of the Family Stress Model. *Current Opinion in Psychology, 13*, 85–90.

Masten, A. S. (2021). Resilience of children in disasters: A multisystem perspective. *International Journal of Psychology, 56*(1), 1–11. https://onlinelibrary.wiley.com/doi/10.1002/ijop.12737

Masten, A. S. (2025). *Ordinary magic* (2nd ed.). Guilford.

Merrick, J. S., Narayan, A. J., DePasquale, C. E., & Masten, A. S. (2019). Benevolent Childhood Experiences (BCEs) in homeless parents: A validation and replication study. *Journal of Family Psychology, 33*(4), 493.

Miller, G.E., Chen, E., Fok, A. K., Walker, H., Lim, A., Nicholls, E.F., Cole, S., & Kobor, M. S. (2009). Low early-life social class leaves a biological residue manifested by decreased glucocorticoid and increased proinflammatory signaling. *Proceedings of the National Academy of Sciences, 106*(34), 14716–14721. https://doi.org/10.1073/pnas.0902971106

Narayan, A. J., Rivera, L. M., Bernstein, R. E., Harris, W. W., & Lieberman, A. F. (2018). Positive childhood experiences predict less psychopathology and stress in pregnant women with childhood adversity: A pilot study of the benevolent childhood experiences (BCEs) scale. *Child Abuse & Neglect*, *78*, 19–30.

Newport, E. L., Bavelier, D., & Neville, H. J. (2001). Critical thinking about critical periods: Perspectives on a critical period for language acquisition. In E. Dupoux (Ed.), *Language, brain, and cognitive development: Essays in honor of Jacques Mehler* (pp. 481–502). The MIT Press.

NSCDC, (2005). National scientific council on the developing child. Excessive stress disrupts the architecture of the developing brain: Working paper #3.

Obradović, J., Burt, K. B., & Masten, A. S. (2009). Testing a dual cascade model linking competence and symptoms over 20 years from childhood to adulthood. *Journal of Clinical Child & Adolescent Psychology*, *39*(1), 90–102.

Rosenzweig, J. M., & Sundborg, S. A. (2022). The neurobiology of toxic stress. *Social Workers' Desk Reference*, p. 278.

Rutter, M. (1979). Protective factors in children's responses to stress and disadvantage. In M. W. Kent & J. E. Rolf (Eds.), *Primary prevention of psychopathology, Vol.3: Social competence in* children (pp. 49–74). University of New England Press.

Shonkoff, J. P., Boyce, W. T., & McEwen, B. S. (2009). Neuroscience, molecular biology, and the childhood roots of health disparities: Building a new framework for health promotion and disease prevention. *Journal of the American Medical Association*, *301*(21); 2252–2259.

Shonkoff, J. P., Garner, A. S., (2012). Committee on psychosocial aspects of child and family health, committee on early childhood, adoption, and dependent care, & section on developmental and behavioral pediatrics (2012). The lifelong effects of early childhood adversity and toxic stress. *Pediatrics*, 129(1), e232–e246. https://doi.org/10.1542/peds.2011-2663

Swedo, E. A., Aslam M. V., Dahlberg L. L., Niolon, P. H., Guinn, A. S., Simon, T. R., &; Mercy, J. A. (2023). Prevalence of adverse childhood experiences among U.S. adults — Behavioral risk factor surveillance system, 2011–2020. *Morbidity and Mortality Weekly Report*, *72*, 707–715. https://dx.doi.org/10.15585/mmwr.mm7226a2

Swedo, E. A., Pampati, S., Anderson, K. N. Thorne, E., McKinnon, I. I., Brener, N. D., Stinson, J., Mpofu, J. J., Niolon, P H. (2024). Adverse childhood experiences and health conditions and risk behaviors among high school students — Youth risk behavior survey, United States, 2023. *MMWR Supplements, 73*(Suppl-4), 39–49. https://dx.doi.org/10.15585/mmwr.su7304a5.

Zeanah, C. H., Gunnar, M. R., McCall, R. B., Kreppner, J. M., & Fox, N. A. (2011). VI. Sensitive periods. *Monographs of the Society for Research in Child Development*, *76*(4), 147–162.

Zelazo, P. D., & Carlson, S. M. (2012). Hot and cool executive function in childhood and adolescence: Development and plasticity. *Child Development Perspectives, 6*, 354–360.

Zhu, W., Chen, Y., & Xia, L. X. (2020). Childhood maltreatment and aggression: The mediating roles of hostile attribution bias and anger rumination. *Personality and Individual Differences*, *162*, 110007.

Part III

Introduction

Global Societal Flashpoints

Thus far, this book has offered insights into the interwoven crises of armed conflict, environmental disasters, and climate change faced by the global community in the 21st century (described in Part I) and a sense of how these adversities may impact children's development (described in Part II). At this point, attentive readers have many of the tools they will need to make child-centered arguments for peace, climate justice, and environmental protections; to grasp the impact of global events (including their own and their communities' actions) on child development; and to focus their attention on children's wellbeing amid local and global challenges.

Part III describes several major global events, trends, and uncertainties from a lens of child development. One may notice, in reading, that many of these "flashpoints" (as argued in Part I) cannot be understood as isolated events or situations, but as manifestations of complex interacting processes across many systems. For example, forced displacement (Chapter 9) and recurring recurring food shortages and conflicts in the Sahel (Chapter 10) are multicausal and play out through bidirectional interactions between environmental factors, conflict, economic health, and community resilience. Understanding ways to protect children from war crimes and genocide (Chapter 11) requires attending to international legal systems. Conversations about children's access to education (Chapter 12) benefit from awareness of the roles that culture, values, and economic mobility play in complex family- and community-level decisions. Discussions about technological innovation and access (Chapter 13) pertain to factors from within-person developmental neurobiology to the chronosphere.

Relatedly, children develop in a world that changes on the scale of days, years, and centuries. Those who hope to support them can benefit from a grasp of the impacts of history on current needs. As a case example, Chapter 14 describes some of the ways in which colonialism can affect Indigenous children's wellbeing in the present, along with approaches to protect and promote their healthy development in the long term amid 21st-century crises. No two children are alike even within the same community, of course, and all adults benefit from attention to these individual differences. As an example,

DOI: 10.4324/9781003488385-11

some children have needs that differ from their same-aged peers (Chapter 15) and deserve targeted resources to help them reach their full potential and thriving.

In some ways, a book like this is often outdated before it has left a printer; at the time of this reading, new conflicts may have started or ended, scientific innovations been publicized, and environmental protections been enacted. This part provides examples of how readers can engage with new and changing events in the world from a child-centered perspective, with attention to the complexity of development, and with appreciation for individual differences, cultural values, community resilience, and equity.

9 Forced Displacement and Migration

9.1 Children on the Move

When a home becomes unsafe or otherwise unlivable, families face the difficult choice to leave behind friends, belongings, and familiar geographies and seek safety and livelihood elsewhere. Since the start of the millennium, there has been an exponential increase in the number of children on the move (Oberg, 2018), young people uprooted from their homes and forced to flee due to conflict, natural disasters, and other social or environmental crises.

The broadest term for a person who has moved away from their home is "migrant," which can describe those who are still on the move, those who have crossed an international border, and those who are still within the nation of their birth, regardless of the reasons for migration. Those who have been forced to leave home but remain in the same country may be called "internally displaced people." The terms "immigrant" and "refugee" refer exclusively to those who have crossed an international border.

Formal refugee status comes with access to legal protection and, often, some practical resources in the resettlement society. A common myth is that refugees are those who have been forced to flee their homes due to danger, while immigrants are those who have left their homes voluntarily and through more or less peaceful routes, possibly in search of economic opportunities, education, or reconnection with family abroad. The reality is more complicated; indeed, the designation of refugee versus immigrant typically rests not on the degree of threat a person has faced in their country of birth, but rather on political decisions in the resettlement society that may be fairly arbitrary (Berthold & Libal, 2016; Sangalang et al., 2019). Indeed, most immigrants face significant adversity before and during their journeys to a new country. As an example, those exposed to gang warfare in Haiti are unlikely to be granted refugee status in most nations, despite serious risks to their safety. Complicating matters further, resettlement nations may assign refugee status by country of origin, with all who move from a given nation granted refugee status, and they may also allow individuals to apply for asylum.

Language like "flight" and "crisis" can evoke images of a displacement experience that is acute and, therefore, short-lived. However, one of the

DOI: 10.4324/9781003488385-12

shocking features of forced displacement is its tendency to affect a group for years on end. Afghanistan's current displacement crisis is in its fifth decade, such that Afghan children born today may be third-generation refugees, their parents and grandparents each affected by unique risks and migration journeys. Meanwhile, the longest ongoing displacement crisis—and the one impacting the largest group of people—is currently occurring in Palestine. For seven decades at the time of this writing, Palestinian people have been relegated to Gaza or the West Bank, or dispersed throughout countries like Syria, Lebanon, or Jordan.

9.2 Scale of Forced Displacement

The scale of forced displacement is staggering, but it is only growing. At the time of this writing, over 114 million people worldwide have been forcibly displaced, more than at any other time in human history (United Nations High Commissioner for Refugees [UNHCR], 2023) and twice the level reported ten years prior (Green, 2024). These numbers do not yet include those displaced due to the Israel-Hamas war. The year-over-year increase in global levels of displacement from 2022 to 2023 was also the largest change on record (UNHCR, n.d.). If these people represented a single country, it would be the 14th most populous nation in the world. One out of every 71 people on the planet has been forced to leave their home.

As with war and climate degradation, the causes of forced displacement originate in the adult world but exert outsized influence on children. Children are disproportionately likely to be forcibly displaced; they currently comprise 40–41% of displaced people and may soon make up the majority, especially after record levels in 2023 (UNHCR Child Protection Unit, 2022; United Nations News, 2022). Already, children comprise the majority of those granted refugee status globally, and there was a 75% increase in the number of global child refugees from 2010 to 2015 (UNICEF, 2016). According to the UN, 400,000 babies are born each year to parents who are themselves forcibly displaced—counting only those whose parents have crossed international borders (i.e., only 43% of displaced people; Green, 2024; UNHCR, n.d.-a, n.d.-b).

9.3 Stages of Vulnerability

Frequently, researchers and practitioners describe forced displacement in three stages, each of which carries unique threats to children: pre-migration, mid-migration, and post-migration. At each stage, risks interact with co-occurring and pre-existing vulnerabilities. For example, among children exposed to forced displacement, girls are more likely to experience educational disruptions, violence, and exploitation (Internal Displacement Monitoring Centre, 2022). Those from minoritized ethnic groups in their nations of origin face additional risks of violence and deprivation while they travel.

One vulnerability that must not be overlooked, of course, is the vulnerability inherent in childhood. It is not a coincidence that children are overrepresented in the global statistics on forced displacement, as they are both exposed to many risks at heightened levels and also unable to respond with the same levels of mobility, autonomy, and agency as adults have. As a result, young age amplifies the vulnerability in each social and environmental adversity (Guha-Sapir & van Panhuis, 2004).

9.4 The Arc of Migration

Figure 9.1 presents a schematic of the transition of families and children from their nations of origin to resettlement societies. As described below, many children do not survive this ordeal, but lose their lives in their country of origin or during their flight.

9.4.1 Pre-Migration

Armed conflict remains the leading cause of worldwide displacement (Bendavid et al., 2021), whether organized and sanctioned by state agents—as has been the case in Syria, Ukraine, Afghanistan, etc.—or civilian in origin, such as gang conflict, femicide, or violence between warring militias (Gutiérrez-Romero, 2022). Refugee status is granted more commonly to those fleeing state-sanctioned violence or warfare than to those fleeing civilian violence.

Increasingly, climate drives forced displacement. Between acute extreme weather events (cyclones, hurricanes, wildfires, etc.) and more gradual degradation (land productivity decline, fauna die-offs, reduced availability of fresh water, rising temperatures, etc.), changes in the environment cause displacement with increasing frequency, especially in regions like South Asia, Central and South America, and Sub-Saharan Africa (Internal Displacement

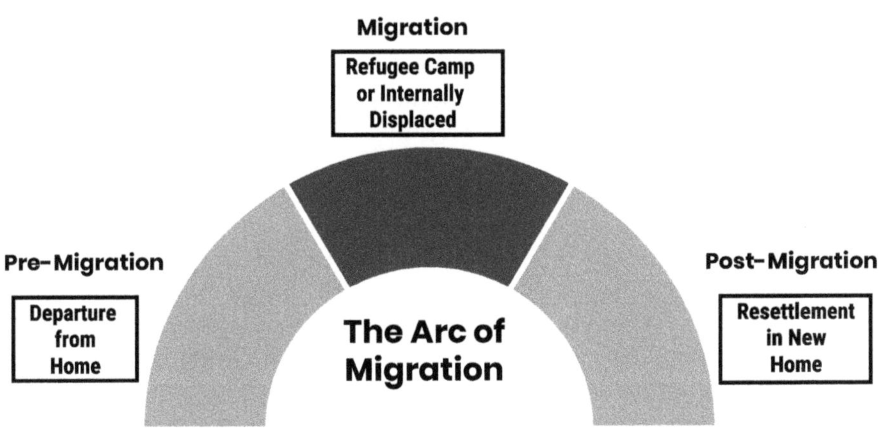

Figure 9.1 The arc of migration.

Monitoring Centre, 2022; Rigaud et al., 2018). In these regions, one in every 36 people may be internally displaced due to climate change by 2050.

Climate crises and conflict, of course, contribute directly to children's risk of displacement; it is not difficult to imagine the rationale for fleeing from the threat of gunfire, chemical weapons, or severe drought. Indirect causes can be similarly pernicious as primary risks undermine the health of essential social structures. Children are dependent on the stability of multiple interdependent systems around them, from healthcare delivery to education to economy. Armed conflict frequently causes indirect risks through disruption of routine and emergency medical care, with cascading impacts for the health of entire families (Guha-Sapir & van Panhuis, 2004). Even living within 30 miles of a conflict zone is associated with adverse effects for maternal and infant mortality and malnutrition (Bendavid et al., 2021). Civilian structures like hospitals and schools may be intentionally targeted, used in civilian shield operations, or damaged in the crossfire of conflicts (UNHCR, 2016). It is all too common for caregivers to die as a result of armed conflict or natural disaster, which is a frequent precipitant of child migration (Oberg et al., 2022).

In addition to armed conflict, climate degradation can disturb economic systems enough that children are compelled to enter the labor force prematurely (Myers & Theytaz-Bergman, 2017; Oberg, Hodges, et al., 2021). Particularly when inequalities and disunity are already present in a society, strains and shocks in the environment can initiate or intensify armed conflict (Ide et al., 2021; Schleussner et al., 2016). Extremist or insurgent groups may recruit with renewed ease (Oberg, Hodges, et al., 2021). In extreme cases, genocide may begin, often from efforts to preserve one group's access to scarce resources or from a growing sense of grievance. One potent example of this phenomenon occurring at the time of this writing is the systematic persecution and killing of the Rohingya people (HRW, 2022).

Any one of these causes alone—drought, lack of access to medical care, loss of economic opportunity, the rise of an extremist organization nearby—would be enough to drive most families to weigh the benefits of a perilous migration journey. But these causes rarely occur alone. Famine, for example, is no longer thought to simply be a caloric crisis but a social one, resulting from the collapse of multiple economic, social, environmental, and infrastructural systems at once. Armed conflict typically reflects a constellation of failures in the structures and systems that, when functioning well, would promote peace and prosperity. Regions already impacted by poverty are the least likely to maintain stability after climate shock (Rigaud et al., 2018). In places like Afghanistan, where the refugee crisis has gone on for five decades, there are few simple causes to reach for. A given Afghan family's reason for leaving may include, at various (and co-occurring) moments, famine, invasion, inter-ethnic conflict, genocide, political oppression, economic collapse, and loss of opportunities for social mobility.

9.4.2 *Mid-Migration*

Regardless of the causes of forced displacement, migration journeys almost invariably entail some degree of danger as children cross deserts, oceans, rivers, and mine fields. Nearly all mothers interviewed after journeying to the southern U.S. border through the desert (90%) report having feared for their children's lives during migration (Ornelas & Perreira, 2011). Families may encounter hostility at transit sites (Ide et al., 2021), and mortality rates are high en route to refugee camps (Spiegel et al., 2011). In camps, families may face overcrowding, poor sanitation, and multiple barriers to healthcare access (Hermans et al., 2017; Martellucci et al., 2021). Crimes against children and exposure to family violence may grow more common due to adults' own vulnerability and to the erosion of protective factors (Ahmad & Nusrat, 2022). While refugee camps may be designed for short-term stays, it is more and more common for people to spend most of their childhoods in these environments (van de Wiel et al., 2021).

Unsurprisingly, between 25 and 87% of children in a given camp may meet criteria for post-traumatic stress disorder (PTSD; Vossoughi et al., 2018). Rates are similarly high for conditions like depression and anxiety. Caregivers frequently show these PTSD symptoms to varying degrees as well, which can limit their abilities to respond proactively and protectively to their children, further exacerbating children's mental health risks through the loss of this powerful relational buffering system (Scharpf et al., 2021; Sim et al., 2018).

Unfortunately, family separation is not uncommon during the migration process. Often, this is unintended and occurs through accidental events or parental death. In 2022, over 150,000 unaccompanied children were encountered at the southern U.S. border (Migration Data Portal, 2024), and in some groups of forcibly displaced people, the majority of children are in transit without adult accompaniment (UNHCR et al., 2023). Even in older children and adolescents, separation from a parent during migration is associated with higher levels of trauma exposure and more severe depression symptoms (Derluyn et al., 2009; Liddell et al., 2021). One reason for this is the role that caregivers play in protecting a child from further trauma exposure during migration, such as exposure to exploitation, malnutrition, and kidnapping. Each of these trauma exposures can amplify the impact of previous trauma exposures (Fazel et al., 2012).

State-sanctioned policies may also contribute to family separation. For example, some resettlement countries are more likely to offer refugee status to single mothers and their children than to two-parent families. Parents may make the difficult choice to divorce, a father remaining behind in the hope of his children securing safety. Those who arrive in resettlement nations through irregular immigration processes or with insufficient documentation face especially steep barriers to reunification with families (Liddell et al., 2021).

Other times, family separation results from intentional processes implemented by resettlement nations to punish immigrants or dissuade immigration.

Separation of children from caregivers at the southern U.S. border is one such policy. This practice is widely believed to go against both the UN General Assembly's guidance and the UN Convention on the Rights of the Child (Waddoups et al., 2019). Among other concerns, administrative officials have stated that the purpose of this policy is to act as a deterrent to immigration, which does not fall under the UN's mandate to use child detention only as a last resort and when it is clearly in a child's best interest. The impacts of family separation on children's mental health, physical health, and neurodevelopment cannot be overstated, and even brief separation from caregivers during these high-stress circumstances can increase lifelong risks of emotional difficulties (Cohodes et al., 2021). Given that family separation induces intense fear and suffering, is intentional, and occurs with the consent and permission of the state, this practice meets international criteria for torture (Oberg, Kivlahan, et al., 2021).

Case Study: Ishmael Beah

Ishmael Beah was still a child when Sierra Leone's civil war broke out in the 1990s. When his hometown, Mogbwemo, was invaded by the Revolutionary United Front (RUF), he was internally displaced and separated from his family. At the age of 13, Mr. Beah was forcibly recruited as a child soldier by government forces. During his time as a soldier, he participated in armed conflict, faced brutal violence, and endured emotional trauma.

Fleeing this violence, Mr. Beah received support from UNICEF and several other organizations and individuals. At a rehabilitation center, he received psychological counseling and education, then moved to New York City at age 18 to complete high school. He later graduated from Oberlin College.

Mr. Beah has become an advocate for peace and for the rights of children affected by conflict. He works with organizations to prevent the recruitment of child soldiers and support post-conflict recovery. His experience exemplifies the vulnerability of children exposed to multisystem crises and forced displacement, as well as the diverse supports that promote resilience: trauma-sensitive care, education, restoration of agency, compassionate individuals, and community belonging.

In 2007, Mr. Beah published his memoir, *A Long Way Gone: Memoirs of a Boy Soldier*, which recounts his experiences and sheds light on the plight of child soldiers globally. His recent novels have touched on some similar themes and also received international acclaim.

9.4.3 Post-Migration

It is a common misconception that resettlement marks the end of the risks of forced displacement. However, the stressors of post-migration life may be responsible for the largest portion of mental health risks faced by immigrants and refugees (Betancourt et al., 2015). To support assessment and research, scholars have grouped the stressors of post-migration into four broad domains: trauma, social isolation, resettlement stress, and acculturative stress (Davis et al., 2021). The following section describes these in more depth.

9.5 Developmental Risks After Displacement

Exposure to trauma is nearly ubiquitous in people exposed to forced migration and includes adversities incurred at each stage of the migration journey, as well as lingering impacts of historical trauma that have impacted families for multiple generations. Caregivers' traumatic stress symptoms and other mental health difficulties can amplify the impact of each new stressor on children's development (Slone & Shoshani, 2017). After displacement, families may be housed in neighborhoods that are subject to discriminatory policing and face high levels of community violence (Ellis et al., 2020; Gillespie et al., 2020; Williams & Collins, 2001; Zeiders et al., 2021). In some cases, immigrants and refugees may be exposed to hate crimes in their resettlement communities (Terrana et al., 2022; Tessler et al., 2020).

Loneliness increasingly affects people of all national identities and legal status, and many nations are beginning to treat this as a public health crisis (Office of the Assistant Secretary for Health, 2023). Numerous studies link loneliness to premature death, with risk quotients comparable to smoking 15 cigarettes a day (Holt-Lunstad, 2017)—to say nothing of mental health costs. Immigrant status consistently emerges as both a predictor of loneliness and a moderator of its health impacts (Lin, 2023; Lin et al., 2020).

Ongoing separation from family members in the nation of origin can beget both new emotional concerns—like worries about loved ones' safety—and also estrange a person from the relationships that would have once helped them process stressful emotional experiences (Miller et al., 2018). Many people also suffer from the effects of status loss after migration, beginning anew without the social standing and work credentials they enjoyed in their nation of origin. Interpersonal discrimination is, sadly, a common experience for immigrants and refugees and may reflect inequity and prejudice around legal status, language abilities, race, ethnicity, income, religion, or any number of other identities and contexts. For youth in particular, discrimination in the resettlement society may be more related to current mental health challenges than are pre-migration stressors (Beiser & Hou, 2016).

Legal status alone often accounts for a great deal of stress for people exposed to forced displacement (Rai et al., 2023). It is challenging in every nation to navigate the process of applying for asylum and long-term residency, and even high-income countries have long backlogs in asylum applications. For example, many Uyghur asylum seekers in the United States have been waiting years for claims to be processed (Szadziewski, 2023). Even in families granted asylum, the fears of deportation and loss of legal status may persist indefinitely (Abisaab et al., 2014; Suárez-Orozco et al., 2018). This fear causes many immigrants and refugees to limit their contact with public agencies, including schools, law enforcement, medical care spaces, and children's schools (León-Pérez et al., 2022).

Access to basic needs is frequently very challenging for immigrants and refugees, since the systems of resettlement societies are not built for them. Figuring out how to enroll a child in school, pay medical bills, and navigate public transportation are challenging for most adults who have grown up in a given nation, but the barriers to building these skills are steeper for those new to a community. Even if families receive financial and practical support as part of refugee resettlement packages, these benefits are typically temporary, and high costs of housing, medical care, transportation, and food can be sources of stress for years after resettlement (Chilton et al., 2018; Rousseau & Frounfelker, 2019). In the meantime, those lacking legal documentation (and, therefore, legal recourse) are vulnerable to labor exploitation (Misra et al., 2021; Nguyen-Ngo, 2020; Pradella & Cillo, 2021). It is important to remember that over three quarters of forcibly displaced people around the world reside in lower- and middle-income countries (UNHCR, n.d.-a). While there are no easy places to live after forced displacement, many of these practical resettlement hassles are most severe for people whose resettlement paths take them to nations and communities already experiencing resource scarcity.

The process of socially and emotionally adjusting to life in a new community, from learning a new language to grasping body language norms, is uniquely associated with mental health risks (Revollo et al., 2011; Sangalang et al., 2019) and physical health risks (Singh et al., 2013). Structural inequities and exposures to discrimination intensify all of these risks, of course (Ferguson et al., 2023). Adults often have more difficulty than children do with becoming competent and comfortable in a new resettlement community, in part because children are quickly given opportunities to learn customs and language through school and friendships (Gil & Vega, 1996; Kia-Keating & Ellis, 2007). Resulting "acculturation gaps" within families can generate both distance and stress across both generations (Hwang & Wood, 2009). Further, these gaps can separate children from some of the sociocultural protective factors present in their heritage cultures (Bas-Sarmiento et al., 2017; Breslau et al., 2007).

9.6 Conclusion

The incidence of forced displacement is accelerating. Thus far, there have been no sufficient or sufficiently coordinated international responses to this crisis. In fact, too often, these trends in migration are met with increasing xenophobia among citizens of resettlement nations. Policy makers may further restrict asylum claims or increase deportations. A growing number of "stateless" children are not safe in their nation of origin and are not welcomed in the country where their exodus ends (Bhabha, 2009). International collaborations can help communities to take a child rights lens to displacement- and resettlement-related supports. Recently, for example, the International Society for Social Pediatrics and Child Health convened a working group of 25 healthcare providers from 15 countries and formulated a *Child Health Action Plan for Children and Youth on the Move.*

Beyond this, adults must work to eliminate the root causes of displacement (such as climate degradation, armed conflict, and social inequality) to protect current and future generations from pre-, mid-, and post-migration risks. Meanwhile, transit and resettlement societies can take steps to prepare for the needs of the populations they expect to welcome in 2030, 2050, and 2070. For example, they may factor climate migration into urban planning and policy development, building the housing, education, and healthcare infrastructures that will holistically support the practical and cultural needs of future immigrant and refugee families.

Reflection Questions

Question 1. What are some refugee and immigrant communities present where you live? What factors led these communities to move? What challenges have they faced during and after migration?

Question 2. Consider one of the following domains of post-migration stress: trauma, acculturation, resettlement, and social isolation. What are three approaches a community can use to support immigrant and refugee children in this domain?

Question 3. What could your local community do now to better support the immigrant and refugee children who will arrive 20 years from now?

References

Abisaab, J., Balsari, S., Siam, Z. A., Fuller, A., Hamill, K., & Leaning, J. (2014). *Syrian refugees in Jordan: Urgent issues and recommendations* [FXB Policy Brief]. Harvard School of Public Health.

Ahmad, M. M., & Nusrat, R. (2022). Human trafficking and crimes in the Rohingya refugee camps in Bangladesh. In *Handbook of research on present and future paradigms in human trafficking* (pp. 26–42). IGI Global. https://doi.org/10.4018/978-1-7998-9282-3.ch003. https://www.igi-global.com/chapter/human-trafficking-and-crimes-in-the-rohingya-refugee-camps-in-bangladesh/303827

Bas-Sarmiento, P., Saucedo-Moreno, M. J., Fernández-Gutiérrez, M., & Poza-Méndez, M. (2017). Mental health in immigrants versus native population: A systematic review of the literature. *Archives of Psychiatric Nursing*, *31*(1), 111–121. https://doi.org/10.1016/j.apnu.2016.07.014

Beiser, M., & Hou, F. (2016). Mental health effects of premigration trauma and postmigration discrimination on refugee youth in Canada. *The Journal of Nervous and Mental Disease*, *204*(6), 464. https://doi.org/10.1097/NMD.0000000000000516

Bendavid, E., Boerma, T., Akseer, N., Langer, A., Malembaka, E. B., Okiro, E. A., Wise, P. H., Heft-Neal, S., Black, R. E., Bhutta, Z. A., Bhutta, Z., Black, R., Blanchet, K., Boerma, T., Gaffey, M., Langer, A., Spiegel, P., Waldman, R., & Wise, P. (2021). The effects of armed conflict on the health of women and children. *The Lancet*, *397*(10273), 522–532. https://doi.org/10.1016/S0140-6736(21)00131-8

Berthold, S. M., & Libal, K. (2016). Migrant children's rights to health and rehabilitation: A primer for US social workers. *Journal of Human Rights and Social Work*, *1*(2), 85–95. https://doi.org/10.1007/s41134-016-0010-3

Betancourt, T. S., Abdi, S., Ito, B. S., Lilienthal, G. M., Agalab, N., & Ellis, H. (2015). We left one war and came to another: Resource loss, acculturative stress, and caregiver–child relationships in Somali refugee families. *Cultural Diversity and Ethnic Minority Psychology*, *21*(1), 114. https://doi.org/10.1037/a0037538

Bhabha J (2009). Arendt's children-do today's children have a right to have rights? *Human Rights Quarterly*, *31*; 410–451

Breslau, J., Aguilar-Gaxiola, S., Borges, G., Kendler, K. S., Su, M., & Kessler, R. C. (2007). Risk for psychiatric disorder among immigrants and their US-born descendants: Evidence from the national comorbidity survey-replication. *The Journal of Nervous and Mental Disease*, *195*(3), 189–195. https://doi.org/10.1097/01.nmd.0000243779.35541.c6

Chilton, M., Mouzon, S., Hager, K., Bovell-Ammon, A., Grimaldi, G., Coleman, S., Cantave, C., & de Cuba, S. E. (2018). *From disparities to discrimination: Getting at the roots of food insecurity*. Drexel University Center for Hunger-Free Communities. https://drexel.edu/hunger-free-center/research/briefs-and-reports/from-disparities-to-discrimination/

Cohodes, E. M., Kribakaran, S., Odriozola, P., Bakirci, S., McCauley, S., Hodges, H. R., Sisk, L. M., Zacharek, S. J., & Gee, D. G. (2021). Migration-related trauma and mental health among migrant children emigrating from Mexico and Central America to the United States: Effects on developmental neurobiology and implications for policy. *Developmental Psychobiology*, *63*(6), e22158. https://doi.org/10.1002/dev.22158

Davis, S. H., Winer, J. P., Gillespie, S. C., & Mulder, L. A. (2021). The refugee and immigrant core stressors toolkit (RICST): Understanding the multifaceted needs of refugee and immigrant youth and families through a four core stressors framework. *Journal of Technology in Behavioral Science*, *6*(4), 620–630. https://doi.org/10.1007/S41347-021-00218-2

Derluyn, I., Mels, C., & Broekaert, E. (2009). Mental health problems in separated refugee adolescents. *Journal of Adolescent Health*, *44*(3), 291–297. https://doi.org/10.1016/j.jadohealth.2008.07.016

Ellis, B. H., Lincoln, A. K., Abdi, S. M., Nimmons, E. A., Issa, O., & Decker, S. H. (2020). "We all have stories": Black Muslim immigrants' experience with the police. *Race and Justice*, *10*(3), 341–362. https://doi.org/10.1177/2153368718754638

Fazel, M., Reed, R. V., Panter-Brick, C., & Stein, A. (2012). Mental health of displaced and refugee children resettled in high-income countries: Risk and protective factors. *The Lancet*, *379*(9812), 266–282. https://doi.org/10.1016/S0140-6736(11)60051-2

Ferguson, G. M., Causadias, J. M., & Simenec, T. S. (2023). Acculturation and psychopathology. *Annual Review of Clinical Psychology*, *19*(Volume 19, 2023), 381–411. https://doi.org/10.1146/annurev-clinpsy-080921-080622

Gil, A. G., & Vega, W. A. (1996). Two different worlds: Acculturation stress and adaptation among Cuban and Nicaraguan families. *Journal of Social and Personal Relationships*, *13*(3), 435–456. https://doi.org/10.1177/0265407596133008

Gillespie, S., Cardeli, E., Sideridis, G., Issa, O., & Ellis, B. H. (2020). Residential mobility, mental health, and community violence exposure among Somali refugees and immigrants in North America. *Health & Place*, *65*. https://doi.org/10.1016/j.healthplace.2020.102419

Green, M. A. (2024). *Numbers in motion, children in motion.* Wilson Center. https://www.wilsoncenter.org/blog-post/numbers-motion-children-motion

Guha-Sapir, D., & van Panhuis, W. G. (2004). Conflict-related mortality: An analysis of 37 datasets. *Disasters*, *28*(4), 418–428. https://doi.org/10.1111/j.0361-3666.2004.00267.x

Gutiérrez-Romero, R. (2022). *Violence in Guatemala pushes adults and children to seek work in Mexico* (arXiv:2212.12796). arXiv. https://arxiv.org/abs/2212.12796

Hermans, M. P. J., Kooistra, J., Cannegieter, S. C., Rosendaal, F. R., Mook-Kanamori, D. O., & Nemeth, B. (2017). Healthcare and disease burden among refugees in long-stay refugee camps at Lesbos, Greece. *European Journal of Epidemiology*, *32*(9), 851–854. https://doi.org/10.1007/s10654-017-0269-4

Holt-Lunstad, J. (2017). The potential public health relevance of social isolation and loneliness: Prevalence, epidemiology, and risk factors. *Public Policy & Aging Report*, *27*(4), 127–130. https://doi.org/10.1093/ppar/prx030

HRW (2022). Myanmar: No Justice, No Freedom for Rohingya 5 Years On. Human Rights Watch News Release. August 24, 2022. https://www.hrw.org/news/2022/08/24/myanmar-no-justice-no-freedom-rohingya-5-years

Hwang, W.-C., & Wood, J. J. (2009). Acculturative family distancing: Linkswith self-reported symptomatology among Asian Americans and Latinos. *Child Psychiatry and Human Development*, *40*(1), 123–138. https://doi.org/10.1007/s10578-008-0115-8

Ide, T., Kristensen, A., & Bartusevičius, H. (2021). First comes the river, then comes the conflict? A qualitative comparative analysis of flood-related political unrest. *Journal of Peace Research*, *58*(1), 83–97. https://doi.org/10.1177/0022343320966783

Internal Displacement Monitoring Centre. (2022). *2022 Global report on internal displacement.* IDMC. https://www.internal-displacement.org/global-report/grid2022/#part2

Kia-Keating, M., & Ellis, B. H. (2007). Belonging and connection to school in resettlement: Young refugees, school belonging, and psychosocial adjustment. *Clinical Child Psychology and Psychiatry*, *12*(1), 29–43. https://doi.org/10.1177/1359104507071052

León-Pérez, G., Patterson, E. J., & Coelho, L. (2022). Legal status history, gender, and the health of Latino immigrants in the US. *International Migration*, *60*(5), 3–22. https://doi.org/10.1111/imig.12925

Liddell, B. J., Byrow, Y., O'Donnell, M., Mau, V., Batch, N., McMahon, T., Bryant, R., & Nickerson, A. (2021). Mechanisms underlying the mental health impact of family separation on resettled refugees. *Australian & New Zealand Journal of Psychiatry*, *55*(7), 699–710. https://doi.org/10.1177/0004867420967427

Lin, S. (Lamson). (2023). The "loneliness epidemic", intersecting risk factors and relations to mental health help-seeking: A population-based study during COVID-19 lockdown in Canada. *Journal of Affective Disorders*, *320*, 7–17. https://doi.org/10.1016/j.jad.2022.08.131

Lin, S. (Lamson), Kobayashi, K., Tong, H., Davison, K. M., Arora, S. R. A., & Fuller-Thomson, E. (2020). Close relations matter: The association between depression and refugee status in the Canadian Longitudinal Study on Aging (CLSA). *Journal of Immigrant and Minority Health*, *22*(5), 946–956. https://doi.org/10.1007/s10903-020-00980-0

Martellucci, C. A., Qaderi, S., Tanimoto, T., & Ozaki, A. (2021). Afghan women and children's health: Three main challenges under Taliban and COVID-19. *Journal of Global Health*, *11*, 03126. https://pmc.ncbi.nlm.nih.gov/articles/PMC8684792/

Migration Data Portal. (2024). *Child and young migrants*. Migration Data Portal, May 21. https://www.migrationdataportal.org/themes/child-and-young-migrants

Miller, A., Hess, J. M., Bybee, D., & Goodkind, J. R. (2018). Understanding the mental health consequences of family separation for refugees: Implications for policy and practice. *American Journal of Orthopsychiatry*, *88*(1), 26–37. https://doi.org/10.1037/ort0000272

Misra, S., Kwon, S. C., Abraído-Lanza, A. F., Chebli, P., Trinh-Shevrin, C., & Yi, S. S. (2021). Structural racism and immigrant health in the United States. *Health Education & Behavior*, *48*(3), 332–341. https://doi.org/10.1177/10901981211010676

Myers, L., & Theytaz-Bergman, L. (2017). *Myers, L., and L. Theytaz-Bergman. "The neglected link: Effects of climate change and environmental degradation on child labour.* Terres des Hommes International Foundation.

Nguyen-Ngo, M. (2020). *Addressing Labor Exploitation: An Examination of Undocumented Asian Americans in the Workplace*. HKS Student Policy Review, June 3. https://studentreview.hks.harvard.edu/addressing-labor-exploitation-an-examination-of-undocumented-asian-americans-in-the-workplace/

Oberg, C. (2018). The rights of *Children on the Move* and the Budapest Declaration. *Children*, 5; 1–5.

Oberg, C., Hodges, H., & Masten, A. (2021). Risk and resilience of Somali children in the context of climate change, famine, and conflict. *Journal of Applied Research on Children: Informing Policy for Children at Risk*, *12*(1). https://doi.org/10.58464/2155-5834.1453

Oberg, C., Hodges, H. R., & Masten, A. S. (2022). Conflict, war, and famine in childhood. In *The Wiley-Blackwell Handbook of Childhood Social Development* (pp. 189–205). John Wiley & Sons, Ltd. https://doi.org/10.1002/9781119679028.ch10

Oberg, C., Kivlahan, C., Mishori, R., Martinez, W., Gutierrez, J. R., Noor, Z., & Goldhagen, J. (2021). Treatment of migrant children on the US southern border is consistent with torture. *Pediatrics*, *147*(1), e2020012930. https://doi.org/10.1542/peds.2020-012930

Office of the Assistant Secretary for Health (OASH). (2023). *New surgeon general advisory raises alarm about the devastating impact of the epidemic of loneliness and isolation in the United States* [Text]. May 3. US Department of Health and Human Services. https://www.hhs.gov/about/news/2023/05/03/new-surgeon-general-advisory-raises-alarm-about-devastating-impact-epidemic-loneliness-isolation-united-states.html

Ornelas, I. J., & Perreira, K. M. (2011). The role of migration in the development of depressive symptoms among Latino immigrant parents in the USA. *Social Science & Medicine*, *73*(8), 1169–1177. https://doi.org/10.1016/j.socscimed.2011.07.002

Pradella, L., & Cillo, R. (2021). Bordering the surplus population across the Mediterranean: Imperialism and unfree labour in Libya and the Italian countryside. *Geoforum*, *126*, 483–494. https://doi.org/10.1016/j.geoforum.2020.06.019

Rai, A., Held, M. L., & Vidal de Haymes, M. (2023). Afghan refugee resettlement in the United States: Implications for service provision. *Families in Society*, *104*(3), 392–396. https://doi.org/10.1177/10443894221122581

Revollo, H.-W., Qureshi, A., Collazos, F., Valero, S., & Casas, M. (2011). Acculturative stress as a risk factor of depression and anxiety in the Latin American immigrant population. *International Review of Psychiatry*, *23*(1), 84–92. https://doi.org/10.3109/09540261.2010.545988

Rigaud, K. K., de Sherbinin, A., Jones, B., Bergmann, J., Clement, V., Ober, K., Schewe, J., Adamo, S., McCusker, B., Heuser, S., & Midgley, A. (2018). *Groundswell: Preparing for internal climate migration*. World Bank. https://doi.org/10.1596/29461

Rousseau, C., & Frounfelker, R. L. (2019). Mental health needs and services for migrants: An overview for primary care providers. *Journal of Travel Medicine*, *26*(2). https://doi.org/10.1093/jtm/tay150

Sangalang, C. C., Becerra, D., Mitchell, F. M., Lechuga-Peña, S., Lopez, K., & Kim, I. (2019). Trauma, post-migration stress, and mental health: A comparative analysis of refugees and immigrants in the United States. *Journal of Immigrant and Minority Health*, *21*(5), 909–919. https://doi.org/10.1007/s10903-018-0826-2

Scharpf, F., Kaltenbach, E., Nickerson, A., & Hecker, T. (2021). A systematic review of socio-ecological factors contributing to risk and protection of the mental health of refugee children and adolescents. *Clinical Psychology Review*, *83*, 101930. https://doi.org/10.1016/j.cpr.2020.101930

Schleussner, C.-F., Donges, J. F., Donner, R. V., & Schellnhuber, H. J. (2016). Armed-conflict risks enhanced by climate-related disasters in ethnically fractionalized countries. *Proceedings of the National Academy of Sciences*, *113*(33), 9216–9221. https://doi.org/10.1073/pnas.1601611113

Sim, A., Bowes, L., & Gardner, F. (2018). Modeling the effects of war exposure and daily stressors on maternal mental health, parenting, and child psychosocial adjustment: A cross-sectional study with Syrian refugees in Lebanon. *Global Mental Health*, *5*, e40. https://doi.org/10.1017/gmh.2018.33

Singh, G. K., Rodriguez-Lainz, A., & Kogan, M. D. (2013). Immigrant health inequalities in the United States: Use of eight major national data systems. *The Scientific World Journal*, *2013*, e512313. https://doi.org/10.1155/2013/512313

Slone, M., & Shoshani, A. (2017). Children affected by war and armed conflict: Parental protective factors and resistance to mental health symptoms. *Frontiers in Psychology*, *8*. https://www.frontiersin.org/articles/10.3389/fpsyg.2017.01397

Spiegel, P. B., Burton, A., Tepo, A., Jacobson, L. M., Anderson, M. A., Cookson, S. T., Bilukha, O. O., Blanton, Navarro-Colorado, C., & Ahmed, J. (2011, August 26). *Notes from the field: Malnutrition and mortality --- Southern Somalia, July 2011*. Centers for Disease Control and Prevention. https://www.cdc.gov/mmwr/preview/mmwrhtml/mm6030a5.htm?s_cid=mm6030a5_w

Suárez-Orozco, C., Motti-Stefanidi, F., Marks, A., & Katsiaficas, D. (2018). An integrative risk and resilience model for understanding the adaptation of immigrant-origin children and youth. *American Psychologist*, *73*(6), 781–796. https://doi.org/10.1037/AMP0000265

Szadziewski, H. (2023). *No time to lose: Uyghurs stuck in the United States asylum system*. Uyghur Human Rights Project. https://uhrp.org/report/no-time-to-lose-uyghurs-stuck-in-the-united-states-asylum-system/

Terrana, A., Ibrahim, N., Kaiser, B., & Al-Delaimy, W. K. (2022). Foundations of Somali resilience: Collective identity, faith, and community. *Cultural Diversity and Ethnic Minority Psychology*, *28*, 533–543. https://doi.org/10.1037/cdp0000536

Tessler, H., Choi, M., & Kao, G. (2020). The anxiety of being Asian American: Hate crimes and negative biases during the COVID-19 pandemic. *American Journal of Criminal Justice*, *45*(4), 636–646. https://doi.org/10.1007/S12103-020-09541-5

UNHCR. (n.d.-a). *Figures at a glance.* UNHCR US. Retrieved June 3, 2024, at https://www.unhcr.org/us/about-unhcr/who-we-are/figures-glance

UNHCR. (n.d.-b). *Refugee Data Finder.* UNHCR. Retrieved June 3, 2024, at https://www.unhcr.org/external/component/header

UNHCR. (2016). *No Protection, No Respect: Health Workers and Health Facilities Under Attack 2015 and Early 2016.* UNHCR. https://www.refworld.org/docid/57441f434.html

UNHCR. (2016). *Global trends in forced displacement in 2015* (Issue brief). The UN Refugee Agency.

UNHCR. (2023). *UNHCR: Forced displacement continues to grow as conflicts escalate.* UNHCR US. https://www.unhcr.org/us/news/press-releases/unhcr-forced-displacement-continues-grow-conflicts-escalate

UNHCR Child Protection Unit. (2022). *UNHCR's child protection data from 2015–2021 – Protecting forcibly displaced and stateless children: What do we know?* United Nations High Commissioner for Refugees. https://www.unhcr.org/sites/default/files/2023-05/child-protection-data-analysis-2015-2021.pdf

UNHCR, UNICEF, & IOM. (2023). *Refugee and migrant children in Europe 2022.* https://eea.iom.int/sites/g/files/tmzbdl666/files/documents/2023-10/refugee-and-migrant-children-in-europe-2022.pdf

UNICEF (2016). Uprooted: The growing crisis for refugee and migrant children. *United Nations Children's Fund (UNICEF). Division of Data, Research and Policy, UNICEF.* 3 United Nations Plaza, New York, NY 10017, USA. ISBN: 978-92-806-4847-8. http://www.unicef.org/publications/index_92710.html

United Nations News. (2022). *UNHCR: A record 100 million people forcibly displaced worldwide.* UN News, May 22. https://news.un.org/en/story/2022/05/1118772

van de Wiel, W., Castillo-Laborde, C., Francisco Urzúa, I., Fish, M., & Scholte, W. F. (2021). Mental health consequences of long-term stays in refugee camps: Preliminary evidence from Moria. *BMC Public Health*, *21*(1), 1290. https://doi.org/10.1186/s12889-021-11301-x

Vossoughi, N., Jackson, Y., Gusler, S., & Stone, K. (2018). Mental health outcomes for youth living in refugee camps: A review. *Trauma, Violence, & Abuse*, *19*(5), 528–542. https://doi.org/10.1177/1524838016673602

Waddoups, A. B., Yoshikawa, H., & Strouf, K. (2019). Developmental effects of parent–child separation. *Annual Review of Developmental Psychology*, *1*(1), 387–410. https://doi.org/10.1146/annurev-devpsych-121318-085142

Williams, D. R., & Collins, C. (2001). Racial residential segregation: A fundamental cause of racial disparities in health. *Public Health Reports*, *116*(5), 404–416.

Zeiders, K. H., Umaña-Taylor, A. J., Carbajal, S., & Pech, A. (2021). Police discrimination among Black, Latina/x/o, and White adolescents: Examining frequency and relations to academic functioning. *Journal of Adolescence*, *90*, 91–99. https://doi.org/10.1016/j.adolescence.2021.06.001

10 Convergence of Conflict and Climate Change in and Around the Sahel

10.1 The Sahel

It is widely known that many of the nations least responsible for rising global temperatures and environmental degradation are those suffering most acutely from the effects of these trends. Many of these nations are in sub-Saharan Africa. Geographers designate the Sahel as a "transition zone" between the dry Sahara desert in the north and the more humid savannahs in central Africa, stretching from the Atlantic Ocean to the Red Sea. It has a semi-arid climate which tends to have high temperatures, a short rainy season, and minimal precipitation overall. These climate and weather trends have, of course, shaped life in the region for many thousands of years, and disruptions in these patterns have the potential to disrupt life in many domains (social, economic, political, etc.). In addition to these environmental and climate similarities, nations in and around the Sahel also have shared histories of colonization by European countries. (Ethiopia was never formally colonized in the ways that other African nations were, though it has experienced economic and political interference from European nations, as well as military occupation by Italy.)

Figure 10.1 depicts an approximate schematic of the Sahel. This chapter considers an expanded notion of the Sahel region, discussing some nations outside of the region indicated in the map but nonetheless connected to the Sahel with regard to proximity, climate impacts, and sociopolitical trends. Readers are encouraged to recall that despite this chapter's emphasis on this particular region as a case study, the principles by which climate vulnerability, environmental degradation, armed conflict, famine, and other social crises interact and amplify one another are, in fact, universal. What is palpably clear to so many families in the Sahel is becoming more obvious worldwide: that a stable climate is critical to the peace, safety, social cohesion, and resource access that make healthy child development possible.

In the 21st century, many countries and communities in the expanded Sahel region have experienced cycles of conflict, drought, and famine that are clearly interrelated and are exacerbated by climate change (Schleussner et al., 2016). In 2022, it was estimated that 18 million persons here were on the brink of starvation (UN, 2022). Meanwhile, this region's population is increasing

DOI: 10.4324/9781003488385-13

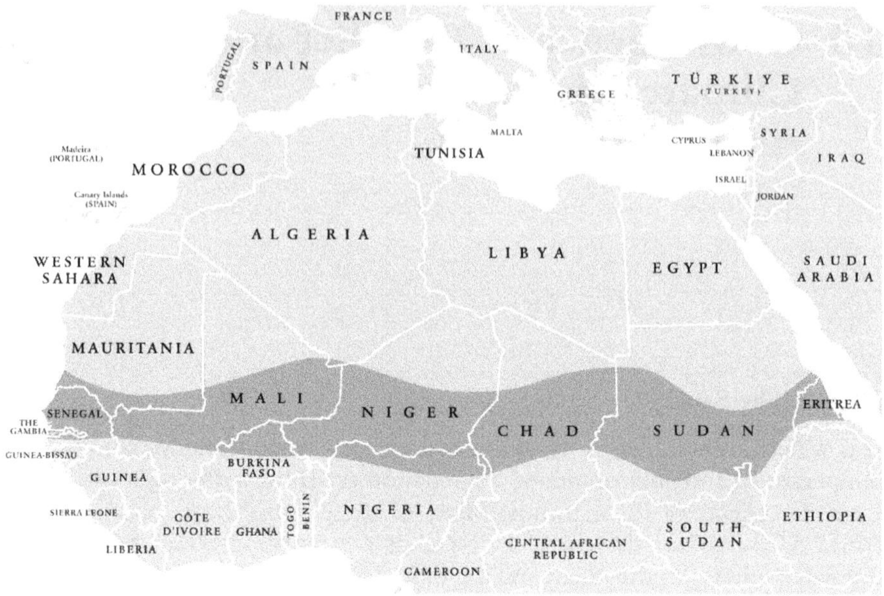

Figure 10.1 The Sahel region and the Horn of Africa.
(*Source:* Shutterstock, Furian, 2023)

rapidly, and in some countries, most people are under the age of 18. All discussions about economics, nutrition, environment, and conflict in the region must pay special attention to the age distribution of its residents. Additionally, productive approaches to supporting the development of children in the Sahel (as elsewhere) must apply multisystem approaches. For example, modern famine is increasingly related to complex social phenomena (e.g., economic downturn, political instability, and armed conflict), and therefore social solutions like promoting equality, peacebuilding, education, and economic resilience can help safeguard food availability in the long term (Oberg et al., 2022).

This chapter examines specific countries in and around the Sahel and some of the multisystem crises they have recently experienced, with an emphasis on climate as a driver and multiplier of these events.

10.2 Mali, Burkina Faso, and Niger

Mali, Burkina Faso, and Niger have seen rising levels of armed conflict in recent years. All three experienced colonization by France that lasted the better part of a century, a period marked by political disenfranchisement and a suite of colonial policies that undermined community sovereignty and social structures. There is, of course, heterogeneity in the levels and types of conflict throughout these countries and in the local resources that protect children. It is notable, though, that in the 2020s, all three countries have seen military coups accompanied by violence and unrest. In Mali, Tuareg separatists in the north of the country battled with other groups, including French forces, and similar conflicts occurred in Niger (e.g., the Tuareg rebellions of 2007). Political instability has left openings for extremist groups to seek power, including Islamic State actors, al-Qaeda, and Boko Haram (Sodik, 2024). For example, in 2024, 86% of Burkina Faso was affected by fighting between Islamist groups and military forces, with widespread forced displacement occurring as a result (Brennan & Durmaz, 2024).

Notably, conflicts in these nations have been partly driven by extreme temperatures and low rainfall. In March and April 2024, the western Sahel faced a heatwave that led to the warmest summer recorded in scientific history. Maximum temperatures reached more than 45°C (113°F) in Burkina Faso and 48.5°C (119.3°F) in Mali (Fraser-Baxter, 2024). This weather caused widespread crop failures that were especially devastating in a region in which 1.7 million people were already experiencing severe hunger and emergency levels of food insecurity (UN, 2022). Scientists concluded that this could not have occurred without the impact of human-caused climate change. Even before this severe heatwave, water shortages, failed crops, and armed conflict (which destroys nutritional infrastructure) had long been converging to cause declines in food availability. A 2021 estimate held that 2.1 million children in Niger were in need of humanitarian aid and 1.6 million were suffering from malnutrition (UNICEF, 2021). In Burkina Faso, moderate and severe malnutrition are similarly widespread (Barba et al., 2020). Forced displacement has, of course, become common as families seek safety, food, and water.

Children in this region also face developmental risks from disruptions to their education and to other rights. These three countries saw 8,400 schools shut down due to violence in 2023 (UNICEF, 2024). In 2021, sixty children in one region of Niger lost their lives as a result of armed conflict (Amnesty International, 2021). In 2023, there were 2,653 grave violations of children's rights across Mali, Burkina Faso and Niger, including recruitment to combat roles, abductions, recruitment, maiming and killing (UNICEF, 2024). In the central Sahel, 7 in 10 girls were married before the age of 18. Globally, the 10 countries with the highest rates of child marriage include Niger and Burkina Faso.

10.3 Nigeria and Boko Haram

The northern portion of Nigeria is part of the Sahel region. British colonization resulted in the formation of Nigeria from many regions that had disparate geographies, ethnicities, languages, and religious faiths. The country has seen long-standing tensions between Christians (who often live in the country's south) and Muslims (who often live in the north).

Boko Haram is a militant organization that aims to spread a strict interpretation of Sunni Islamist law and eradicate Shia Islam, and to establish an Islamic caliphate in the north of Nigeria. The group opposes influence from the

West, especially through education. Boko Haram has expanded its territory through the escalation of violence, and there is widespread speculation that the group is linked to al-Qaeda and al-Shabaab. The group's activity has proliferated since the summer of 2009, when they clashed with Nigerian security forces. This group has since expanded its influence into neighboring countries and is responsible for armed conflict, terror activities, and forced displacement in Chad, Cameroon, and Niger. Their activities also contribute to regional food availability decline. Boko Haram has frequently been involved in kidnapping and killing of civilians, as well as the use of children as suicide bombers.

Case Study: The Abduction of Schoolgirls by Boko Haram

On April 14–15, 2014, 276 schoolgirls in Chibok, Nigeria were sitting for their final exams at the Government Girls Secondary School when they were abducted by Boko Haram. From there, they were transported to the Sambisa Forest, a known stronghold for the extremist group. The girls were used as leverage for potential prisoner swaps, as human shields, and/or sold into marriage.

Over 50 girls were able to escape from captivity shortly after abduction. Others have escaped or been rescued in the years since. However, around 82 are still unaccounted for. The Nigerian government's initial response was criticized as slow, and parents and local groups launched search efforts before official military action was taken. In an early example of digitally facilitated activism, a group of Nigerian activists launched the #BringBackOurGirls campaign, which drew widespread international support and brought attention to the issues of terrorism, gender-based violence, and the right to education in conflict zones (though it is difficult to determine the extent to which this campaign resulted in Chibok schoolgirls being freed).

The girls and young women who have exited captivity have often reported both physical and emotional trauma including hard labor, forced conversions, beatings, and sexual assaults. Many had children against their will. Reintegration has been challenging, and some report stigmatization and social rejection. It is also notable that many young women who have survived this ordeal have gone on to have meaningful roles in their families, to express hope about the future, and to participate in healing activities. Several have been pursuing academic degrees.

Armed conflict within Nigeria parallels a period of increasingly harsh droughts driven by climate change. One in six of the country's children (15.6 million) faced hunger in 2024, with close to a half a million facing catastrophic levels of hunger. These incidence rates have increased drastically over the years, driven both by climate factors and by the hikes in food prices that accompany armed conflict in a region (Save the Children, 2024). Meanwhile, while primary education is free and presumably compulsory in Nigeria, 10.5 million children are not in school. In northern Nigeria, around a third of Muslim children receive Qur'anic education but no additional schooling (i.e., they are not taught numbers or basic literacy skills); the government considers these children to be out-of-school (UNICEF-Nigeria, 2024). Notably, in these states, more than half of all girls do not attend school. These low attendance rates are partly driven by gender norms, social barriers, economic disparities, security fears around school attendance, and the destruction of national state-sponsored schools by groups like Boko Haram. In three northeastern conflict-affected states (Borno, Yobe, and Adamawa), 802 schools are closed, 497 classrooms are destroyed, and 1,392 classrooms are damaged.

10.4 Sudan, South Sudan, and Darfur

Sudan and South Sudan were under British colonial rule from the end of the 19th century until 1956, with South Sudan becoming its own nation through referendum in 2011. Within and between these nations, there is vast heterogeneity in ethnicities, languages, and religious beliefs. In Sudan, over two thirds of the population is of Arab descent, and Islam is the predominant religion. Most people in South Sudan are from Indigenous African groups. This country has a Christian majority, with substantial practice of traditional faiths. Both nations have young populations, though total fertility rates have declined in recent decades.

Civil war and armed conflict have occurred several times since Sudanese independence. The First Sudanese Civil War (1955–1972) centered around the southern region's desire for more autonomy. Failure to fully address these issues led to the Second Sudanese Civil War (1983–2005), which was fought between the central Sudanese government in the North and the Sudan People's Liberation Army of the south and resulted in the eventual establishment of South Sudan as an independent nation in 2011. During this conflict, Colonel Omar al-Bashir led a bloodless military coup in 1989, with his military government then dissolving political parties. He maintained power for 30 years before being deposed and convicted of corruption by the International Criminal Court (ICC). Roughly two million people died while he was in charge of Sudan as a result of the convergence of war, famine, and disease. At least four million more have been displaced.

Darfur is in the western part of Sudan and experienced its own conflict with the Sudanese government. The War in Darfur began in 2003 and lasted until 2010, with conflict primarily occurring between the Sudanese government and a group of rebel forces (including the Janjaweed militia group and forces from the Sudan Liberation Movement [SLM] and the

Justice and Equality Movement [JEM]). The rebel forces of Darfur started fighting due to their concern that the Sudanese government was oppressing Darfur's non-Arab population. This conflict entailed high amounts of civilian deaths, with 200,000–400,000 civilians estimated to have died over a three-year period. In 2008, the ICC filed genocide charges against al-Bashir. In the 2000s, observers had already labeled the War in Darfur the "first climate change conflict," driven as it was by rapid desertification, loss of arable land, decreases in rainfall, and lowering of the water table (Sova, 2020). In fact, the Sahara desert extended southward by additional one mile each year for the decades leading up to the 2003 war, while rainfall declined. Livestock herders (who are most often of Arab descent in Sudan) and farmers (who are most often from African ethnic groups) began to see diminishing supplies of usable land and water. Land productivity is expected to decline further in the coming decades.

Civil war arose again in Sudan in 2023, with international groups warning of genocide. Internal displacement is estimated to have affected 10 million, and reports have emerged of civilian killings and kidnappings. In addition, the United Nations Population Fund (UNFPA) estimated that 6.7 million Sudanese people, primarily women, are at risk of gender-based violence (Think Global Health, 2024).

10.5 Somalia

For over three decades, Somalia has faced famine, conflict, and environmental crises, all of which influence and exacerbate one another (Oberg et al., 2021). One in six Somali people lives in a city, and most of the rest of the population is involved in livestock herding and farming. As a result, the country's economy is closely tied to the health of the climate and the environment (UNDP, 2021). Somalia historically has had fairly predictable monsoon seasons, but its rainfall has been decreasing in recent decades and now occurs erratically, with droughts becoming more frequent and intense (NAPA, 2013). Meanwhile, the nation is experiencing rapid warming, with a 4.3°C increase in mean temperatures expected before the 21st century ends (IPCC, 2007). As soil has dried out and deforestation has accelerated, the land itself has become less resilient to extreme weather events; for example, rainfalls now commonly result in floods as parched soil fails to absorb water (FAOUN, 2013).

Complicating (and bidirectionally influencing) these environmental and climate crises, Somalia has faced civil war for decades that has eroded many of the social, economic, and ecological resilience resources it used to enjoy (Kinyangi et al., 2009; Oberg et al., 2021). Famines in the 1990s and early 2010s killed half a million people, half of whom were under the age of five (BBC, 2013; Hansch et al., 1994). When another drought struck the country in 2016–2017, Somalia's humanitarian networks and government partnered with international actors to develop a prevention plan that successfully averted a famine (UNOCHA, 2017).

In Somalia, as elsewhere, resource scarcity brought about by climate degradation intensifies conflict, and vice versa. Access to food, arable land, and water is often at the root of violence, and conflict, in turn, levies huge environmental tolls (SPIRI, 2019). In fact, Al-Shabaab has taken control of water rights in many regions, restricting both drinking water and irrigation to those who do not give them financial support (Zimmerman, 2021). In the 2020s, drought has displaced more than 1 million Somali people, many of whom are women and children suffering from severe malnutrition (McFadden, 2022).

10.6 Successful Initiatives in the Sahel

There are a number of initiatives underway to improve the lives of children in the Sahel, including government interventions, educational and economic initiatives, and NGO activities. The Sahel Alliance is made up of 27 nations and organizations including the African Development Bank, the West African Development Bank, the European Union, the United States, Canada, and the World Bank. The Alliance has five "fields of action": promoting access to basic services, increasing access to sustainable energy, promoting civic participation and confidence, supporting education and employment, and developing sustainable agriculture and nutrition systems (Alliance Sahel, 2025). For example, in July of 2024, the Alliance launched an education initiative to support primary school attendance, with funding support from Germany and the World Bank—an especially critical mission when one considers that nearly half of the Sahel's population is under 15 years of age (UN, 2021).

Another major intervention over the last decades was undertaken by the Food and Agriculture Organization of the United Nations (FAOUN), Helen Keller International (HKI), the Micronutrient Initiative (MI), UNICEF, and the World Food Programme (WFP), which launched an initiative to support infant and child nutrition in the Sahel. The initiative's aim was to achieve optimal feeding of >80% of children 0–24 months in the region (Wuehler et al., 2011). Meanwhile, UN-affiliated programs have backed local efforts in the Sahel to improve agricultural sustainability and increase people's access to livelihoods that will be resilient to climate change (UNEP, 2024). Educational access is associated with the likelihood of sustainable peace amid armed conflict (Hima, 2025). Locally led efforts to promote school enrollment and attendance, especially for children who face barriers to schooling (e.g., girls, youth from impoverished families, and displaced children), are likely to be responsive to cultural and contextual needs in affected communities.

10.7 Conclusion

These are but a few examples of the convergence of climate and conflict in the Sahel and the Horn of Africa. Climate scientists speculate that seasonal temperatures well past 40–48°C may well be the "new normal" for the region.

Sustained and long-term planning is necessary, in addition to rapid international responses to emergent crises. It is particularly important for solutions to apply lenses of equity—for example, to ensure that distribution of aid reaches those with limited transportation resources and that educational initiatives are culturally and contextually tailored to support schooling in children who face barriers to school involvement. All responses benefit from local and sub-regional leadership, of course.

Climate mitigation at the international level is imperative in the coming decades, as is climate adaptation at the regional, country and local levels. As evidence emerges of the interconnectedness of armed conflict and climate change, damage from armed conflict could justifiably be included in calculations of the global cost of climate change. International agreements on climate finance responsibilities, coupled with legislative actions to hold parties accountable for damage to the global climate, may be a part of protecting the development of children in the Sahel and elsewhere. As discussed in Section IV, a child rights approach may offer shared language to local, regional, and international actors and equip decisive actions in the domains of climate justice, education, gender equity, nutrition, and safety.

Reflection Questions

Question 1. Which of the crises (and response strategies) in this chapter were you aware of prior to reading it? What do you think shaped your awareness?

Question 2. What are the benefits and challenges of international involvement in addressing some of the crises discussed above?

Question 3. How do education and employment opportunities shape resilience to climate change and armed conflict in the Sahel? What about in your own region?

References

Alliance Sahel (2024). Alliance Sahel. https://www.alliance-sahel.org/en/sahel-alliance/

Amnesty International (2021). "Niger: Increasing number of children killed and recruited by armed groups in Sahel's Tri-Border area – new report", 12 September. https://www.amnesty.org/en/latest/news/2021/09/niger-increasing-number-of-children-killed-and-recruited-by-armed-groups-in-sahels-tri-border-area-new-report/.

Barba, F., Huybregts, L., & Leroy, J. L. (2020). Incidence correction factors for moderate and severe acute child malnutrition from 2 longitudinal cohorts in Mali and Burkina Faso. *American Journal of Epidemiology, 189*(12), 1623–1627.

BBC (2013). Somalia famine killed 260,000 people. *BBC Africa*, May 2. https://www.bbc.com/news/world-africa-22380352

Brennan, H., & Durmaz, M. (2024). Conflict zones grow by two thirds globally since 2021, covering 6 million km^2. *Verisk Maplecroft*. https://www.maplecroft.com/

products-and-solutions/geopolitical-and-country-risk/insights/conflict-zones-grow-by-two-thirds-globally-since-2021-covering-6-million-km2/

FAOUN (2013). Food and Agriculture Organization of the Unite Nations. *Resilient livelihoods-disaster risk reduction for food and nutrition security*, April.

Hansch, S., Lillibridge, S., Egeland, G., Teller, C., & Toole, M. (1994). *Lives lost, lives saved: Excess mortality and the impact of health Interventions in the Somali Emergency.* Center for Policy Analysis and Research on Refugee Issues.

Hima, H. (2025). Learning on the move: Facilitating the continuation of learning for children in conflict-affected settings in the Sahel. *Center for Universal Education at The Brookings Institution.* https://eric.ed.gov/?id=ED666600

Intergovernmental Panel on Climate Change (IPCC), AR4 Climate Change 2007: Synthesis Report, Contribution of Working Groups I, II and III to the Fourth Assessment Report of the Intergovernmental Panel on Climate Change [Core Writing Team, Pachauri, R. K. and Reisinger, A. (eds)] (IPCC: Geneva, 2007); and Ministry of National Resources (note 32), p. 28.

Kinyangi, J., Herrero, M., Omolo, A., Steeg. J., & van de Thornton, P. K. (2009). *Scoping study on vulnerability to climate change and climate variability in the greater Horn of Africa: Mapping impacts and adaptive capacity* (87p). International Livestock Research Institute.

McFadden, K. (2022). In Somalia, women and children are bearing the brunt of the Horn of Africa drought. World Food Program, USA. https://www.wfpusa.org/articles/somalia-women-children-bearing-brunt-of-drought/

NAPA, 2013. *National adaptation programme of action on climate change.* Ministry of National Resources, Federal Republic of Somalia: Mogadishu, p. 14, April.

Oberg, C. N., Hodges, H. R., & Masten, A. (2022). Conflict, war, and famine in childhood: Risks and resilience for social development. In Peter K. Smith & Craig H. Hart (Eds.), *The Wiley-Blackwell handbook of childhood social development* (3rd ed.). John Wiley & Sons Ltd.

Oberg, C. N., Hodges, H. R., & Masten, A. (2021). Risk and resilience of Somali children in the context of climate change, famine, and conflict. *Journal of Applied Research on Children, 12*(1), 1–26. https://digitalcommons.library.tmc.edu/childrenatrisk/vol12/iss1/10/.

Save the Children (2024). Nigeria: One in six children set to go hungry as kidnappings, conflict and rising prices push food out of reach. https://www.savethechildren.org/us/about-us/media-and-news/2024-press-releases/nigeria-one-six-children-set-to-go-hungry

Schleussner, C. F., Donges, J. F., Donner, R. V., & Schellnhuber, H. J. (2016). Armed-conflict risks enhanced by climate-related disasters in ethnically fractionalized countries. *Proceedings of the National Academy of Sciences, 113*(33), 9216–9221. https://doi.org/10.1073/pnas.1601611113

Sodik, K. O. (2024). Dynamic of conflict in the Sahel: Mali, Burkina Faso and Niger. *FUOYE International Journal of Criminology and Security Studies, 3*(2), 58–79. ISSN: 2786–9636.

Sova, C. (2020). The first climate change conflict. World Food Program, USA. https://www.wfpusa.org/articles/the-first-climate-change-conflict/

SPIRI (2019). Stockholm International Peace Research Institute (SIPRI), Climate change challenges the future success of peacebuilding. Policy Paper, No. 53, October 2019.

Think Global Health (2024). Bodies into Battlefields: Gender-based violence in Sudan. March 25. https://www.thinkglobalhealth.org/article/bodies-battlefields-gender-based-violence-sudan

UN (2022). UN News-Global perspective human stories. 18 million in Africa's Sahel on the brink of starvation. May 20. https://news.un.org/en/story/2022/05/1118702

UN Environment Programme. (2024). *Climate change and adaptation.* UNEP. https://www.unep.org/sudan/climate-change-and-adaptation

UNICEF (2021). United Nations children's fund, "more than 2.1 million children caught up in a humanitarian crisis in Niger", Press Release, July 1. https://www.unicef.org/niger/press-releases/more-21-million-children-caught-humanitarian-crisis-niger.

UNICEF (2024). Escalating crisis in the central Sahel-advocating for children's rights, August. https://www.unicef.org/reports/escalating-crisis-central-sahel

UNICEF-Nigeria (2024). Education. https://www.unicef.org/nigeria/education

United Nations (2021). *The Sahel: Land of opportunities.* United Nations Africa Renewal. https://www.un.org/africarenewal/sahel

United Nations Development Program (UNDP) Climate Change Adaptation. (2021). https://www.adaptation-undp.org/explore/eastern-africa/somalia

UNOCHA (2017), Somalia operational plan for famine prevention (Jan–Jun 2017), February.

Wuehler, E., Hess, S. Y., & Brown, K. H. (2011). Accelerating improvements in nutritional and health status of young children in the Sahel region of Sub-Saharan Africa: Review of international guidelines on infant and young child feeding and nutrition. *Maternal & Child Nutrition*, *7*(1), 6–34. https://onlinelibrary.wiley.com/doi/full/10.1111/j.1740-8709.2010.00306.x

11 Genocide, War Crimes, and Crimes against Humanity

11.1 Introduction: History, Definitions, and Legislation

Genocide is an ancient and persistent phenomenon. Sources as diverse as the Hebrew Bible and the annals of Rome describe the intentional destruction of entire nations or identity groups, and colonizing forces have routinely eradicated Indigenous populations through state-sanctioned murder or lethal labor conditions. While often associated with war, genocide may occur independently of officially declared conflict, as was the case in the systematic killing of California's Indigenous peoples during the U.S. Gold Rush and the surrounding years. The deadliest genocidal activities, by sheer numbers, occurred during the Second World War, with the Nazi regime taking the lives of an estimate 6 million Jewish Europeans, of whom 1.5 million were children, in addition to several million who were killed because they were Polish, Roma, Sinti, or from other marginalized groups (e.g., gay people).

Though ancient and persistent, genocide is far from inevitable. Members of victimized, perpetrating, and bystander groups have always worked to counteract these violent crimes through resistance and advocacy. In fact, the founding of the United Nations (UN) in the immediate aftermath of the Second World War came largely out of a desire to prevent future wars and preserve human rights worldwide. In 1948, the UN passed the Universal Declaration of Human Rights (UDHR) stating, for example, that "Everyone has the right to life, liberty and security of person," that "No one shall be subjected to torture or to cruel, inhuman or degrading treatment or punishment," and that human rights extend to all regardless of race, ethnicity, national origin, or other identities. The same year, the UN passed the Convention on the Prevention and Punishment of the Crime of Genocide (CPPCG), defining genocide as intentional efforts to "destroy, in whole or in part, a national, ethnic, racial or religious group" by, for example, killing people, causing serious physical or mental harm, inflicting lethal or dangerous life conditions, attempting to prevent births, and removing children to another group. Intentional efforts at eradication of a culture—for example, through forced assimilation, destruction of significant sites, or deportations designed to separate communities—may be considered cultural genocide as well.

DOI: 10.4324/9781003488385-14

Case Study: Dr. Korczak

When he was not providing pediatric medical care, writing books for young readers, or penning guidance on pedagogy and parenting, Dr. Janusz Korczak (born in Poland in the 1870s) used the written word and the radio to spread awareness of children's rights. Seventy years before the ratification of the UN Convention on the Rights of the Child, Dr. Korczak argued that adults are responsible for, among other things, respecting children's bodies and self-determination.

Particularly dedicated to children on the margins, Dr. Korczak helped to found an orphanage (Nasz Dom, or "Our House") that was designed to foster children's sense of agency and empowerment. As Poland grew more dangerous for people with Jewish ancestry like himself, Dr. Korczak was given many opportunities to seek safety. Instead, living in an attic room above the orphanage, he continued serving the young people in his care.

Eventually, Dr. Korsczak was forced to relocate his orphanage, moving with nearly 200 orphaned Jewish children to the Warsaw ghetto. Even amid the chaos of this environment, he and the other orphanage staff worked hard to support the children's healthy development through education, routines, and play. In early August of 1942, occupying Nazi forces ordered the entire orphanage to be deported to the death camp at Treblinka. Refusing all those who offered him reprieve and sanctuary, Dr. Korczak walked hand in hand with the children onto the trains that led them to their deaths. When encouraged to seek safety and leave the orphans behind, he is credited with saying, "You do not leave a sick child in the night, and you do not leave children at a time like this."

(Oberg, 2008; Syrkin, 1988)

The Geneva Conventions had existed for some time by the end of the Second World War. These international agreements established that soldiers who were sick or wounded, including prisoners of war, had a right to care and protection. In the late 1940s, these agreements were expanded to describe detailed protections for noncombatants (Miles, 2016), with other child-relevant protocols adopted in 1977. Meanwhile, Geneva defined war crimes for which combatants could be held accountable, including inhumane treatment toward protected people, forced conscription of them, willfully causing them death or serious injury, taking hostages, and destroying civilian property without military justification. More recent rulings have established that these grave violations of rights can be prosecuted whether armed conflict is occurring between nations or within a nation. These Conventions also state that civilian populations must have their basic needs met, including food, clothing, and medicine, and that if an occupying or combatant force cannot meet these needs, it must accept other parties' help to ensure that these necessities are available to civilians. These and other international treaties and humanitarian laws are intended to protect those who are most vulnerable during armed conflict, such as children.

Despite resounding international agreement about the severity of genocide and war crimes, these atrocities have continued in staggering scales. The following section describes a select number of episodes of genocide and war crimes impacting children in recent decades and elucidates themes in these events (Oberg, 2008).

11.2 Crimes against Children in the 21st Century

As described in Chapter 1 of this textbook, modern armed conflict increasingly occurs in urban settings, with battle erupting in the places where children play, study, and grow. In fact, the civilian status of children regularly appears to confer minimal protection from exposure to combat, and the majority of people injured or killed in modern wars are noncombatants. There is dangerous potential for combatants to perpetrate war crimes against children.

Armed conflict, environmental crises, and climate shocks may provide new openings for extremist leaders or organizations to rise to power. Furthermore, the resource scarcity brought about by these adversities can increase fractionalization within communities and intensify mistrust and hatred toward "the other." Discourse may proliferate that casts members of minority groups as "subhuman." These risk factors, coupled with the erosion of social protective buffers, can increase the risk that societal strain escalates into genocidal activity.

Additionally, it is all too common for international communities to acclimate to these atrocities; to deny their magnitude; or to interpret them as simply part of the horrors of war, glossing over the fact that these crimes target children and others who have not taken up arms (Oberg, 2008; Powers, 2003).

Genocide and war crimes not only exert direct harm toward children, but also harm survivors indirectly. Children left without caregivers are vulnerable to poverty, neglect, and exploitation. The infrastructures that should protect them, such as education, healthcare, and food supplies, may be severely disrupted. Meanwhile, traumatic stress in caregivers may make it harder for the family to buffer children's stress (Christie et al., 2019).

11.2.1 Sexual and Gender-Based Violence

War crimes frequently entail disproportionate harm toward girls and women. As described in previous chapters, many of the social systems that ordinarily protect girls and women can become eroded during armed conflict, and perpetrators may exploit pre-existing power differentials with impunity. In addition, groups may inflict gendered violence as a way of preventing future births in a cultural community and of inflicting additional terror on victimized communities. These themes were evident in what is now Bangladesh in the early 1970s when, following serious flooding and famine, the West Pakistani army engaged in genocide toward the Bengali people in the east. Efforts to eliminate Bengali people included large-scale sexual violence and physical violence toward women of this community (Jones, 2006). Armies of Pakistan sexually assaulted hundreds of thousands of women and also kidnapped large groups of young women, including female university students, for sexual exploitation and abuse.

More recently, the wars in the Democratic Republic of the Congo have seen high levels of sexual assault, trafficking, forced marriages, and exploitation (Freedson & Singh, 2006; UN News, 2025). Women and girls who are victimized in these ways are at particular risk of physical health problems like infections with HIV and other sexually transmitted infections, difficulty having children in the future, unwanted pregnancies, and gynecological fistulas (Mathias et al., 2008). Many concurrently experience humiliation, ostracization from families and communities, and disruption of education.

For a long time, sexual violence was seen as an inevitable side effect of war. However, this idea has been challenged, with advocates pointing out that sexual and gendered violence are commonly used as a strategy of perpetrators and combatants to elicit additional terror and humiliation (Machel, 2000). In June of 2008, in fact, the UN Security Council officially classified rape as a weapon of war, reiterating that sexual violence is a crime against humanity and a form of torture, and that it can be treated as a constituent act of genocide.

11.2.2 Targeting of Children

Frequently, children are targeted in genocide and other crimes against humanity. During Cambodia's brutal Khmer Rouge regime of the 1970s, children and youth were systematically killed at concentration camps, including the notorious Tuol Seng, a former high school in the capital of Phnom Penh (Kiernan, 2004). Other times, children were exploited for use in agricultural labor, where they often died of exhaustion and starvation. The U.S. invasions of Iraq and Afghanistan involved a series of massacres and murders that targeted women and children. One, in Kandahar, involved the brutal and premeditated murder of 16 Afghan civilians, including 11 children. In Mahmudiyah, Iraq, U.S. soldiers sexually assaulted 14-year-old Abeer Qassim Hamza al-Janabi, then murdered her, her parents, and her six-year-old sister. U.S. military personnel covered up these crimes until they were exposed several months later.

Russia's 2022 invasion of Ukraine has resulted in widespread destruction of civilian sites, including places that serve children. Under the Geneva Conventions' "rules of war," the loss of civilian life (collateral damage) must be proportional to the value of a military objective. In contrast to this principle, Russia has bombed sites like the Maternity and Children's Hospital in Mariupol and similar locations throughout Ukraine, locations with no discernible military objectives. Violence directed at medical facilities disrupts children's access to routine and emergency care alike. One surgeon in Ukraine reported enduring a bombing while operating on a child (Amnesty International, 2024). These actions have resulted in the death of hundreds of children (Ukraine, 2022). The International Criminal Court (ICC) issued a warrant for the arrest of Russian President Vladimir Putin for war crimes, genocide, and crimes against humanity (ICC, 2023).

11.2.3 Children in Combat Roles

Another grave violation of international human rights law is the conscription of children into combat roles. This occurred frequently during the Khmer Rouge in Cambodia, where children were often asked specifically to kill other children who were viewed as not representing the peasantry class. In the 1990s and 2000s, civil war in Sierra Leone claimed close to a quarter of a million lives and displaced around 1.3 million individuals, with half the country estimated to have experienced homelessness (Medeiros, 2007). Both rebel and government forces abducted children as young as six for use in combat roles, with over 10,000 children forced to participate in the conflict. At one point, half of the individuals fighting with the rebel forces were between 8 and 14 years of age (Sesay, 2003). Often tortured, indoctrinated, and forced to take drugs, these children were used to commit indiscriminate killings and other atrocities, including amputating civilians' limbs. Some survivors report being put on the front lines against government forces in high-risk military operations (Wilson, 2001). Meanwhile, many girls were sexually exploited by combatants.

In 2024, Haiti saw a 70% increase in the incidence of children being abducted or forcibly recruited to participate in armed violence, with up to half of all members of armed groups estimated to be under the age of 18. Family separation, poverty, and infrastructure damage render children especially vulnerable to this atrocity (UNICEF, 2024).

11.2.4 Cascading Effects on Children

War crimes frequently target civilians and civilian structures that support children's development. Following the genocide in the mid-1990s, Rwanda had close to 100,000 orphans (Geltman & Stover, 1997). It became common for children to grow up in households headed by youth, which comes with known mental and physical health risks, as well as barriers to education (Boris et al., 2006). In the conflict in Darfur, Sudan in the early 2000s, militia groups engaged in genocidal violence in the form of a scorched earth campaign, often burning villages or poisoning wells that supplied children with fresh water (Steidle, 2007). Millions of people were displaced as a result of these actions. A resumption of violence in 2023 has resulted in Sudan becoming the site of the world's largest child displacement crisis, with over seven million children fleeing their homes for safety (UNICEF, 2025). Meanwhile, 19 million children are out of school, and four million children under age five are projected to suffer from acute malnutrition this year (UNHCR, 2024).

A similar scorched earth campaign has occurred in Gaza, where Israeli response to the October 2023 Hamas attacks and abductions has resulted in destruction of homes, supply lines, and transportation infrastructure. The Israeli military has targeted places that shelter civilians, such as internal displacement camps, shelters, and children's hospitals. At times, this has been justified as part of efforts to target Hamas strongholds hidden in civilian locations, but there is frequently little evidence to support this claim. Within eighteen months, this war had killed or injured more than 50,000 children (UNICEF, 2025). Supply blockages and violence at distribution sites has resulted in severe shortages of food, fuel, and medicine. In four months alone, 19,000 children were hospitalized for acute malnutrition (Lederer, 2025). Children are overrepresented in Gaza's death toll. In November of 2024, the ICC issued an arrest warrant for Israel President Benjamin Netanyahu and his defense minister, accusing them of crimes against humanity, including targeting civilians and using starvation as a weapon of war.

11.2.5 Cultural Genocide and Separation of Families

The intentional eradication of a culture often precedes or accompanies violence. Perpetrators may attempt to destroy a culture by destroying sites of significance to members of a given group or by forcing them to assimilate to a culture that is not their own. Another pernicious tool of cultural genocide is the separation of families, which prevents the transmission of culture through child-rearing. For example, during the California Genocide of the 19th century, thousands of Indigenous children were separated from their families, enslaved, and forbidden to practice their heritage cultures. The Khmer Rouge regime frequently separated children from their families as well. In these and other cases, children are often raised by members of the very same communities who separated them from their families. One other notable example occurred in Argentina in the 1970s and 1980s, when hundreds of babies were abducted shortly after birth, including from mothers who gave birth in concentration camps, and raised by families affiliated with the military dictatorship. Many of these children have never been accounted for, though ongoing advocacy efforts persist in Argentina, often led by women whose children or grandchildren disappeared during the Dirty War (Taylor, 2001).

Separation of families is still used as a weapon of war. As of the spring of 2025, Russian forces removed at least 19,000 children from their families in Ukraine and subjected them to re-education, along with forced and illegal adoptions by Russian families (Yale School of Medicine, 2025). Many of these children's families continued searching for them, and at the time of this writing, Russia has not complied with international laws dictating that they help facilitate these searches.

Case Study: The Tamil Genocide in Sri Lanka

Following many decades of ethnic tension, Sri Lanka suffered through a civil war that lasted from 1983 to 2009, in which the military of the nation (which had a Sinhalese majority) fought with the Liberation Tigers of Tamil Eelam (LTTE). Over 100 massacres occurred during this war in which Tamil civilians were killed, and there were also widespread reports of indiscriminate bombings, random shootings, and physical mutilation. Human rights investigators uncovered events in which women and children lining up at food distribution shelters were killed with shelling. Meanwhile, government security forces engaged in attempts to erase Tamil culture and history, including by burning the Jaffna Public Library (which contained countless manuscripts and pieces of art that documented Tamil history and culture). The Sri Lankan government also supported colonization of Tamil lands by Sinhalese people.

In 2013, a tribunal unanimously concluded that the Sri Lankan government was guilty of genocide against the Tamil population, with the United States and United Kingdom listed as complicit in these crimes (Veerassingham, 2013). The road to social healing has been long, including in national political discourse, and the destruction of the 2004 tsunami has further complicated this process. One of the greatest casualties of the civil war was the erosion of protective social and family structures in Tamil communities (Somasundaram, 2007). For example, social trust has been harmed in communities where one person was expected to report on another. Some adults have reported having difficulty with their parenting and with navigating family conflict. Recovery efforts there have taken a multisystem approach and have included diverse forms of social and emotional support (e.g., support groups for widows, delivering mental health training for teachers, reconnecting people to cultural coping strategies). For many Tamil people, identity is closely shaped by the environment in which one lives, and these environments were frequently damaged by the conflict. Environmental justice organizations have partnered with local Sri Lankan communities to promote sustainable economic activities (farming, fishing, etc.) and protect against pollution and land exploitation (Camisani, 2018). There is a strong potential for environmental justice work to support Tamil communities in strengthening a sense of collective agency and place-based identity after decades of violence and displacement.

11.3 Limitations of International Humanitarian Law

As mentioned, a suite of international declarations, treaties and laws has been put in place to address and prevent the worst aspects of combat on the lives of children. International Humanitarian Law (IHL) is the field that attempts to regulate the actions of parties engaged in war in order to protect both military and civilian individuals. In theory, children are entitled to special protections under IHL, ***including family reunifications, exchange of family news between separated relatives, and protection against any form of assault*** (Plattner, 1984).

In general, it is not the task of IHL bodies to carry out prosecutions and sanctions when these principles are violated. Instead, this task is typically appointed to international criminal law (ICL) bodies and to the ICC, which was established in 2002 by the UN Security Council (Gegout, 2013). The ICC has jurisdiction over genocide, crimes against humanity, war crimes, and crimes of aggression, which occur when one state uses armed force in a way that violates another state's sovereignty. Several countries, like the United States, have never ratified the ICC.

There are limits to ICL and to the activities of the ICC. First, the ICC can only investigate crimes committed after July 1st, 2002, when the Court was established. Additionally, many international legal bodies are vague in their discussion of intra-state armed conflict, like civil wars and insurrections (Alexander, 2015). The ICC's prosecuting power may be constrained in these cases, even when other nations become involved in an intra-state conflict.

11.4 Conclusion

Effective advocacy for children often involves addressing and preventing genocide, war crimes, and crimes against humanity. First, education about genocide and war crimes in classrooms and in other spaces can help young people to learn to respond collectively to this threat and, importantly, to recognize the warning signs, such as marginalization of a group, hate speech, dehumanization, or framing a group as a threat. Some nations have worked to prevent genocide through measures like policy blueprints and committees (like the United States' interagency Atrocities Prevention Board) that meet regularly to assess the risk of possible crimes against humanity worldwide, share strategies between networks, and augment the capacity of international partners like the UN to address these risks (Albright & Cohen 2008). Additionally, bodies like the UN have worked to create early warning and rapid response systems that can help identify where unrest, conflict, and marginalization are likely to escalate into genocide and other crimes against humanity. Unfortunately, these systems failed to prevent mass atrocities in places like Rwanda, Ethiopia, Côte d'Ivoire, and Darfur; despite early warnings, political will did not move international bodies to sufficient action (McLoughlin et al., 2023). An informed population that holds each member state accountable will likely be essential in the prevention of future atrocities.

As described in other chapters, many approaches to preventing genocide are also promotive of wellbeing in general. These include access to education, opportunities for positive civic engagement, economic resilience, and a culture that supports interdependence and respect across lines of difference.

Meanwhile, for those children and families already affected by these grave human rights violations, every effort must be made to restore physical, social, emotional, relational, and environmental health. Reunification efforts with family and community are critical, as is restoration of social and political agency, individually and collectively. International efforts, delivered through organizations within affected communities, can ensure that interventions are responsive to the changing needs of participants and closely informed by local contexts and cultures.

Reflection Questions

Question 1. Do you ever feel as if there is nothing you can do about crimes against humanity? Can you name one thing you could do to make a difference?

Question 2. Hatred toward the "other" has persisted across time and in many different societies. Using Bronfenbrenner's socio-ecological framework, can you think of factors in each sphere that might contribute to the occurrence of this hatred? What might protect against it?

References

Albright, M. K., & Cohen, W. S. (2008). *Preventing genocide-A blueprint for US policy makers*, the US Holocaust Memorial Museum, the Academy of Diplomacy, and the Endowment of the Unites States Institute of Peace.

Alexander, A. A. (2015). Short history of international humanitarian law. *The European Journal of International Law*, *26*, 109–138.

Amnesty International (2024). Ukraine: Russian strikes amounting to war crimes continue to kill and injure children. *Amnesty International.* https://www.amnesty.org/en/latest/news/2024/11/ukraine-russian-strikes-amounting-to-war-crimes-continue-to-kill-and-injure-children/

Boris, N. W, Thurman, T. R., Snider, L., Spenser, E., & Brown, L. (2006). Infants and young children in youth-headed households in Rwanda: Implication of Emerging Data. *Infant Mental Health Journal*, *27*, 584–602.

Camisani, P. B. (2018). Sri Lanka: A political ecology of socio-environmental conflicts and development projects. *Sustainability Science*, *13*(3), 693–707.

Christie, H., Hamilton-Giachritsis, C., Alves-Costa, F., Tomlinson, M., & Halligan, S. L. (2019). The impact of parental posttraumatic stress disorder on parenting: A systematic review. *European Journal of Psychotraumatology*, *10*(1), 1–13.

Freedson, J., & Singh, S. (2006). Children and armed conflict in the democratic republic of the Congo. *UN Chronicle*, *4*, 35–37.

Gegout, C. (2013). The International Criminal Court: Limits, potential and conditions for the promotion of justice and peace. *Third World Quarterly*, *34*(5), 800–818. https://doi.org/10.1080/01436597.2013.800737

Geltman, P., & Stover, E. (1997). Genocide and the plight of children in Rwanda, *Journal of the American Medical Association*, *227*, 289–294.

ICC (2023). Situation in Ukraine: ICC judges issue arrest warrants against Vladimir Vladimirovich Putin and Maria Alekseyevna Lvova-Belova. ICC Press Release: 17 March 2023. https://www.icc-cpi.int/news/situation-ukraine-icc-judges-issue-arrest-warrants-against-vladimir-vladimirovich-putin-and

Jones, A. (2006). *Genocide—a comprehensive introduction*. Routledge Press.

Kiernan, B. (2004). The Cambodian genocide—1975–1979. In *Century of Genocide*. 363–398. Routledge.

Lederer, E. M. (2025). Devastating toll for Gaza's children: Over 13,000 killed and an estimated 25,000 injured, UN says. AP. https://apnews.com/article/un-gaza-war-children-killed-malnutrition-israel-bef00a350a7fbe5a33dfb2c9883803ce

Machel, G (2000). Chapter 5: "Ending gender-based violence and sexual exploitation" in the impact of armed conflict on children: A critical review of progress made and obstacles encountered in increasing protection for war-affected children. *International Conference on War-Affected Children* (pp. 18–21). Winnipeg, Canada.

Mathias, O., Solbjorg, S., Luhirri, R., & Mukwege, D. (2008). Sexual violence related fistulas in the Democratic Republic of Congo. *International Journal of Gynecology and Obstetrics, 193*, 265–269.

McLoughlin, S., Gifkins, J., & Bellamy, A. J. (2023). The evolution of mass atrocity early warning in the UN secretariat: Fit for purpose? *International Peacekeeping, 30*(4), 477–505.

Medeiros, E. (2007). Integrating mental health into post-conflict rehabilitation-the case of Sierra Leonean and Liberian "Child Soldiers". *Journal of Health Psychology, 12*, 498–504.

Miles, N. (2016). *International humanitarian law-a comprehensive introduction*. International Committee of the Red Cross. ISBN: 9782940396467. August.

Oberg, C. N. (2008). Children of genocide—A legacy of lost dreams. *Pediatrics, 121*, 611.

Plattner, D. (1984). Protection of Children in International Humanitarian Law. International Review of the Red Cross, 24(240), 140–152. doi:10.1017/S002086040006993X

Powers, S. (2003). *A problem from hell—American and the age of genocide* (p. 50). Harper Perennial.

Sesay A. (Ed.). (2003). *Civil wars, child soldiers and post conflict peace building in West Africa*. AFSTRAG.

Somasundaram, D. (2007). Collective trauma in northern Sri Lanka: a qualitative psychosocial-ecological study. *International journal of mental health systems, 1*(1), 5. https://doi.org/10.1186/1752-4458-1-5

Steidle, B. (2007). *The devil came on Horseback—bearing witness to the genocide in Darfur*. Public Affairs.

Syrkin, M. (1988). The King of Children: a Biography of Janusz Korczak. *The New Republic, 198*(23), 44–49.

Taylor, D. (2001). Making a spectacle: The mothers of the Plaza de Mayo. *Journal of the Association for Research on Mothering, 3*, 97–109.

Ukraine(2022).287childrenkilledinUkrainesinceRussianinvasionBegan.June11.https://www.ndtv.com/world-news/287-children-killed-in-ukraine-since-the-russian-invasion-began-report-3057853

UNHCR (2024). Sudan conflict: 24 million children exposed to a year of brutality and rights violations, UN Committee says. March 18, 2024. Retrieved March 13, 2024, at https://www.ohchr.org/en/press-releases/2024/03/sudan-conflict-24-million-children-exposed-year-brutality-and-rights https://gsp.yale.edu/case-studies/cambodian-genocide-program.

UNICEF (2024). *Number of children in Haiti recruited by armed groups soars by 70 per cent in one year.* UNICEF. https://www.unicef.org/press-releases/number-children-haiti-recruited-armed-groups-soars-70-cent-one-year-unicef

UNICEF (2025). Two Years On: Children in Sudan are living through one of the world's worst crises. https://www.unicef.org/sudan/two-years-children-sudan-are-living-through-one-worlds-worst-crises

UNICEF (2025). *'Unimaginable horrors': More than 50,000 children reportedly killed or injured in the Gaza Strip.* UNICEF. https://www.unicef.org/press-releases/unimaginable-horrors-more-50000-children-reportedly-killed-or-injured-gaza-strip

United Nations News. (2025). *Sexual violence systematically used as a weapon of war in the DR Congo.* United Nations. https://news.un.org/en/story/2025/04/1162536

Veerassingham, R. (2013). Sri Lanka guilty of genocide against Eelam Tamils with UK, US complicity: PPT. *Journalist for Democracy in Sri Lanka (JDS),* December 11. https://www.jdslanka.org/index.php/news-features/human-rights/426-sri-lanka-guilty-of-genocide-against-tamils-with-uk-us-complicity-ppt-rules

Wilson, R. A. (2001). Children and war in Sierra Leone: A West African diary. *Anthropology Today, 17*(5), 20–22. https://www.jstor.org/stable/2678293.

Yale School of Medicine (2025). Fact sheet: Russia's kidnapping and re-education of Ukraine's children. Yale school of medicine. https://medicine.yale.edu/news-article/fact-sheet-russias-kidnapping-and-re-education-of-ukraines-children/

12 Child Labor and Its Impact on Education

12.1 Introduction: What Is Child Labor?

Hundreds of millions of children today work outside of the home, representing approximately 17% of the world's children (International Labor Organization [ILO], 2015). There is substantial heterogeneity in their experiences, though. Some types of employment have the potential to be beneficial to development, such as part-time jobs on the weekends or during school breaks. These activities can help build young people's sense of agency, provide them with skills that will help them in future education and employment, and cover some of their costs of living. In fact, one study based in Boston with primarily teenagers from lower-earning families found that students assigned by lottery to engage in supervised summer employment were more likely to graduate on time, develop mentorship relationships, have essential work skills (e.g., asking for help, managing emotions, and keeping a schedule), and even contribute to college savings accounts (Modestino & Paulsen, 2023). Critically, this work promotes healthy development because it is appropriate for children—that is, it is safe; tailored to their age level; offers scaffolding of skills; and does not interfere with critical developmental tasks like education, sleep, or time with family. Labor like this does not need to be eliminated, but nonetheless requires thoughtful monitoring by families, employers, and policymakers to ensure that it continues to promote healthy development.

As can be seen in Figure 12.1, there is an interrelationship between the economic stability of families and children's access to education. Unfortunately, the forms of labor available to most children can cause serious harm to personal development. These jobs include employment that is exploitative, dangerous, and harms their ability to meet developmental tasks. Unsurprisingly, the prevalence of exploitative child labor is difficult to establish, but reports estimate that between 138 and 160 million children are currently engaged in developmentally inappropriate work (UNICEF, 2025). Of these, an estimated 79 million are working in highly hazardous conditions (ILO, 2021). These jobs need to be eliminated as a matter of urgency. The vast majority of children working in hazardous conditions are employed in the agricultural sector, which is also the most dangerous type of labor for children

DOI: 10.4324/9781003488385-15

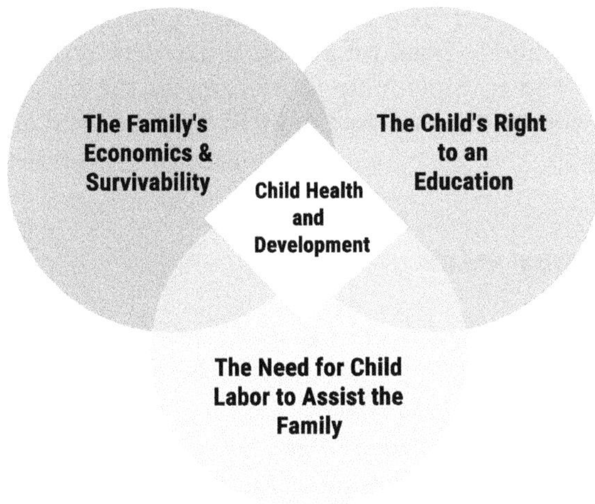

Figure 12.1 Poverty, education, and child labor.

(Dreier et al., 2023). Many others work in mining, construction, manufacturing, and domestic labor.

Child labor is associated with a number of adverse health outcomes, including restricted growth, malnutrition, infectious diseases, and behavioral and emotional disorders (Ibrahim et al., 2018). There is also significant risk of serious injury, including hearing loss, bone fractures, organ damage, and permanent disability (Ambadekar et al., 1999; Hosseinpour et al., 2014). Many others experience chronic conditions like watery eyes, diarrhea, and respiratory diseases. Child labor frequently makes it impossible or very difficult for children to attend school (ILO, 2021).

12.2 Worst Forms of Child Labor

The International Labor Organization (ILO) identifies a few forms of child labor as the most severe and dangerous, representing flagrant and inherent violations of the rights of children that, by definition, harms their safety and development (ILO, C182, 1999). These include forced recruitment for use in armed conflict; slavery and similar circumstances (including trafficking, debt bondage, and compulsory labor); and use in the production of child abuse imagery (sometimes called "child pornography").

12.2.1 Forced and Bonded Child Labor

Parents and caregivers facing extreme poverty may offer the work of a child as collateral on a loan, frequently to afford basic needs like food and healthcare or to finance weddings or funerals. Frequently, a child must work as a result of the debt of an entire family. In fact, bonded labor may be an intergenerational phenomenon: If a parent dies or is unable to work, it may become the responsibility of a child to work off a debt. While debt bondage is banned by international law and by most nations, it is among the most common forms of forced labor worldwide, estimated in 2016 to affect over 21 million people (Bhoola, 2016).

Case Study: Iqbal Masih

Iqbal Masih was born in a Catholic Pakistani family in 1983. His father was a laborer, and his mother worked as a house cleaner. In 1986, one of his older brothers was to marry, but the family lacked the funds to finance the wedding, and banks would not offer the family a loan. Instead, Iqbal was indentured to the owner of a carpet factory as collateral for a loan totaling 600 rupees. He was four years old. Because this was an illegal and informal arrangement, the interest rate was exorbitantly high, and the loan ballooned to 13,000 rupees. Meanwhile, Iqbal was physically abused, starved, and chained to a carpet loom for up to 14 hours at a time. He earned one rupee each day.

When he was 10, Iqbal learned that bonded labor was illegal. He reported his employer to the police, but they returned him to the factory owner for a finder's fee. After escaping a second time, Iqbal attended school and advocated for the rights of other Pakistani children involved in forced labor. He hoped to be a lawyer when he grew up. However, he was assassinated at age 12, on Easter Sunday, by the "carpet mafia," a group that hunted down people who escaped indentured servitude in carpet factories.

12.2.2 Sexual Trafficking

Sexual trafficking of children occurs in all parts of the world, the second largest criminal enterprise globally (after the drug trade) and the fastest growing. Many countries consider trafficking to occur any time that a child is involved in commercial sex, whether or not a third party benefits from their exploitation. Children make up over 25% of those who suffer sexual trafficking worldwide (ILO, 2022). Unfortunately, the internet has opened up many new opportunities for exploitation of children, including through the creation and transmission of online materials depicting the sexual abuse of children (ILO et al., 2022). Unsurprisingly, those most vulnerable to sexual trafficking are people already facing marginalization due to immigration status, race, gender, poverty, and other aspects of their context and identity. For example, in the United States, one of every six children who have run away from home is estimated to have been victimized through sex trafficking (Safe House, 2024).

12.2.3 Forced Recruitment to Combat Roles

Over 105,000 children were found to have participated in armed conflict between 2005 and 2022, though this likely represents an underestimate (UNICEF, 2021). In addition to being forced into combat roles, children may be used in military support roles (cooks, guards, messengers, etc.) and in other highly dangerous roles like human shields, spies, or suicide bombers. Frequently, armed groups perpetrate sexual violence towards children (UN, 2023). In addition to suffering serious injuries or death, children forced into combat roles often live in unsafe circumstances, face frequent exposure to violence, and may be made to engage in substance use. They are also separated from the family and school communities that usually support their development. Unfortunately, these crimes may have become more frequent in recent years.

12.3 Vulnerabilities to Child Labor

Exploitative or hazardous child labor most often arises out of multisystem vulnerabilities in families and communities. At their core, though, the causes of child labor amount to poverty, the breakdown of the systems that usually protect children, and, above all, the exploitation of vulnerabilities by those with more power and resources.

Individual factors can make children more vulnerable to certain types of forced labor. For example, girls are more likely to be compelled to enter domestic work, while boys are more likely to be involved in agricultural and construction work (UNICEF, 2025). Older siblings in some communities are more likely to leave school at an early age to support younger children in the family (Patrinos and Psacharopoulos, 1997). Meanwhile, children with disabilities may already face barriers to accessing education, so they may be more vulnerable to labor exploitation (ILO et al., 2022). In the microsystem, factors like orphanhood and separation from caregivers make children more vulnerable to labor exploitation (ILO et al., 2022). In some cases, cultural factors also contribute, such as a belief that girls' education is less important than boys' education and, therefore, that it may be more acceptable for girls to enter the labor force as children. Further, when families have faced multiple generations of education disruption and economic marginalization, their employment opportunities may be limited, increasing their children's vulnerability to labor exploitation (Jensen & Nielsen, 1997).

As is likely already clear, though, children's vulnerability to labor is best understood as a structural and multisystem phenomenon. Marginalization of people with minoritized social identities, such as Indigenous people and those from ethnic or religious minority groups, spans socio-ecological spheres like culture and economy, such that children from groups that are already subject to marginalization are also more vulnerable to labor exploitation (ILO et al., 2022). This includes individuals and communities with limited legal protections, including those who have low literacy and those with marginalized legal status (e.g., people who are stateless or undocumented). Above all, greed—especially in wealthy nations—results in willingness to ignore or violate human rights across supply chains.

Case Study: *Ruferitos*

Children working on construction sites have six times the mortality rates of children laboring in other sectors. Roofing in particular is the second most dangerous work for child laborers, surpassed only by agriculture (Moskowitz et al., 2021). For this reason, many states and countries prohibit minors from roofing work. However, this is not uncommon labor for children who arrive in the United States as undocumented immigrants. Often starting as young teens or earlier (and as young as elementary school), these youth may scale roofs for up to 12 hours at a time to support relatives locally and abroad. The motives of contractors who hire them are varied; some hope to reduce costs of a project, while others report trying to help out children in need by giving them opportunities to earn money (Dreier et al., 2023).

The consequences for children can be severe. Most, of course, miss out on developmental opportunities like time with friends, extracurriculars, and education. For others, unsafe working environments (including insufficient numbers of harnesses, lack of training, and minimal oversight) leads to permanent injury and death. One youth, Antoni Padilla, began working as a roofer in South Carolina after immigrating alone from Honduras. At age 15, he fell 30 feet and suffered a skull fracture, punctured lung, massive internal bleeding, and severe brain trauma. He was unable to receive rehabilitation care because he did not have health insurance, and the contractors who hired him have not paid his medical bills either.

For many *ruferitos*, multiple intersecting vulnerabilities make them more likely to experience labor exploitation: undocumented status, language barriers, social isolation, poverty. There is also vulnerability inherent in adolescence, of course, as youth are increasingly motivated to contribute, show competence, and take calculated risks, but still depend on adults around them to help them do so safely (Moskowitz et al., 2021). Developmentally and contextually sensitive policies in labor, education, and healthcare should afford additional protections to youth experiencing these compounded vulnerabilities.

Efforts to reduce child labor have stalled after two decades of progress. There are several reasons for this, some of which reflect the multisystem crises described in this book. First, the economic strain resulting from the

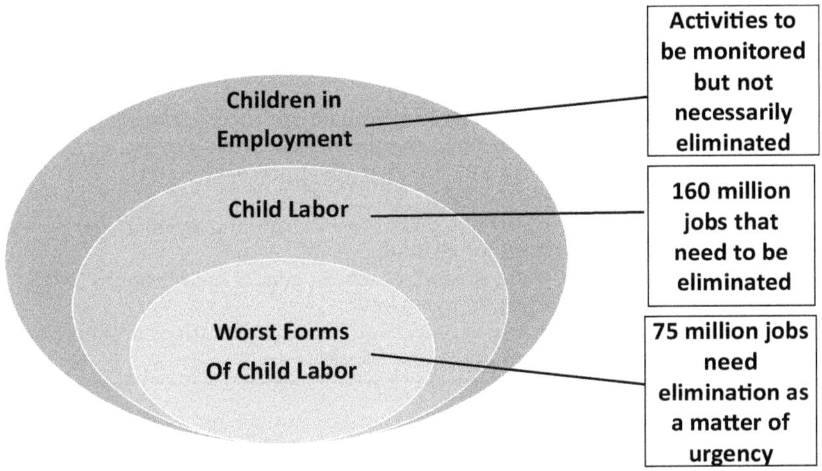

Figure 12.2 Types of child labor.

COVID pandemic, coupled with the breakdown in children's usual support resources, is thought to have plunged many more children into labor (Habib et al., 2024). Escalation and proliferation of armed conflict represents another risk factor (Naufal et al., 2019). Finally, climate change and damage to the environment can also increase family poverty and social inequities, all known risk factors for child labor (Mwendwa et al., 2024). There is a dynamic interplay between a child's right to an education, a family's resources, and pressure for the child to assist the family by working (Brando, 2022; Figure 12.2).

12.4 Advocacy and Legislation

The Universal Declaration of Human Rights was written in 1948. Since then, over 30 international treaties and agreements have established and re-established children's rights to education and to protection from child labor. One of the most important, the UN Convention on the Rights of the Child (CRC, 1989), became a part of international law in 1991. The Convention lays out 39 specific rights of children, including protection from economic exploitation and from engagement in work that could be harmful to their health or interfere with education (Article 32). Health, here, is understood to include optimal physical, mental, spiritual, and social development. In addition, Article 28 of the CRC recognizes "the right of the child to education." The Millennium Development Goals operationalized these rights in 2000 (followed by the 2020 "Sustainable Development Goals," intended to be reached by 2030). For example, these goals expressed the aim of ensuring that all boys and girls worldwide will complete a full course of primary school, and that all children will have access to inclusive, equitable, and high-quality education. UN agencies like the ILO provide guidance to member nations on

Table 12.1 The Dakar Framework for Action Goals (2000), summarized

1. Expand access to quality early childhood education, especially in communities facing multiple vulnerabilities
2. Secure access to free, compulsory, and high-quality primary education for all children, especially girls and people from minoritized ethnic groups, by 2015
3. Provide learning and life skills programs that are appropriate to the needs and abilities of all young people and adults
4. See adult literacy improve by 50% by 2015, for women in particular, and provide basic and continuing education for all adults
5. By 2005, eliminate primary and secondary school gender inequities; by 2015, achieve gender equity in education as a whole
6. Improve educational quality and excellence in accordance with established learning outcomes, especially in math, literacy, and life skills

prioritizing children's educational access and work to establish labor standards that advance social and economic justice (ILO, 1999).

Importantly, while child labor remains too common, several countries have managed to virtually eliminate this violation of children's rights over the course of the last century. Ensuring that adults have diverse economic opportunities (through continuing education, microloans, fair trade practices, etc.) has been a critical part of this effort. Protecting children's access to free education has also been key. In 2000, the United Nations launched the Education for All (EFA) assessment, the largest evaluation of global education access and quality ever conducted. This assessment gave rise to the World Economic Forum's (WEF) Dakar Framework for Action, a set of six goals in the domains of educational excellence and equity (Table 12.1; UNESCO, 2000).

The WEF adopted several strategies to achieve these goals, including generating buy-in from national governments around basic education investments; linking educational goals to economic development strategies; generating civic and community investment in educational goals at the local and national level; enhancing the status of teachers; relying creatively on new technologies; tying education goals to peace strategies; and promoting education systems' resilience to conflict and disaster (UNESCO, 2000).

12.5 Conclusion

The ILO emphasizes that it is the responsibility of member states to "ensure access to free basic education" and protect children from the worst forms of child labor (ILO, 1999). Any work that precludes a child from obtaining an education has adverse long-term impacts on their health and development. Child labor can also itself be a contributor to intergenerational transmission of adversities like poverty, as its damage to children's development and education may exacerbate vulnerabilities in families over time. Multisystem responses to children at risk of labor exploitation can include oversight on worksites, investment in communities' access to education, and awareness campaigns that help consumers to advocate for child-friendly supply chains. Young girls and adolescents in particular may benefit from local campaigns and initiatives to improve their health and nutrition (Parker et al., 2005).

Needless to say, the Millennium Development Goals, Sustainable Development Goals, and Dakar Framework for Action have not yet been realized. In many nations, girls are still much less likely than boys to attend school. Contexts like conflict, environmental degradation, poverty, and discrimination continue to force children's early entry into the labor force. COVID brought much of the progress in educational equity to a standstill. The remainder of the century requires renewed commitment to children's right to a childhood, including education and freedom from exploitation. Part IV of this book—in particular, Chapters 16 (Child Rights), 19 (Advocacy), and 21 (Promoting Peace)—offers tools and frameworks to help adults safeguard children's healthy development amid complex global and local challenges.

Reflection Questions

Question 1. Where is child labor occurring in your own community?
Question 2. Within a community, what can help facilitate a philosophical shift toward prioritizing education over the need for child labor?
Question 3. What factors make it possible for children in your community to attend school instead of working? List as many as you can.

References

Ambadekar, N. N., Wahab, S. N., Zodpey, S. P., & Khandait, D. W. (1999). Effect of child labour on growth of children. *Public Health*, *113*(6), 303–306.

Bhoola, U. (2016). Debt bondage remains the most prevalent form of forced labour worldwide. *United Nations Human Rights*. https://www.ohchr.org/en/press-releases/2016/09/debt-bondage-remains-most-prevalent-form-forced-labour-worldwide-new-un

Brando, N. (2022). Child work and education, a global perspective. In *Handbook of Philosophy of Education* (pp. 209–220). Routledge.

CRC (1989). United Nations General Assembly. Assembly resolution 44/25: Convention on the Rights of the Child, November 20 [cited 2005 July 26].

Dreier, H., McDonald, B., Salazar, N., Correal, A., & Kessler, C. (2023). Children risk their lives building America's roofs. *New York Times*. https://www.nytimes.com/interactive/2023/12/14/us/roofing-children-immigrants.html

Habib, R. R., El Khayat, M., Ghanawi, J., Katrib, R. S., Hneiny, L., & Halwani, D. A. (2024). Child labor and associated risk factors in the wake of the COVID-19 pandemic: A scoping review. *Frontiers in Public Health*, 11, 1240988. https://doi.org/10.3389/fpubh.2023.1240988

Hosseinpour, M., Mohammadzadeh, M., & Atoofi, M. (2014). Work-related injuries with child labor in Iran. *European Journal of Pediatric Surgery*, *24*(01), 117–120.

Ibrahim, A., Abdalla, A. M., Jafer, M., Abdelgadir, J., & de Vries, N. (2018). Child labor and health-a systematic literature review of the impacts of child labor on child's health in low- and middle-income countries. *Journal of Public Health*, *41*, 18–26. https://doi.org/10.1093/pubmed/fdy018

ILO (1999). International Labour Organization. Convention 182: Worst forms of child labour. Convention. https://normlex.ilo.org/dyn/nrmlx_en/f?p=NORMLEXPUB:12100:0::NO::P12100_ILO_CODE:C182

ILO (2015). *World report on child labour 2015: Paving the way to decent work for young people / International Labour Office*. ILO. ISBN 978–92-2–129689-8 (Print); 978–92-2–129690-4. https://ourworldindata.org/child-labor

ILO (2021). International labour office and united nations children's fund, child labour: Global estimates 2020, trends and the road forward, ILO and UNICEF. License: CC BY 4.0. https://www.ilo.org/publications/major-publications/child-labour-global-estimates-2020-trends-and-road-forward

International Labour Organization (ILO), Walk Free, and International Organization for Migration (IOM). (2022). Global estimates of modern slavery: Forced labour and forced marriage. https://www.ilo.org/wcmsp5/groups/public/---ed_norm/---ipec/documents/publication/wcms_854733.pdf

Jensen, P., & Nielsen, H. S. (1997). Child labor or school attendance? Evidence from Zambia. *The Journal of Population Economic, 10*, 407–424.

Modestino, A. S., & Paulsen, R. (2023). Year-round benefits from summer jobs. *Education Next, 23*(4), 1–1.

Moskowitz, A. F., Ramirez, M. R., Ryan, A. D., McGovern, P. M., Schofield, K. E., & Zaidman, B. A. (2021). What are the risks to minors who work in the construction industry? *Journal of occupational and Environmental Medicine, 63*(7), e462–e463. https://doi.org/10.1097/JOM.0000000000002273

Mwendwa, K. A., Aurah, C. M., Atieno Opiyo, R., & Warria, A. (2024). Climate change, environmental stressors, and child labor: The (In) visible links. In *The Palgrave handbook on modern slavery* (pp. 31–51). Palgrave Macmillan.

Naufal, G., Malcolm, M., & Diwakar, V. (2019). Armed conflict and child labor: Evidence from Iraq. *Middle East Development Journal, 11*(2), 236–250. https://doi.org/10.1080/17938120.2019.1672020

Parker, D. L., Leinberger, A., & Oberg, C. N. (2005). Child labor, gender & health. *Public Health Reports, 120*(6), 642–647.

Patrinos, H. A., & Psachropoulos, G. (1997). Family size, schooling, and child labor in Peru—and child labor in Peru—an empirical analysis. *The Journal of Population Economics, 10*, 387–405.

Safe House (2024). Child trafficking-every 2 minutes a child is sold. *Safe House Project*, April 4. https://www.safehouseproject.org/blog/child-trafficking-every-2-minutes-a-child-is-sold/

UN (2004). United Nations Security Council. Children in Armed Conflict. The report of the Secretary-General. June 5.

UNESCO (2000). Dakar framework for action, education for all: Meeting our collective commitments. Conference proceeding adopted by the World Education Forum; 2000 Apr 26–28; Dakar, Senegal. https://www.portal.oas.org/LinkClick.aspx?fileticket=M/7kIZ0taMw%3D

UNICEF (2021). Children recruited by armed forces or armed groups. https://www.unicef.org/protection/children-recruited-by-armed-forces

UNICEF (2025). What is child labor? UNICEF. https://www.unicef.org/protection/child-labour

UNICEF Data (2024). Child labor data. July. https://data.unicef.org/topic/child-protection/child-labour/#:~:text=Main%20indicators&text=UNICEF's%20standard%20indicator%20for%20child,unpaid%20household%20services%20per%20week

13 Technological Innovation

13.1 Introduction

The text to this point has covered features of the 21st-century socio-political landscape that make this period an unprecedented one in which to develop, including increasing political polarization, the expansion of armed conflict in civilian zones, and climate degradation. One obvious additional domain of change is the proliferation of new technologies and the growing access individuals have to these resources. This chapter discusses impacts of technological innovations on children's development and wellbeing. While innovations continue to proliferate in domains like medicine, transportation, and sustainable building design, this chapter predominantly focuses on digital technologies in order to maintain a manageable scope. Due to the rapid pace of change in this area, some of the specific technologies discussed here may be on their way to obsolescence before this volume has left the printer. For this reason, an attempt has been made to address *themes* in technology use and access that will continue to be relevant regardless of particular innovations in question.

13.2 The Promise of Digital Technologies

Every domain of life in the 21st century has been impacted by innovation and expanding access to digital technologies. This section describes some of the sectors in which technology is already being used to create a better world for children and families.

13.2.1 Healthcare

Smartphones and wearable devices are already a part of preventative healthcare for many individuals, allowing users to track health behaviors like diet and physical activity, as well as physiological measures such as blood pressure, blood glucose levels, and heart rate (Ferreira et al., 2021; Sharma et al., 2022). Some researchers and interventionists have begun examining these devices' potential to promote physical activity in children, track mood, and deliver micro-interventions for depression (Creaser et al., 2021; Sequeira et al., 2020).

DOI: 10.4324/9781003488385-16

If distributed with an eye to equity, these technologies can support mobility, health, and longevity for children and the adults who love them.

Electronic health record systems allow providers to review patients' medical history and plan interventions even a thousand miles from that patient's primary care clinic. Thanks to telehealth, families in rural communities or who lack the means to travel for specialty care may participate in services like developmental assessments, sleep tracking, and psychotherapy from their homes.

Meanwhile, digital technologies are expanding global capacity for disease detection and monitoring. A new suite of smartphone-based imaging devices is reducing the need for microscopes in the field, allowing public health teams to scan samples of blood or stool for flatworms or pathogens causing malaria, and even aiding in the diagnosis of conditions like iron-deficiency anemia, sickle cell disease, and certain tumor conditions (Yu et al., 2022). These devices can support care for individuals and communities who face transportation challenges, who live in healthcare deserts, and whose environments otherwise present barriers to care (Banik et al., 2021). For example, there is the potential for large numbers of children in refugee camps to receive fully mobile, same-day diagnosis of parasite-related diseases. Mobile diagnostic technology increasingly benefits from artificial intelligence (AI) software (Molani et al., 2024). Many technologies that once seemed like science fiction are growing more and more accessible in some healthcare settings. The cost of sequencing an individual's genome, for example, declined from $100 million in 2001 to under $1,000 in 2022, and it is declining by the year (Caulfield et al., 2013).

Mental health researchers have identified biomarkers of hypothalamic-pituitary-adrenal (HPA) axis activity that may predict an individual's response to a certain treatment (Klimes-Dougan et al., 2018). One pilot program with college students generates a "personal feedback profile" that, based on personality and behavioral markers with established genetic associations, describes participants' individual-level risks and protective factors around problematic substance use (Dick et al., 2022). As these innovations become less expensive and more accessible, their use could reduce the amount of time and money required for successful treatments, allowing health systems to serve more patients.

Digital technologies also have the potential to help a growing number of young people and families participate in research. Due to structural and historic factors influencing trust in and access to research institutions, many members of marginalized groups are given few viable or appealing opportunities to participate in research, which represents an equity issue (Hodges et al., 2024). Relying on digital technologies may reduce barriers to participating in research. There is the potential for app-based data collection, ecological momentary assessment (EMA), and wearable devices to produce longitudinal and contextually valid findings on young people's life experiences, health behaviors, and emotional wellbeing (Russell & Gajos, 2020). An equity lens is still essential, of course—for example, studies have found that recruiting people for research through social media channels frequently generates under-representative samples (Whitaker et al., 2017), and families with higher socioeconomic status may be more likely to enroll children in technology-assisted research (Kim et al., 2023). This said, thoughtful incorporation of digital strategies into research agendas may help a growing number of diverse youth and families shape their worlds through health research.

13.2.2 Education

During the COVID-19 pandemic, millions of children worldwide relied on internet technologies to access educational material and virtual classrooms. To be sure, there were substantial challenges with implementing distance learning, especially for communities new to this modality (Azhari & Fajri, 2022; Dietrich et al., 2020), with the greatest difficulties felt in groups that faced existing inequities (Oberg et al., 2022). At the same time, the software, resource guides, infrastructure, and best practices guidance that emerged from this period will benefit future students whose schooling is interrupted by disease, political instability, natural disasters, and other challenges. Outside the classroom, supplemental learning supports like virtual tutoring or educational apps may help to narrow achievement gaps among groups facing barriers to educational access (Gortazar et al., 2024).

Child-serving professionals frequently face shortages of time and resources. Educators present a clear example of this dynamic: Those who perceive that their time is scarce experience higher levels of burnout (Skaalvik & Skaalvik, 2020), which is associated with absenteeism, job turnover, lower-quality teacher-student relationships, and reduced learning (Madigan & Kim, 2021; Saloviita & Pakarinen, 2021). Some have proposed that technological solutions may mitigate teacher burnout. For example, generative AI can be used to help teachers complete first drafts of syllabi, lesson plans, slideshows, and exams (Hashem et al., 2024). Of course, biases in AI's source material and inequity in access limit its usefulness in many ways at present, and these technologies cannot replace the wisdom, instincts, and community-responsiveness of experienced professionals (Baidoo-Anu & Ansah, 2023; Celi et al., 2022; Ferrara, 2024). Nonetheless, prudent use of AI has the potential to ease the administrative burdens of child-serving professionals, potentially freeing up their time to engage in direct service and advocacy.

13.2.3 Social Connection

Social support promotes healthy development in both periods of difficulty and relative ease (Masten & Barnes, 2018). Digital spaces can reduce barriers to building and maintaining relationships and, as such, may grow in importance amid challenges like resource scarcity, bereavement, and forced displacement (Finucane et al., 2024). In one study of U.S. adults who earned very low incomes, those with the lowest social support saw the greatest boost in wellbeing when given cell phone access (Read et al., 2022).

People facing identity-related marginalization, such as LGBTQ+ youth, may be particularly likely to find meaningful community online, and even to use these digital spaces to access information about health and wellness issues pertinent to their identity groups (Berger et al., 2022). Meanwhile, young people from religious groups with low representation in a given region can use social media and online communities to connect from afar with others who share their beliefs (Bahfen, 2018).

13.2.4 Potential for Equity

Any technological advance that facilitates human connection can likely be leveraged to promote equitable developmental opportunities. Telehealth technology can be thought of as "promotive" of healthcare access, in that it facilitates care regardless of a person's level of risk. These tools are also "protective," having their greatest impact on health and quality of life for people who face the greatest barriers to accessing care (e.g., those who live in healthcare deserts, have transportation or mobility challenges, have low healthcare literacy, or feel unsafe attending clinics). Digital connection opportunities also promote equity in indirect ways. Interpretation services, for example, are frequently hard to find, especially when service users are members of small language communities in an area or face emergent levels of need. Mobile apps and remote interpretation services can help individuals communicate while they ride in an ambulance or attend parent-teacher conferences (Ji et al., 2021). Meanwhile, hybrid or virtual licensure, supervision, and training programs can accelerate communities' capacity to deliver services (e.g., special education, first aid, and mental health interventions; Rose-Clarke et al., 2020).

People with diverse disabilities and medical conditions have always relied on technologies to support their independence and quality of life while they navigate societies that are not built to reflect their needs. Assistive technologies range from simple (e.g., canes, ramps) to cutting-edge (e.g., neuroprosthetics, artificial organs). Digital technologies across the spectrum of complexity, often made by and for people with disabilities, are useful for building relationships, pursuing vocational goals, and enjoying hobbies (Burgstahler et al., 2011). A growing suite of apps, for example, connects the smartphone cameras of blind and vision-impaired users to volunteers with typical eyesight, supporting users in real time as they check the expiration dates of products, read news articles, sort money, or plan outings with friends over text (Akkara & Kuriakose, 2019; Senjam, 2021). Of course, technological advances are not a substitute for justice or equity—for example, teachers must be aware of the ways that their students using hearing-assistive devices have inequitable experiences of various classroom activities.

A more connected world has the potential to be a more responsible world, and social media is credited with connecting users to causes of importance for child rights (McCabe & Harris, 2021). There are, of course, some limitations to reliance on the internet for social connectivity, given the high potential for "echo chambers" and the chances that activism and advocacy fail to leave the online space. This said, time spent online may help expand the community to which a person feels obligation.

13.3 Potential Harms to Child Development

In general, the regulatory capacity of the adult world has not caught up with young people's access to digital technologies and social media platforms. For example, professional guidelines on children's recommended daily screen time are rarely met in practice (Ponti, 2023). The adverse effects of childhood exposure to screen media are still becoming clear, but a growing body of data already suggests that without proper protections and buffers, children are at risk of both direct and indirect harm as they attempt to navigate the digital world.

13.3.1 Mental Health

Screen time relates bidirectionally to mental health problems and reduced wellbeing in youth (Cai et al., 2023). Some of the same neurobiological mechanisms and risk factors may impact these processes as impact other addictive challenges, such as problematic substance use (Sigman, 2017). In particular, excessive screen time is associated with damage to reward systems in the brain, such as dopaminergic circuits, blunting the natural pleasure response to experiences like social interaction or academic achievement and increasing risk of anhedonia and isolation. Stress regulation capacities may also be impeded (Lissak, 2018).

Social connectedness, one of the most important resilience factors for people of any age, suffers as a result of technology dependence. Youth with excessive screen use frequently show reduced social functioning and are less able to rely on others to cope with life's challenges (Lissak, 2018). They also report inclinations toward escapism (Hamad et al., 2023) and are more likely to feel lonely (Ge et al., 2023). Over time, they may show reduced empathy (Lissak, 2018). Social media use (especially for girls) can harm self-esteem and increase depressed mood (Santos et al., 2023).

Digital devices emit stimulating content, bright lights, and noises that can delay sleep onset or reduce the depth of sleep (Lissak, 2018). Furthermore, media content may increase a child's activation as they try to fall asleep. In fact, the mental health risks associated with problematic screen use are exacerbated in the context of sleep disturbances (Santos et al., 2023).

13.3.2 Delayed Development

By and large, children do not learn efficiently during passive engagement with screen media (Ponti, 2023). When children use screens, they miss out on opportunities to engage in developmentally critical activities like experimentation through play, conversations with adults, and peer interactions. In fact, preschoolers with greater exposure to screen media as infants and toddlers show delays in daily living skills, problem-solving, and verbal communication (Sugiyama et al., 2023; Takahashi et al., 2023). These associations are driven, at least in part, by reductions in the time that children spend outside, with their caregivers, and in exploration. In school-aged children, internet dependence may contribute to reduced academic achievement (Hamad et al., 2023).

Granular cognitive skills can also be damaged through excessive screen use. Some sensory processing skills, such as perceptual-motor integration, may be damaged or delayed (Korcz et al., 2023). Cognitive control appears to also be diminished in people with screen dependence, with impacts felt in domains like emotion regulation and executive functioning (Sigman et al., 2017). In fact, excessive time spent on screens is associated with the emergence and intensification of attentional and impulsivity challenges that resemble attention deficit hyperactivity disorder (ADHD; Lissak, 2018).

13.3.3 Physical Health

Screen use can indirectly impact the body through reduced participation in activities that support physical health, like exercise and social contact. Overall, screen use is associated with more sedentary behavior and reduced motor skills (Felix et al., 2020; Sallis et al., 2020). The use of screens during mealtimes has been associated with poorer nutrition intake and less healthy eating practices (Litterbach et al., 2023); meanwhile, young people who play video games show increases in food consumption over and above their bodies' physiological needs (Chaput et al., 2011). Children with excessive media exposure have increased risks of cholesterol, metabolic, and cardiovascular challenges (Lissak, 2018).

13.4 Equity and Inequity

Social, political, and economic factors consistently moderate the impacts of digital technologies on child development. These relationships can run in at least two directions. First, technological innovations do not reach children evenly, such that those from more advantaged communities or from higher-income countries are most likely to benefit from these resources. Second, "vulnerability amplifies vulnerability," such that those already affected by higher levels of risk and lower levels of resources are most likely to suffer adverse effects in relation to technology access. As technologies advance in the coming century, these themes will likely remain—and, barring structural intervention, accelerate.

13.4.1 Digital Poverty

Even for those who live in areas with cell service infrastructure, costs of devices, internet access, and cellular data are often prohibitive, and access to these resources increasingly predicts a person's ability to receive healthcare (Gonzales et al., 2014). Phone and internet service disconnection can make patients unreachable for scheduling and follow-up care, for example, and at least one study has found that cellphone access is causally related to health outcomes for over the course of seven months for adults experiencing poverty (Read et al., 2022).

Similar patterns occur in education, employment, and access to social welfare programs, where disconnected phone lines or devices that are lost and not yet replaced may interfere with a family's ability to attend healthcare appointments and education-related meetings or apply for services like housing. Digital poverty, as it is sometimes called, may limit families' economic opportunities, prohibiting adults from accessing continuing education and job training materials (Butcher & Curry, 2022; Leidig & Teeuw, 2015). As digital technology becomes more and more central to the functioning of medical, educational, and other social systems, structural gaps in technology access and maintenance will grow more pronounced.

One other domain emerges commonly in the research on digital poverty and its risks: disaster preparedness and response. In the case of rapidly developing crises like active shooter threats or tornado warnings, access to up-to-date safety information may make the difference between life and death. In 2023, as war was escalating in Sudan, two university students in Khartoum turned their car into an unpaid humanitarian taxi service. Responding to distress calls via text messages and WhatsApp, Sami al-Gada and Hassan Tibwa wove through gunfire and artillery in and around the country's capital to rescue at least 60 people, including United Nations workers, diplomats, and teachers (Walsh, 2023). It is no small matter that these students were able to receive these calls in the first place: The volume of data usage during a crisis (as people search for updated information, seek to reunite with loved ones, and coordinate emergency services) frequently strains and slows service (Leidig & Teeuw, 2015).

Access to cell and internet service continues to matter in the post-disaster period. Following crises, psychological support resources may be distributed online as well, such as through digital libraries like the National Child Traumatic Stress Network (NCTSN) resource page (https://www.nctsn.org/resources). Through sites like this, caregivers may learn about signs of traumatic stress in toddlers or preschoolers, the importance of keeping family routines after a tragedy, and asking thoughtful questions about children's feelings.

Case Study: Trinka and Sam

U.S. psychologist Dr. Chandra Ghosh Ippen has helped develop and disseminate innovative therapy modalities for children and families exposed to trauma. In addition, she authors books for caregivers and children to read together, which are intended to support processing, dialogue, and emotional validation in the context of caregiver-child relationships. One book series, *Trinka and Sam*, is about two young mice and their experiences during and after various natural disasters. Following crises around the globe, the team behind *Trinka and Sam* rapidly translates, culturally adapts, prints, and distributes copies of these books for communities affected by natural disasters, partnering with local organizations and often relying on virtual collaboration (Piplo Productions, 2024). As a result, versions of these books are now translated into languages like Spanish, Cebuano, Waray, and Albanian, each dealing with the specific disaster (pandemic, earthquake, hurricane, tornado, or wildfire) that impacted a community. Communities that receive *Trinka and Sam* books report that these resources (and their accompaniments: a guide for parents, a coloring book, and other useful items) facilitate healing and connection within families that helps people process the frightening events and their aftermath.

Of note, the *Trinka and Sam* program has reached communities that, owing to infrastructural factors or post-disaster damage, do not have consistent access to digital resources. The "active ingredient" in the *Trinka and Sam* intervention is a physical book—and, more importantly, the compassionate presence of loved ones who read the story. Groups of children can gather around a single copy of the book, or around overhead transparencies of the story projected onto a wall. Once, donkeys delivered thousands of copies of a *Trinka and Sam* book to children affected by an earthquake in rural, mountainous Nepal.

13.4.2 *Vulnerability to Negative Experiences*

Young children commonly see violent themes and images on television, even small amounts of which can harm the quality and quantity of sleep (Lissak, 2018). Screen exposure to simulated violence has some shared impacts with exposure to real-life violence, increasing the risk that children may later engage in aggressive behavior (Ybarra et al., 2022). In fact, a longitudinal birth cohort study found that exposure to violent media in preschool predicted academic and social functioning at age 12 (Pagani et al., 2023). Several mediating steps are likely implicated in these long-term associations, such as increases in anxiety and depression. Risks are likely enhanced when media portrayals document real-life events with implications for the safety and wellbeing of viewers, as in the case of young Black American men viewing footage of anti-Black community violence (Motley et al., 2020).

The internet plays an ever-expanding role in sexual abuse of children. Several reasons account for this trend. First, perpetrators take advantage of the anonymity of online environments, the reduced vigilance that many users feel in these spaces, and the high likelihood that young people are unmonitored there, especially at nighttime (Hamilton-Giachritsis et al., 2020). Beyond this, there is a risk of child exploitation in any place children are present, and the internet is such a place today. In the United States, young people who spend time online report that strangers and acquaintances alike have nonconsensually shared inappropriate content, pressured them to share sexual content, or shared private images without consent (Finkelhor et al., 2022). Young internet users also report grooming by known adults, solicitation of sexual acts, and commercial exploitation. All in all, 22.5% of U.S. youth report some form of online solicitation in their childhood, with 1.7% reporting commercial exploitation.

Online childhood abuse and exploitation must, of course, be met with fierce public health prevention campaigns and legislative measures (Ali et al., 2023; Hamilton-Giachritsis et al., 2020). Some curricula and training programs have shown success at helping youth identify "red flags" of exploitation, including online, and also reduced the likelihood of young people harming others through these behaviors (Jones et al., 2024). Meanwhile, young people who experience online abuse and exploitation may face blame from themselves and others due to misunderstandings and misinformation (Hamilton-Giachritsis et al., 2020). Mental health needs may also be inadvertently overlooked for young people victimized online (Joleby et al., 2021). Communities can benefit from educational resources that help them to support children and youth harmed in these ways.

Online spaces are increasingly implicated in young people's paths to engaging in violent acts. On large scales, social media has been named as a major driver of genocidal acts, such as the genocide of Rohingya people in Myanmar (Schissler, 2024). Facebook posts calling for "Burmese racial purity" and action against the "Muslim threat" disseminated misinformation and hateful messaging, inciting some of the platform's 20 million users in the country to engage in violence against Rohingya people. In many cases, the government created or shared these posts, with senior military leaders using the platform to encourage others to take direct action to protect the interests of majority ethnic and religious groups (Rapp, 2021). Social media companies and the countries they come from are rarely held accountable for inciting wide-scale violence.

The spread of misinformation and hate speech online is associated with patterns in individual acts of violence as well. During the COVID-19 pandemic, political polarization and conspiracy theories spread on social media spurred an increase in violence toward healthcare workers (Bhatti et al., 2021). In 2024, in the United States, baseless rumors on social media about Haitian immigrants in Springfield, Ohio—repeated and amplified by major candidates for office—incited residents to threaten violence against their Haitian neighbors (Hesson et al., 2024). These threats were sometimes directed at schools, community centers, and places of worship, harming children's access to some of the spaces that can best support their positive development.

Some social media sites have become havens for people to air grievances or frustrations about their social positions; occasionally, sub-communities online incite people to violence, including at schools (Hoffman et al., 2020; Suzor et al., 2019). Youth with vulnerabilities like exposure to discrimination and low social support may themselves be vulnerable to recruitment from extremist or radical groups online (Ellis et al., 2021; Hollewell & Longpré, 2021).

13.4.3 Disproportionate Exposure to Risks: Screen Dependence

Another relationship between inequity and technology can emerge in less advantaged areas within middle- to upper-income countries (e.g., public housing blocks in cities like Madrid or Houston). Here, wealth and resource limitations may actually be associated with higher risks of screen dependence in children. The underlying causes reflect structural adversity in the form of discriminatory policing, childcare deserts, segregationist housing policies, and economic disinvestment, which can all be associated with community disorganization and community violence. While wealthier families and communities may be able to enroll children in extracurricular activities, facilitate playdates, and spend time outdoors together, practical factors like lack of safe public spaces, busy parental work schedules, mistrust of local institutions, and transportation barriers may constrain families' choices of activities. For families facing these structural barriers, it may not feel safe to bring children outside to play (Felix et al., 2020). Organized neighborhood activities may not be available or affordable, and informal childcare networks may be small or difficult to access. Youth in economically marginalized families may be at particular risk for early or excessive screen use, given that non-screen options for entertainment and play are less available. In fact, parents who have had fewer economic and educational opportunities report feeling less confident that they can offer their children entertainment and activities that do not include screens (Sallis et al., 2020).

Finally, adolescents with higher exposure to adverse childhood events are at greater risk of developing problematic screen use habits (Raney et al., 2023). Traumatic stress symptoms can include low mood, social withdrawal, low self-esteem, and increased anxiety, all of which can increase a child's reliance on screens.

13.5 Conclusion

The prologue to this book noted that the creations of the human mind have great potential, both for social good and for social evil—that the same species has designed both penicillin and sarin. This principle is also true in the case of digital technologies. After all, a location-sharing feature on a cellphone may be used for a wide range of purposes: to ensure a teenager's bus makes it safely home from school, to locate a friend in a crowded place, or more nefarious purposes such as stalking. As technology continues to develop rapidly, a set of broad guiding principles may help adults to support the children in their lives.

13.5.1 *Balanced Orientation*

There are two common errors that persist in adults' conversations about children's use of digital technologies, whether around dinner tables or in legislative offices. The first could be described as "reactive alarmism," an instinctive rejection of novel tools without openness to considering their potential for supporting development. The second is, perhaps, a sort of negligence, a failure to reflect on ways that new technologies may be used to amplify or exploit the innate vulnerabilities of children. In many cases, in homes and governments alike, a nuanced perspective is most helpful: an orientation toward technology that combines hopefulness, openness, and vigilance. In other words, adults may ask: What is the best possible fruit of children engaging with this innovation? What is the worst possible outcome?

13.5.2 *Involving Developmentalists*

Decisions about technology access can benefit from the guidance of pediatricians, developmental psychologists, and other advocates for children. Neuroscientists may point to addictive components of cell phone technologies that can exploit developing dopaminergic systems in adolescents' brains. Developmental psychologists may be able to inform the public about ways that online communities can both support a teenager's identity formation through connection with peers, while also allowing others to exploit this process by offering belonging in antisocial groups. Ideally, policies and guidelines for social media sites and other digital resources will be informed by knowledge about the needs and vulnerabilities of children at each stage of development.

13.5.3 *Staged Implementation*

Young people are generally more adept than adults are with new technologies, having grown up as digital natives. In an unregulated and unmonitored digital world, children are likely to be among the first to discover both benefits and risks of every new technology. On an app that allows adults and children to message with each other, a video-sharing platform, or an AI-assisted chat feature, a lot may go wrong for children before adults have discovered these downsides. Families and regulatory bodies may consider setting aside time for developmentalists, child advocates, and other trusted adults to explore new innovations with an eye to developmental opportunities and vulnerabilities before releasing it to younger people.

13.5.4 *Proportional Oversight*

In most areas of life, children receive monitoring and guidance that is proportional to their independent decision-making capacity. If a preschooler hopes to bake, an adult will undoubtedly be involved in every step, whereas

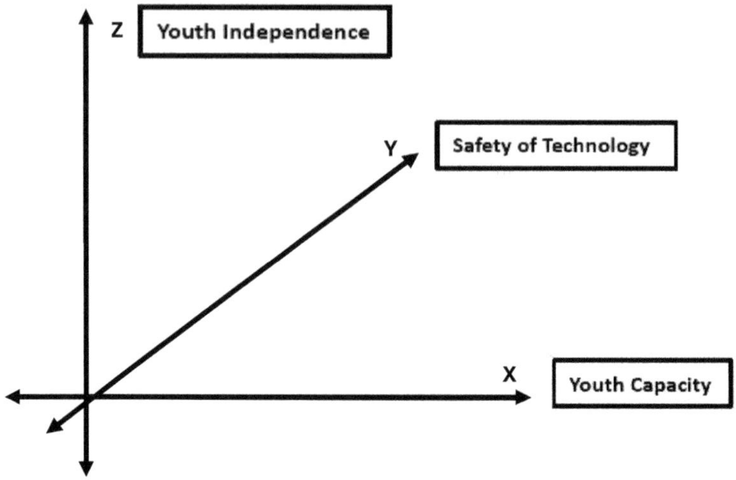

Figure 13.1 Proportional independence for children's digital technology use.

a fourteen-year-old may only need help with driving to the grocery store and purchasing ingredients. Many jurisdictions have implemented graduated drivers' license processes in support of this paradigm. However, adults may have more trouble applying this principle of gradual independence when it comes to digital media use, perhaps because many people think of online spaces as being lower risk than real-life spaces. Adults—whether they work as caregivers, app developers, educators, or regulators—are encouraged to offer children freedom to explore technologies in proportion to two factors: the youth's capacity to make informed and safe decisions, and the risk of adverse outcomes (both the likelihood and severity of harm).

Figure 13.1 shows a three-dimensional graph in which the *x*-axis represents young people's capacity to make informed decisions around technology use, the *y*-axis represents the safety and child-friendliness of the technology, and the *z*-axis represents the amount of independence afforded to youth with regard to the technology.

13.5.5 *Legal Oversight*

As described, digital technologies are often subject to minimal oversight by regulatory bodies. Creativity and innovation can flourish in such spaces of freedom, and there is likely no particular regulatory strategy that should be universally applied to digital tools. Instead, an attention to child rights in the online space can shape adults' decision making. For example, these principles can spur legal and legislative bodies to establish recourse for instances in which children are harmed, directly or indirectly, through exposure to violence or abuse perpetrated online, facilitated through digital means, or incited through the action or inaction of digital media and communication companies.

Such inquiries are rife with legal complications and challenges. At the same time, online spaces are not, in the end, vastly different from schools, parks, playgrounds, or town halls; all are places where child development can be either harmed or hindered, and all are places where responsible adults have obligations to foster children's health.

13.5.6 Equity

In many ways, technological innovations can act as equalizers, allowing people in healthcare deserts to access needed services through telehealth or building caring communities among youth with minoritized identities. In other ways, the benefits and risks of technological innovations are unevenly distributed. Online abuse can be particularly likely and damaging for youth whose caregivers lack the language skills or bandwidth to engage in co-use of technologies. Radicalization to extremist violence is most probable when young people have experienced early–life adversity. Meanwhile, youth from wealthier families with more educational resources often have an easier time connecting to effective digital resources that promote their learning.

Those who develop and disseminate technologies are encouraged to apply equity lenses. In other words, when one is considering the best and worst possible outcomes of a new technology, one must also ask *for whom* each outcome is the most likely. The result is a world in which new technological innovations reduce children's barriers to thriving and increase their connections to developmental resources.

Reflection Questions

Question 1. What are two positive impacts that digital technology had on your development? What are two negative impacts?

Question 2. If you were advising policymakers on how to regulate a new digital technology, what steps would you recommend they take to protect children's wellbeing?

Question 3. Think of six factors that could help protect young people from developing problematic screen dependence. Try to name factors across individual, family, and structural levels.

References

Akkara, J. D., & Kuriakose, A. (2019). Smartphone apps for visually impaired persons. *Kerala Journal of Ophthalmology*, *31*(3), 242. https://doi.org/10.4103/kjo.kjo_81_19

Ali, S., Haykal, H. A., & Youssef, E. Y. M. (2023). Child sexual abuse and the internet—A systematic review. *Human Arenas*, *6*(2), 404–421. https://doi.org/10.1007/s42087-021-00228-9

Azhari, B., & Fajri, I. (2022). Distance learning during the COVID-19 pandemic: School closure in Indonesia. *International Journal of Mathematical Education in Science and Technology*, *53*(7), 1934–1954. https://doi.org/10.1080/0020739X.2021.1875072

Bahfen, N. (2018). The individual and the ummah: The use of social media by Muslim minority communities in Australia and the United States. *Journal of Muslim Minority Affairs*, *38*(1), 119–131. https://doi.org/10.1080/13602004.2018.1434939

Baidoo-anu, D., & Ansah, L. O. (2023). Education in the era of generative artificial intelligence (AI): Understanding the potential benefits of ChatGPT in promoting teaching and learning. *Journal of AI*, *7*(1), Article 1. https://doi.org/10.61969/jai.1337500

Banik, S., Melanthota, S. K., Arbaaz, Vaz, J. M., Kadambalithaya, V. M., Hussain, I., Dutta, S., & Mazumder, N. (2021). Recent trends in smartphone-based detection for biomedical applications: A review. *Analytical and Bioanalytical Chemistry*, *413*(9), 2389–2406. https://doi.org/10.1007/s00216-021-03184-z

Berger, M. N., Taba, M., Marino, J. L., Lim, M. S. C., & Skinner, S. R. (2022). Social media use and health and well-being of lesbian, gay, bisexual, transgender, and queer youth: Systematic review. *Journal of Medical Internet Research*, *24*(9), e38449. https://doi.org/10.2196/38449

Bhatti, O. A., Rauf, H., Aziz, N., Martins, R. S., & Khan, J. A. (2021). Violence against healthcare workers during the COVID-19 pandemic: A review of incidents from a lower-middle-income country. *Annals of Global Health*, *87*(1), 41. https://doi.org/10.5334/aogh.3203

Burgstahler, S., Comden, D., Lee, S.-M., Arnold, A., & Brown, K. (2011). Computer and cell phone access for individuals with mobility impairments: An overview and case studies. *NeuroRehabilitation*, *28*(3), 183–197. https://doi.org/10.3233/NRE-2011-0648

Butcher, J., & Curry, G. (2022). Digital poverty as a barrier to access. *Widening Participation and Lifelong Learning*, *24*(2), 180–194. https://doi.org/10.5456/WPLL.24.2.180

Caulfield, T., Evans, J., McGuire A., McCabe, C., Bubela, T., Cook-Deegan, R., Fishman, J., Hogarth, S., Miller, F. A., Ravitsky, V., Biesecker, B., Borry, P., Cho, M. K., Carroll, J. C., Etchegary, H., Joly, Y., Kato, K., Lee, S. S., Rothenberg, K., Sankar, P., Szego, M. J., Ossorio, P., Pullman, D., Rousseau, F., Ungar, W. J., Wilson, B. (2013). Reflections on the cost of "low-cost" whole genome sequencing: Framing the health policy debate. *PLoS Biology*, *11*(11), e1001699, 2013-11-05. https://journals.plos.org/plosbiology/article?id=10.1371/journal.pbio.1001699

Cai, Z., Mao, P., Wang, Z., Wang, D., He, J., & Fan, X. (2023). Associations between problematic internet use and mental health outcomes of students: A meta-analytic review. *Adolescent Research Review*, *8*(1), 45–62. https://doi.org/10.1007/s40894-022-00201-9

Celi, L. A., Cellini, J., Charpignon, M.-L., Dee, E. C., Dernoncourt, F., Eber, R., Mitchell, W. G., Moukheiber, L., Schirmer, J., Situ, J., Paguio, J., Park, J., Wawira, J. G., Yao, S., & Data, for M. C. (2022). Sources of bias in artificial intelligence that perpetuate healthcare disparities—A global review. *PLOS Digital Health*, *1*(3), e0000022. https://doi.org/10.1371/journal.pdig.0000022

Chaput, J.-P., Visby, T., Nyby, S., Klingenberg, L., Gregersen, N. T., Tremblay, A., Astrup, A., & Sjödin, A. (2011). Video game playing increases food intake in adolescents: A randomized crossover study. *The American Journal of Clinical Nutrition*, *93*(6), 1196–1203. https://doi.org/10.3945/ajcn.110.008680

Creaser, A. V., Clemes, S. A., Costa, S., Hall, J., Ridgers, N. D., Barber, S. E., & Bingham, D. D. (2021). The acceptability, feasibility, and effectiveness of wearable activity trackers for increasing physical activity in children and adolescents: A systematic review. *International Journal of Environmental Research and Public Health, 18*(12), 6211. https://doi.org/10.3390/ijerph18126211

Dick, D. M., Saunders, T., Balcke, E., Driver, M. N., Neale, Z., Vassileva, J., & Langberg, J. M. (2022). Genetically influenced externalizing and internalizing risk pathways as novel prevention targets. *Psychology of Addictive Behaviors: Journal of the Society of Psychologists in Addictive Behaviors, 36*(6), 595–606. https://doi.org/10.1037/adb0000759

Dietrich, N., Kentheswaran, K., Ahmadi, A., Teychené, J., Bessière, Y., Alfenore, S., Stéphanie Laborie, S., Bastou, D., Loubière, K., Guigui, C., Sperandio, M., Barna, Paul, E., Cabassud, C., Liné, A., Hébrard, G., & Hébrard, G. (2020). Attempts, successes, and failures of distance learning in the time of COVID-19. *Journal of Chemical Education, 97*(9), 2448–2457.

Ellis, B. H., Miller, A. B., Sideridis, G., Frounfelker, R., Miconi, D., Abdi, S., Aw-Osman, F., & Rousseau, C. (2021). Risk and protective factors associated with support of violent radicalization: Variations by geographic location. *International Journal of Public Health, 66*, 617053. https://doi.org/10.3389/ijph.2021.617053

Felix, E., Silva, V., Caetano, M., Ribeiro, M. V. V., Fidalgo, T. M., Rosa Neto, F., Sanchez, Z. M., Surkan, P. J., Martins, S. S., & Caetano, S. C. (2020). Excessive screen media use in preschoolers is associated with poor motor skills. *Cyberpsychology, Behavior, and Social Networking, 23*(6), 418–425. https://doi.org/10.1089/cyber.2019.0238

Ferrara, E. (2024). Fairness and bias in artificial intelligence: A brief survey of sources, impacts, and mitigation strategies. *Science, 6*(1), Article 1. https://doi.org/10.3390/sci6010003

Ferreira, J. J., Fernandes, C. I., Rammal, H. G., & Veiga, P. M. (2021). Wearable technology and consumer interaction: A systematic review and research agenda. *Computers in Human Behavior, 118*, 106710. https://doi.org/10.1016/j.chb.2021.106710

Finkelhor, D., Turner, H., & Colburn, D. (2022). Prevalence of online sexual offenses against children in the US. *JAMA Network Open, 5*(10), e2234471. https://doi.org/10.1001/jamanetworkopen.2022.34471

Finucane, A., Canny, A., Mair, A. P. A., Harrop, E., Selman, L. E., Swash, B., Wakefield, D., & Gillanders, D. (2024). A rapid review of the evidence for online interventions for bereavement support. *Palliative Medicine*, 02692163241285101. https://doi.org/10.1177/02692163241285101

Ge, M.-W., Hu, F.-H., Jia, Y.-J., Tang, W., Zhang, W.-Q., Zhao, D.-Y., Shen, W.-Q., & Chen, H.-L. (2023). The relationship between loneliness and internet or smartphone addiction among adolescents: A systematic review and meta-analysis. *Psychological Reports*, 00332941231180119. https://doi.org/10.1177/00332941231180119

Gonzales, A., Ems, L., & Suri, V. (2014). Cell phone disconnection disrupts access to healthcare and health resources: A technology maintenance perspective. *New Media & Society, 18*. https://doi.org/10.1177/1461444814558670

Gortazar, L., Hupkau, C., & Roldán-Monés, A. (2024). Online tutoring works: Experimental evidence from a program with vulnerable children. *Journal of Public Economics, 232*, 105082. https://doi.org/10.1016/j.jpubeco.2024.105082

Hamad, N. I., Eweida, R. S., Rashwan, Z. I., Menessy, R. F. M., & Khaled, A. M. S. (2023). Compulsive digital use among school-age children and association with escapism and feeling of loneliness: A call for action. *Journal of Pediatric Nursing*, *73*, e227–e235. https://doi.org/10.1016/j.pedn.2023.09.015

Hamilton-Giachritsis, C., Hanson, E., Whittle, H., Alves-Costa, F., & Beech, A. (2020). Technology assisted child sexual abuse in the UK: Young people's views on the impact of online sexual abuse. *Children and Youth Services Review*, *119*, 105451. https://doi.org/10.1016/j.childyouth.2020.105451

Hashem, R., Ali, N., El Zein, F., Fidalgo, P., & Khurma, O. A. (2024). AI to the rescue: Exploring the potential of ChatGPT as a teacher ally for workload relief and burnout prevention. *Research & Practice in Technology Enhanced Learning*, *19*, 1–26. https://doi.org/10.58459/rptel.2024.19023

Hesson, T., Sullivan, A., & Borter, G. (2024). *Haitian Americans fear for their safety after Trump repeats false claims about immigrants and pets | Reuters*. Reuters, September 13. https://www.reuters.com/world/us/haitian-americans-fear-their-safety-after-trump-repeats-false-claims-about-2024-09-11/

Hodges, H. R., Gillespie, S. C., Cherubini, F. D. S., Ibrahim, S. A., Gibson, H., Ali Daad, A. M., Davis, S. L., Abdi, S. M., Senesathith, V., Food, Culture, and Health Study Data Collection Team, & Ferguson, G. M. (2024). Ethical applications of digital community-based research with black immigrant and refugee youth and families. *American Psychologist*. https://doi.org/10.1037/amp0001191

Hoffman, B., Ware, J., & Shapiro, E. (2020). Assessing the threat of incel violence. *Studies in Conflict & Terrorism*, *43*(7), 565–587. https://doi.org/10.1080/1057610X.2020.1751459

Hollewell, G. F., & Longpré, N. (2021). Radicalization in the social media era: Understanding the relationship between self-radicalization and the internet. *International Journal of Offender Therapy and Comparative Criminology*, *66*(8), 896–913. https://doi.org/10.1177/0306624X211028771

Ji, X., Chow, E., Abdelhamid, K., Naumova, D., Mate, K. K. V., Bergeron, A., & Lebouché, B. (2021). Utility of mobile technology in medical interpretation: A literature review of current practices. *Patient Education and Counseling*, *104*(9), 2137–2145. https://doi.org/10.1016/j.pec.2021.02.019

Joleby, M., Landström, S., Lunde, C., & Jonsson, L. S. (2021). Experiences and psychological health among children exposed to online child sexual abuse – a mixed methods study of court verdicts. *Psychology, Crime & Law*, *27*(2), 159–181. https://doi.org/10.1080/1068316X.2020.1781120

Jones, L. M., O'Brien, J. E., Colburn, D., McKinney, K., & Martin, L. (2024). Youth attitudes toward commercial sexual exploitation and help-seeking: An analysis of data collected by the not a number trafficking prevention program. *Research in Human Development*, *21*(2–3), 159–178. https://doi.org/10.1080/15427609.2024.2412427

Kim, E. H., Jenness, J. L., Miller, A. B., Halabi, R., de Zambotti, M., Bagot, K. S., Baker, F. C., & Pratap, A. (2023). Association of demographic and socioeconomic indicators with the use of wearable devices among children. *JAMA Network Open*, *6*(3), e235681. https://jamanetwork.com/journals/jamanetworkopen/fullarticle/2802895

Klimes-Dougan, B., Westlund Schreiner, M., Thai, M., Gunlicks-Stoessel, M., Reigstad, K., & Cullen, K. R. (2018). Neural and neuroendocrine predictors of pharmacological treatment response in adolescents with depression: A preliminary study. *Progress in Neuro-Psychopharmacology and Biological Psychiatry*, *81*, 194–202. https://doi.org/10.1016/J.PNPBP.2017.10.015

Korcz, A., Krzysztoszek, J., Bronikowski, M., Łopatka, M., & Bojkowski, Ł. (2023). Associations between physical activity, screen time, sleep time and selected academic skills in 8/9-year-old children. *BMC Public Health*, *23*(1), 1335. https://doi.org/10.1186/s12889-023-16230-5

Leidig, M., & Teeuw, R. M. (2015). Quantifying and mapping global data poverty. *PLOS ONE*, *10*(11), e0142076. https://doi.org/10.1371/journal.pone.0142076

Lissak, G. (2018). Adverse physiological and psychological effects of screen time on children and adolescents: Literature review and case study. *Environmental Research*, *164*, 149–157. https://doi.org/10.1016/j.envres.2018.01.015

Litterbach, E., Laws, R., Zheng, M., Campbell, K. J., & Spence, A. C. (2023). "That's the routine": A qualitative exploration of mealtime screen use in lower educated Australian families with young children. *Appetite*, *180*, 106377. https://doi.org/10.1016/j.appet.2022.106377

Madigan, D. J., & Kim, L. E. (2021). Does teacher burnout affect students? A systematic review of its association with academic achievement and student-reported outcomes. *International Journal of Educational Research*, *105*, 101714. https://doi.org/10.1016/j.ijer.2020.101714

Masten, A. S., & Barnes, A. J. (2018). Resilience in children: Developmental perspectives. *Children*, *5*(7), Article 7. https://doi.org/10.3390/children5070098

McCabe, A., & Harris, K. (2021). Theorizing social media and activism: Where is community development? *Community Development Journal*, *56*(2), 318–337. https://doi.org/10.1093/cdj/bsz024

Molani, A., Pennati, F., Ravazzani, S., Scarpellini, A., Storti, F. M., Vegetali, G., Paganelli, C., & Aliverti, A. (2024). Advances in portable optical microscopy using cloud technologies and artificial intelligence for medical applications. *Sensors*, *24*(20), Article 20. https://doi.org/10.3390/s24206682

Motley, R. O., Jr., Chen, Y.-C., Johnson, C., & Joe, S. (2020). Exposure to community-based violence on social media among black male emerging adults involved with the criminal justice system. *Social Work Research*, *44*(2), 87–97. https://doi.org/10.1093/swr/svaa002

Oberg, C., Hodges, H. R., Gander, S., Nathawad, R., & Cutts, D. (2022). The impact of COVID-19 on children's lives in the United States: Amplified inequities and a just path to recovery. *Current Problems in Pediatric and Adolescent Health Care*, *52*(7), 101181. https://doi.org/10.1016/j.cppeds.2022.101181

Pagani, L. S., Bernard, J., & Fitzpatrick, C. (2023). Prospective associations between preschool exposure to violent televiewing and psychosocial and academic risks in early adolescent boys and girls. *Journal of Developmental & Behavioral Pediatrics*, *44*(1), e1. https://doi.org/10.1097/DBP.0000000000001135

Piplo Productions. (2024). Trinka and Sam in action. *Piplo Productions*. https://piploproductions.com/stories/trinka-and-sam/trinka-and-sam-in-action/

Ponti, M. (2023). Screen time and preschool children: Promoting health and development in a digital world. *Paediatrics & Child Health*, *28*(3), 184–192. https://doi.org/10.1093/pch/pxac125

Raney, J. H., Al-shoaibi, Abubakr. A., Ganson, K. T., Testa, A., Jackson, D. B., Singh, G., Sajjad, O. M., & Nagata, J. M. (2023). Associations between adverse childhood experiences and early adolescent problematic screen use in the United States. *BMC Public Health*, *23*(1), 1213. https://doi.org/10.1186/s12889-023-16111-x

Rapp, K. (2021). Social media and genocide: The case for home state responsibility. *Journal of Human Rights*, *20*(4), 486–502. https://doi.org/10.1080/14754835.2021.1947208

Read, G. L., Yan, H. Y., Anderson, P. B., Partain, L. P. B., Vaughn, Z., Semivolos, A., Kim, Y., & Gonzales, A. L. (2022). Making stability dependable: Stable cellphone access leads to better health outcomes for those experiencing poverty. *Information, Communication & Society*, *25*(14), 2122–2139. https://doi.org/10.1080/1369118X.2021.1928263

Rose-Clarke, K., Pradhan, I., Shrestha, P., B. K., P., Magar, J., Luitel, N. P., Devakumar, D., Rafaeli, A. K., Clougherty, K., Kohrt, B. A., Jordans, M. J. D., & Verdeli, H. (2020). Culturally and developmentally adapting group interpersonal therapy for adolescents with depression in rural Nepal. *BMC Psychology*, *8*(1), Article 1. https://doi.org/10.1186/s40359-020-00452-y

Russell, M. A., & Gajos, J. M. (2020). Annual Research Review: Ecological momentary assessment studies in child psychology and psychiatry. *Journal of Child Psychology and Psychiatry*, *61*(3), 376–394. https://doi.org/10.1111/jcpp.13204

Sallis, J. F., Conway, T. L., Cain, K. L., Geremia, C., Bonilla, E., & Spoon, C. (2020). Electronic devices as correlates of sedentary behavior and screen time among diverse low-income adolescents during the school year and summer time. *Journal of Healthy Eating and Active Living*, *1*(1), 27–40.

Saloviita, T., & Pakarinen, E. (2021). Teacher burnout explained: Teacher-, student-, and organisation-level variables. *Teaching and Teacher Education*, *97*, 103221. https://doi.org/10.1016/j.tate.2020.103221

Santos, R. M. S., Mendes, C. G., Sen Bressani, G. Y., de Alcantara Ventura, S., de Almeida Nogueira, Y. J., de Miranda, D. M., & Romano-Silva, M. A. (2023). The associations between screen time and mental health in adolescents: A systematic review. *BMC Psychology*, *11*(1), 127. https://doi.org/10.1186/s40359-023-01166-7

Schissler, M. (n.d.). Beyond hate speech and misinformation: Facebook and the Rohingya genocide in Myanmar. *Journal of Genocide Research*, 1–26. https://doi.org/10.1080/14623528.2024.2375122

Senjam, S. S. (2021). Smartphones as assistive technology for visual impairment. *Eye*, *35*(8), 2078–2080. https://doi.org/10.1038/s41433-021-01499-w

Sequeira, L., Perrotta, S., LaGrassa, J., Merikangas, K., Kreindler, D., Kundur, D., Courtney, D., Szatmari, P., Battaglia, M., & Strauss, J. (2020). Mobile and wearable technology for monitoring depressive symptoms in children and adolescents: A scoping review. *Journal of Affective Disorders*, *265*, 314–324. https://doi.org/10.1016/j.jad.2019.11.156

Sharma, A., Singh, A., Gupta, V., & Arya, S. (2022). Advancements and future prospects of wearable sensing technology for healthcare applications. *Sensors & Diagnostics*, *1*(3), 387–404. https://doi.org/10.1039/D2SD00005A

Sigman, A. (2017). Screen dependency disorders: A new challenge for child neurology. *Journal of the International Child Neurology Association*, *1*(1). https://doi.org/10.17724/jicna.2017.119

Skaalvik, E. M., & Skaalvik, S. (2020). Teacher burnout: Relations between dimensions of burnout, perceived school context, job satisfaction and motivation for teaching. A longitudinal study. *Teachers and Teaching*, *26*(7–8), 602–616. https://doi.org/10.1080/13540602.2021.1913404

Sugiyama, M., Tsuchiya, K. J., Okubo, Y., Rahman, M. S., Uchiyama, S., Harada, T., Iwabuchi, T., Okumura, A., Nakayasu, C., Amma, Y., Suzuki, H., Takahashi, N.,

Kinsella-Kammerer, B., Nomura, Y., Itoh, H., & Nishimura, T. (2023). Outdoor play as a mitigating factor in the association between screen time for young children and neurodevelopmental outcomes. *JAMA Pediatrics*, *177*(3), 303–310. https://doi.org/10.1001/jamapediatrics.2022.5356

Suzor, N., Dragiewicz, M., Harris, B., Gillett, R., Burgess, J., & Van Geelen, T. (2019). Human rights by design: The responsibilities of social media platforms to address gender-based violence online. *Policy & Internet*, *11*(1), 84–103. https://doi.org/10.1002/poi3.185

Takahashi, I., Obara, T., Ishikuro, M., Murakami, K., Ueno, F., Noda, A., Onuma, T., Shinoda, G., Nishimura, T., Tsuchiya, K. J., & Kuriyama, S. (2023). Screen time at age 1 year and communication and problem-solving developmental delay at 2 and 4 years. *JAMA Pediatrics*, *177*(10), 1039–1046. https://doi.org/10.1001/jamapediatrics.2023.3057

Walsh, D. (2023, May 5). 'Only word for them is heroes': How 2 students rescued dozens in Sudan. *The New York Times*. https://www.nytimes.com/2023/05/05/world/africa/sudan-fighting-evacuations-rescue.html

Whitaker, C., Stevelink, S., & Fear, N. (2017). The use of Facebook in recruiting participants for health research purposes: A systematic review. *Journal of Medical Internet Research*, *19*(8), e290. https://doi.org/10.2196/JMIR.7071

Ybarra, M. L., Mitchell, K. J., & Oppenheim, J. K. (2022). Violent media in childhood and seriously violent behavior in adolescence and young adulthood. *Journal of Adolescent Health*, *71*(3), 285–292. https://doi.org/10.1016/j.jadohealth.2022.03.003

Yu, Z., Li, Y., Geng, D., & Wu, P. (2022). A wide-field microscope utilizing two cellphones for health-care applications. *Journal of Biophotonics*, *15*(2), e202100200. https://doi.org/10.1002/jbio.202100200

14 Indigenous Populations

14.1 Introduction: Overview of Indigenous Peoples

Today's world is globally connected through, among other things, the "Four Ts" of globalization: trade, tourism, technology, and transnationalism (Eales et al., 2020). While the 21st century has brought about changes in the methods and scale of such globalization, the fact of such connection is hardly new. Vast trade networks predate the existence of nations as nations are understood today. Ships and caravans have allowed regions of the world to contact and learn from one another across gulfs of seas and deserts. Unfortunately, when combined with intentions to subjugate, exploit, or expand political and economic reach, the tools and technologies of connection and travel have too often given rise to patterns of colonization, where a foreign power indelibly (and often permanently) exerts cultural, economic, and political control over the people already living in a region. One form of colonization, sometimes called *settler colonialism*, occurs when the foreign power does not simply exert control from a distance but moves its own members to the colonized region in large enough numbers that these newcomers comprise the numerically and culturally dominant group. Together with their descendants, those present before colonization made their group non-dominant are often broadly referred to as *Indigenous*.

People have endured colonization on every continent except Antarctica. The phases of colonization have been described as following a familiar trajectory of exploration, expropriation, appropriation, exploitation and justification (Mengara, 2019), though these stages may happen in any order or concurrently to each other. In the first, colonizing powers assay a land they have not yet entered and declare it to be uninhabited and/or unused (and, by extension, its inhabitants non-human). Next, existing power structures in the land are undermined through force, coercion, or sham treaties. Culture, religion, ecology, and economy are gradually transformed to reflect the image of the colonizing force (e.g., through religious evangelism or schooling practices that replace communities' languages and epistemologies with those of the colonizers). Concurrently, but especially after this stage, human and natural

DOI: 10.4324/9781003488385-17

resources are extracted for the benefit of colonizing forces. Meanwhile, colonizing forces engage in justification (which may be ideological or religious, such as a doctrine like Manifest Destiny or a desire to spread Christianity) to explain the rationale or the necessity of inhabiting and benefiting from the land in this way. At each stage, colonizing practices disrupt and dehumanize the Indigenous populations that they encroach upon, frequently denying their right to exist as they have existed before, or to exist at all. Genocide is not uncommon as a result of colonization.

This chapter will describe the impacts of conflict, climate change, cultural marginalization, and environmental degradation on children and youth in Indigenous communities in the 21st century. As in other chapters, it is difficult to adequately cover these issues and their history in the space of a chapter. Additionally, it is irresponsible to elide variation in the culture and history of the world's distinct Indigenous ethnic groups, which number more than 5,000. For this reason, this chapter attends to vulnerabilities common across many Indigenous groups today, as well as approaches that have promise for promoting the healthy development of children exposed to the stressors of past, present, and ever-present colonization.

Case Study: The Yawanawá Life Plan

The Amazon basin continues to face deforestation and a threat to the Yawanawá traditional ways of life. The Yawanawá communities in the Brazilian Amazon have built a plan to protect their long-term wellbeing. Leaders, including Chief Tashka and Laura Yawanawá, have helped to develop **The Yawanawá Life Plan**, a living document that guarantees the existence of the Yawanawá people on their territory (UNESCO, 2023). It lays frameworks for the adaptation of this community into the future, grounded in their worldview and history, describing roadmaps for strengthening cultural identity, preserving traditions, building a sustainable economy, protecting local environments, and flourishing alongside the forest. This effort has been supported by a collaborative called Forest Trends. A participatory approach was used throughout the creation of this living document, with attention to representation across genders, generations, and villages. One strategy that emerged from this collaboration is a priority project involving the community's participation in the national and global açaí trade. The project team also addressed themes of education, sustainable development, biodiversity, climate change, food insecurity, and gender equality.

14.2 Vulnerabilities of Indigenous Children

By most metrics, in most countries, Indigenous children face stark challenges to their development, challenges that are inherent (and often intentional) parts of the colonial machine. This section describes some of the ways in which colonization can complicate children's completion of developmental tasks and impede their access to developmental resources.

This volume has explored forms of structural violence like racial disparities in housing safety, policies that overlook police brutality, or economic practices that allow child labor to proliferate. Colonization is one such form of structural violence. Because of its pervasive impact on the identities of an entire community, and its interference with the transmission of cultural and familial resources through multiple generations, Indigenous peoples' experiences of settler colonialism are often described using the language of *Historical trauma* (Brave Heart, 1998; Smallwood et al., 2021). The word "historical" here merits special attention. In many other contexts, this word may imply that something has happened in the past and is no longer occurring in the present. In the case of colonization, historical trauma refers to ongoing harms that began with colonization and persist into the present. The term historical trauma has been used to emphasize that even when colonizing processes were ostensibly "over" long ago (for example, with the departure of colonizers, with a nation's independence, or with constitutional and legal victories that enshrine an Indigenous group's sovereignty), many aspects of the damage done to a people group may persist. *Historical trauma* can be said to encompass at least two forms of harm: *presences* and *absences.* The *presences* of historical trauma refer to intrusions of colonial violence into consciousness, including family stories of violence, parenting practices that have been shaped by fear and loss, and the flow of unhealthy nutritional options into a community. The *absences* of historical trauma include experience of lack and loss resulting from colonialism, such as estrangement from cultural protective practices, gradual loss of fluency in the heritage language, unfamiliarity with family stories, and a sense of being cut off from the land and community that could be foundational for one's identity and health. Of course, there is no uniform experience of such traumas; factors like proximity in time and space to the activities of colonization, duration and extent of cultural subjugation, and the continuity of protective factors across generations impact an individual's or group's experience of colonization (Gone et al., 2019).

14.2.1 Colonial Practices of Evasion and Denial

One of the most sinister vulnerabilities that affects Indigenous people worldwide is the tendency for colonizing societies to choose not to see Indigenous people. From the earliest moments of colonization, colonizers' myth of an uninhabited land (or a land inhabited only by individuals characterized as "subhuman") begins to train the eyes of settlers to not see the humans who are there. This selective vision evolves over time: Indigenous people may be driven from the land in advance of new waves of settlement, as occurred during the expansion of the United States across North America, such that settlers could choose not to be reminded of the land's rightful inhabitants. Historical narratives, written by colonizers, conveniently neglect these details or report them with narratives that justify or mask their violence. Frequently, forced assimilation is also responsible for hiding the presence of Indigenous people. The Sámi of northern Scandinavia, for example, were subject to forced assimilation measures by Swedish and Norwegian governments from the 17th century onward and were unable to speak Sámi languages or wear Sámi clothing. Other times, the erasure of Indigenous people occurs through intentional genocide. Well into the 20th century, South Africa's government issued "hunting licenses" allowing European settlers to kill San people for sport. Similar dynamics played out during the United States' frontier era and the Gold Rush. Another type of erasure takes the form of stereotypical and dehumanizing portrayals, such as through "human zoo" exhibits that promoted social Darwinism in the 19th and 20th centuries, or caricature-like depictions of Indigenous people.

As a result of such ongoing processes, many non-Indigenous people have not learned to *see* the presence of Indigenous communities. Some readers may be surprised to hear that Indigenous peoples make up about 6.2% of the world's population, or over 476 million people (Amnesty International, 2024). Figure 14.1 depicts the percentage of countries' land held by Indigenous groups worldwide.

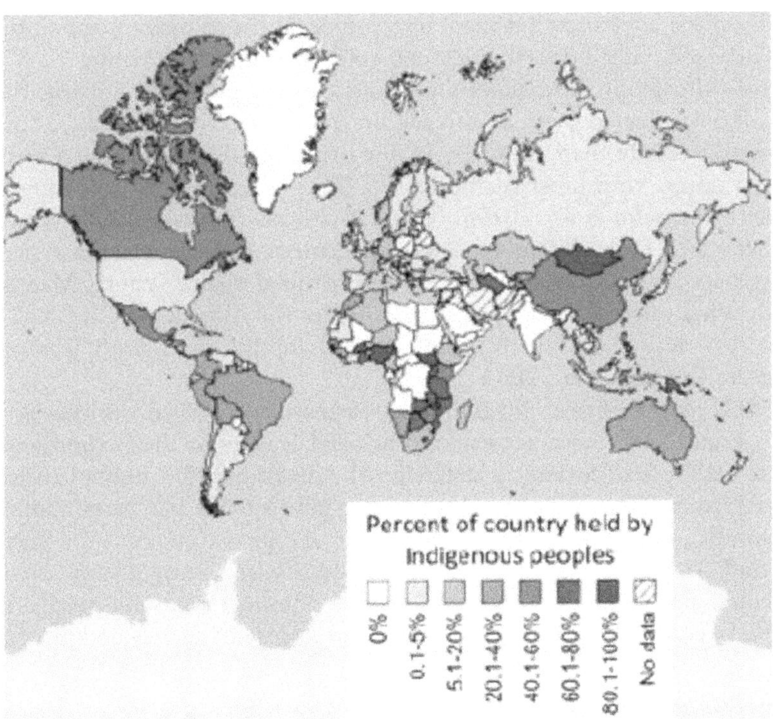

Figure 14.1 Land held by Indigenous populations around the world.

Source: Dubertret F and Wily LA. 2015. Percent of Indigenous and Community Lands. Data file from LandMark: The Global Platform of Indigenous and Community Lands. Available at: http://www.landmarkmap.org

Meanwhile, the tendency for colonial processes to obscure the existence of Indigenous peoples is replicated even in demography: A 2011 analysis of census records from 231 countries and regions found systematic homogenization and undercounting of Indigenous groups (Peters, 2011; Smylie & Firestone, 2015), which can be responsible for shortages in child-serving workforces (e.g., nurses, teachers, and pediatricians).

14.2.2 Legal Vulnerabilities

One of the vulnerabilities that commonly affects Indigenous groups and individuals is lack of legal protection and recourse. Many Indigenous peoples, such as Pygmies of Central Africa, are still denied citizenship in the nations they inhabit. In other cases, citizenship was granted only recently—for example, Aboriginal and Torres Strait Islanders became Australian citizens by referendum in 1967. Frequently, the protections and privileges of citizenship are easier to access in theory than in practice. In Australia's Indigenous communities, many births go unregistered due to a range of structural disparities and cultural practices. Other times, the cost of purchasing birth certificates is prohibitive for families. As a result, Indigenous people may be unable to vote or obtain a driver's license (Gibberd et al., 2016). Their children, unsurprisingly, may suffer as a result, given that they depend on the adults around them to transport them to medical appointments, access new economic opportunities, and voice needs through voting.

Across the globe, Indigenous peoples are barred from realizing the full rights that are due to them as citizens. In the United States, Indigenous people are more likely than members of any other racial group to be a victim of a violent crime, with most such crimes (70%) perpetrated by non-Indigenous people (Monchalin et al., 2019). Native Americans are more likely than peers of other races to be killed by law enforcement officials and to experience adverse outcomes across all sectors of the criminal justice system. Meanwhile, despite being offered special protections under the Affordable Care Act, many Native Americans lack health insurance, and children frequently lack reliable healthcare (Empey et al., 2021).

In 2021, approximately 90 Indigenous activists were killed worldwide (FLD, 2022). Frequently, these activists are beloved leaders in their communities—such as Father Stan Swamy, a defender of Adivasi people's rights in India, or Sandra Liliana Peña Chocué, who was the governor of her Nasa community in Colombia, a mother of two, and a leader of efforts to disrupt the impact of drug trafficking in her community. These deaths frequently go un- or under-prosecuted and have ripple effects on the development of young people, taking from them community mentors, parents, and a sense of agency and justice.

14.2.3 Land-Based Violence

When colonizing powers claim ownership and use of land held by Indigenous peoples, the residents and stewards of the land are often displaced. These new "homes" are likely to be in areas that have few natural resources. Newer analyses suggest that the regions assigned to displaced Indigenous peoples are often more vulnerable to climate shocks and ecological degradation (Farrell et al., 2021). For example, in the United States, Indigenous communities have frequently been displaced to places with lower average precipitation, more extreme heat, and a heightened risk of wildfire. Furthermore, laws around land usage and rights have impeded the relationship between land productivity and community wealth in some Indigenous communities (Leonard et al., 2020). Large industrial projects like mining, logging, and power infrastructure frequently occur close to rural Indigenous communities, where they may introduce health risks (e.g., from chemical runoff and noise pollution; Blåhed & Sebastián, 2021; Lewis et al., 2017).

In addition to introducing new risks to health and safety, displacement and damage to the land separate Indigenous communities from the place-based protective factors that had helped them to thrive before. For example, mining projects in northern Sweden have interfered with Sámi peoples' reindeer herding. This loss has directly impacted adult herders' mental health, and it has also posed a new obstacle to parents, given that herding has historically been a prominent modality for parenting and enculturation of children (Blåhed & Sebastián, 2021). When Co-tu communities in Vietnam were compelled to move their villages elsewhere to make room for hydroelectric dam projects, they faced challenges like longer ripening times for crops (due to lower land fertility), reduced availability of fish (Singer et al., 2015), and some childhood malnutrition attributable to fewer vegetables in the diet. Meanwhile, Co-tu adults hunted less often after the move. With declining income from agriculture, fewer festivals were held. While Co-tu people often showed positive adaptation in response to the move, "social disarticulation" was fairly widespread. Many felt cut off from the sense of community they had enjoyed before displacement. In the United States, some Indigenous commenters have noted that connection to and respect for the land is foundational for children's development of identity and agency, as well as connection to culture, including through attending specific ritual sites and caring for ancestors' burial places.

Disconnection from ancestral lands has implications at the level of identity and health, with implications for mental wellbeing (Walters et al., 2010). The Alaskan island city of Shishmaref, whose residents are primarily Inupiat, is faced with rising coastal erosion and the melting of permafrost that has already damaged the city's infrastructure. The community plans to move to the mainland.

14.3 Health Disparities

Many health conditions are more common in Indigenous communities than in non-Indigenous people residing in the same country (Gilmour et al., 2023). Children in Indigenous communities of Central and South America are disproportionately affected by anemia, with the disease impacting more than 40% of young children in some communities (Rosas-Jiménez et al., 2022). Structurally embedded malnutrition is frequently to blame. An assessment of Indigenous communities in Attappadi, India, found rates of stunting that exceeded 40% in children, and anemia in 91.2% of young children (Jaleel et al., 2023). In Canada and the United States, Indigenous youth develop diabetes and related complications at rates far exceeding those of the general population (Cheran et al., 2023; Lucero & Roubideaux, 2022). Of course, underlying health vulnerabilities impact adults as well as children, rendering them more vulnerable to disease and death. American Indian children were 4.5 times more likely to lose a primary caregiver to COVID-19 than their White counterparts due to the underlying health vulnerabilities caused by economic marginalization, stress, trauma, and disparities in care access (Hillis et al., 2021).

In discussing physical and mental health, it is especially clear that the historical trauma of colonization does its damage through two routes simultaneously (i.e., the *presence* of risks and the *absence* of protective factors). American Indians, for example, face an onslaught of health insults, such as food deserts and "food swamps" (Liddell et al., 2022; Love et al., 2019; O'Connell et al., 2011); the toxic stress of discrimination (Blume et al., 2019); and violence from outside their communities (Monchalin et al., 2019). They are also frequently cut off from traditional health practices that would ordinarily promote wellbeing and reduce the risk of diseases. For example, the Pima people of North America had developed irrigation systems that allowed them to farm fresh vegetables, catch fish, and hunt game in the desert around the Gila River. Settlers in the area gradually diverted water from this irrigation system, such that Pima people have had to eat mostly processed foods; they now have among the highest per capita rates of Type II diabetes in the world, with rates climbing the fastest among young people (Booth et al., 2017). Similarly, mentoring practices are commonly identified as a protective factor for Indigenous youth's mental health (Sanchez et al., 2023), but factors like displacement-related community disconnection and shortened lifespans among elders may make it harder for young Indigenous people to find these relationships.

14.4 Impacts of Historical Trauma on Indigenous Children

As noted, prior to colonization, Indigenous communities have access to a suite of practices, beliefs, and relationships that buffer young people from the effects of stress and also help them to reach developmental milestones. In Yup'ik culture, hunting practices traditionally help adolescents foster relationships with elders, learn problem-solving, and build a sense of collective mastery, all of which are protective against mental health risks like suicide and alcohol misuse (Allen et al., 2018). Across several Indigenous communities in Nigeria, age cohorts are a potent social affiliation; people born within a few years of each other frequently form "clubs" to take on projects together, filling potholes, renovating schools, buying classroom supplies, and covering groceries for one another's families, to the clear benefit of children (Mokomane et al., 2021). At the same time, these highly protective groups are often overlooked in development initiatives.

Prior to European colonization of Aotearoa (New Zealand), Maori culture was known for respect for women and children; transgressions against their spiritual and physical wellbeing were addressed quickly by community leaders (Wilson et al., 2021). The imposition of British culture, which prized the autonomy of nuclear families as decision-making units (as opposed to broader community networks) and did not hold women to be the equals of men, eroded the cultural protective factors that had kept women and children safe from abuse. Today, 57–80% of Maori women have suffered violence in an intimate relationship, with the vast majority having children at home with them during these experiences.

The microsystem comprises the most direct sphere of influence on child development. It has also been, across the globe, a major target of the weapons of colonization. From North America to New Zealand, colonizing governments have forcibly separated children from their families, often through removal to boarding schools or "training homes" designed to force their acculturation to the values of the colonizers (Menzies, 2019). Scholars and practitioners often argue that over time, these practices have lived on in the functioning of child welfare institutions that rely on family separation rather than holistic health as a tool for keeping children safe (Leckey et al., 2022). In Austrlia, Aboriginal and Torres Strait Islander children are eleven times more likely to be placed in out-of-home care than their non-Aboriginal counterparts (Lima et al., 2024).

The grief associated with losing one's child is, of course, a risk to a parent's own health, sense of identity, and agency. Such a separation also challenges children's own development of attachment, self-regulation skills, and identity while disconnecting them from the systems of meaning-making and self-efficacy that would serve to protect their development into the future. Meanwhile, children may miss out on chances to experientially learn the parenting skills that may help them raise healthy children of their own someday (Whitesell et al., 2012). Table 14.1 describes examples of the ways in which the effects of colonization may impact the development of Indigenous children in the present.

Table 14.1 Possible impacts of historical trauma on indigenous children's attainment of developmental competencies

Developmental Task	*"Presence" Risk Factor*	*"Absence" Risk Factor*
Formation of stable family relationships	Parental mental health challenges resulting from structural and intergenerational stressors (Richards et al., 2021)	Separation from nuclear and extended family networks through discriminatory practices like boarding school placement and child removal to foster homes (Gatwiri et al., 2019)

(*Continued*)

Table 14.1 (Continued)

Developmental Task	*"Presence" Risk Factor*	*"Absence" Risk Factor*
Identity development	Challenges to psychosocial functioning resulting from discrimination (e.g., Blume et al., 2019)	Disconnection from physical spaces and land-based practices of historical and cultural significance (Walters et al., 2010)
Development of agency	Harm toward Indigenous community advocates and activists (FLD, 2022)	Diminished opportunities to pursue competence in traditional community roles (Allen et al., 2018; Crooks et al., 2010)
School success	Low expectations from educators based on stereotypes (Uink et al., 2022); bullying (Blume et al., 2019); funding disparities	Lack of assessment of and education in the skills that do matter in a child's context

14.5 Steps Forward for Indigenous Children

Clearly, the world is overdue for concerted actions to protect and promote healthy development among Indigenous children. This goal, while lofty, is attainable. This section describes several approaches that can orient adults' actions.

14.5.1 Truth-telling and Truth-listening

As described above, one of the earliest casualties of colonization is awareness of Indigenous peoples' lived experiences. Historical narratives, cultural mythology, popular media, lack of political representation, and systematic errors in census-level data may perpetuate this damage (Peters, 2011). Indigenous communities around the world have long attempted to teach others about their histories and their present experiences. In 2021, Simon Kofe, the foreign minister of Tuvalu, stood in knee-deep seawater while he told attendees of the United Nations Climate Change Conference about the ways rising ocean levels were already impacting his community.

Another important form of storytelling is the collection, interpretation, and dissemination of data. A lens of Indigenous data sovereignty (IDS) throughout this process can help ensure that research narratives are accurate to, beneficial to, and owned by the Indigenous communities that generate this information (Lovett et al., 2019). The Yawuru people of western Australia, after noticing the ways in which census data failed to capture their community's lived experience (and numbers), have led an effort to collect data that are locally useful, merging assessment processes with community development activities (Taylor et al., 2012). Relatedly, the activity of telling and listening to stories through research, combined with the design of interventions, must involve *local* truths (Morriseau, 2022). For example, it is rarely advisable or possible to generalize solutions from one Indigenous community to another.

Readers are encouraged to seek out Indigenous perspectives on their local histories, as well as information about colonial incursions in their region and the impacts these have today. At the same time, the re-centering of Indigenous stories in popular awareness is not merely an individual endeavor. When communities wish to listen to Indigenous peoples' experiences, this commitment will emerge in their school curricula, political campaigns, funding for public art, program budgets, and more.

14.5.2 Rights-based Approaches

In 2007, the United Nations adopted a Declaration on the Rights of Indigenous Peoples. This document affirmed, among many other principles, the rights of Indigenous peoples to self-determination, freedom from discrimination, and agency in how children are raised (United Nations Office of the High Commissioner for Human Rights, 2007). Of note, four nations (Australia, Canada, New Zealand, and the United States) initially voted against the Declaration but have since endorsed it. See Chapter 17 for more information on child rights orientations.

Many declarations are difficult to enforce. One powerful strategy for increasing the probability of rights being protected is to combine international agreement with international collaboration. For example, in 2023, after Foreign Minister Tofe of Tuvalu's rousing speech in knee-deep seawater, Australia and Tuvalu put in place the Falepili Union, a cooperative agreement that provides Tuvaluans a path to permanent residency in Australia in light of imminent climate displacement. A plan like this is protective of child development, not only mitigating the physical risks that children can suffer as a result of rising sea levels (e.g., drinking unsafe water) but also preventing rushed or chaotic relocation, which can separate communities and even families. Needless to say, though, this relocation will come with the loss of connections to Tuvalu's place-based heritage and history (Farbotko & Lazrus, 2012).

14.5.3 Land and Climate Protection

Effective national and international collaborations around environmental and climate protections are a prerequisite for protecting Indigenous children's development in the 21st century. Indigenous communities contribute the lowest amount globally to emissions—and are often living in the most ecologically critical regions in the world (Ram & Shahzar, 2024)—but are frequently the first to experience the effects of climate change. Three distinct approaches can protect children from the direct and indirect damage of climate degradation.

First, Indigenous communities often have generations of experience managing a given ecosystem. Honoring Indigenous sovereignty in land management can lead to adoption of effective practices like controlled burns, managed fishing, and sustainable farming practices that preserve the health of the ecosystem as a whole (World Bank, 2023; Neubacher, n.d.). Control over collection and management of ecological data is also a critical part of this goal (Olson et al., 2016). Meanwhile, educating Indigenous children and youth about their community's land stewardship practices can leverage the resilience factors of cultural belonging, agency, and intergenerational relationships.

Second, Indigenous communities must have full enfranchisement and legal recourse in light of ongoing damages to their environments. Industrial activities like mining, logging, drilling, and natural gas pipeline installation cause direct and indirect damage to developing children. Families and communities need legal recourse for the activities that impact their environments. Where damage has occurred beyond repair or in ways that imminently harm children's health, community sovereignty and child developmental needs can help to inform child-friendly resettlement plans, bolstered by financial compensation (Singer et al., 2015).

Third, to safeguard the development of Indigenous children, climate change must be halted and reversed. Worldwide, Indigenous people are seven times more likely to face climate-related displacement (Ram & Shahzar, 2024). Local causes of displacement may include droughts, the bursting of glacial lakes, or the salination of groundwater. The underlying cause, though, is almost invariably the shift in global climate due to human activities. Climate justice and Indigenous child rights are inextricably linked.

14.5.4 Keeping Families Together

Implementing supportive services for families during infancy (and even the prenatal period) can reduce the likelihood of out-of-home care for children (Lima et al., 2024). These programs are most likely to be successful when they are led by communities and are informed by knowledge both of trauma related to colonization and also of community strengths. Multidisciplinary teams that center Indigenous leaders' voices are often better equipped to make decisions about what is in the best interest of a child and a family during child welfare cases (Ettinger, 2022). In cases in which children's safety does require a removal from their home, placement with safe relatives (as defined by the community) is an important priority deserving of structural supports that help caregivers navigate housing, healthcare, education, and childcare costs (Burke et al., 2023). In general, prioritizing children's psychological safety and cultural connectedness during out-of-home care is associated with better outcomes (Ettinger, 2022; Gatwiri et al., 2021; Leckey et al., 2022). Some nations have legally asserted the right of Indigenous communities to manage their own child welfare systems, an encouraging trend that responds to both empirical evidence and Indigenous community wisdom about the primacy of cultural and relational assets in development.

It is worth noting that for some Indigenous communities, connection to ancestral lands can be thought of as a family bond. Ongoing estrangement from these lands may be held to pose similar risks to child development and family functioning as, say, estrangement from a close relative. The topic of land return may justifiably be a part of conversations about Indigenous sovereignty in child welfare—that is, the right of a child to be connected to the maximal number of cultural and relational developmental resources.

14.5.5 Health Sovereignty

As described above, many of the health burdens faced by Indigenous communities worldwide emerge through either the *presence* of the toxins of colonization (e.g., the stress of discrimination, parental trauma exposure, and structural disparities in nutrition access) or the *absence* of protective factors that had been a part of their heritage (e.g., close relationships, food sovereignty, and parenting practices). Worldwide, Indigenous communities must have access to the appropriate resources to co-design and co-lead healthcare, public health, and research structures that are most likely to be effective and culturally harmonious in their settings. Such models have already shown success in shaping pandemic responses, mental health interventions, and more (Joseph, 2024; Petrov et al., 2023).

These efforts rely on supportive policy, such as governmental funding allocation practices that promote community sovereignty in health system design and management (Bell et al., 2021). Non-Indigenous parties involved in these systems must also be prepared to act with humility, responsiveness, and community-centeredness at each level—for example, by avoiding pan-Indigenous approaches, advocating for community-prioritized policies, and integrating diverse community voices in planning discussions (Morriseau, 2022).

14.5.6 Restore and Amplify Cultural Connectedness

As argued throughout this book, the resources that promote children's development are diverse and ever-changing as the child grows and contexts change. Indigenous communities have access to a wealth of these protective factors. Caregivers, healthcare professionals, educators, infrastructure developers, and others who serve children must make every effort to amplify children's connection to these resources in their environments. This may include design of culturally centered primary care, mental health, and home-visiting programs (Bell et al., 2021; Whitesell et al., 2012); provision of funding for community spaces (Singer et al., 2015); connecting youth to mentorship programs (Sanchez et al., 2023); infusing cultural values into activities like sports (Bruner et al., 2016); and inviting youth to apply traditional wisdom in arenas as diverse as farming, activism, and science (World Bank, 2023).

In recent years, many regions of the world have seen growth in Indigenous language reclamation movements. These efforts are marked by creativity and commitment to "go where the learners are." Coming from Montana, Christian Parrish Takes His Gun (also known as Supaman) uses the media of rap music and fancy dancing to share Apsáalooke language and culture. He has also founded a hip-hop collective called Rezawrecktion. Children and youth are a particular focus of Supaman's work, and he often hosts performances and conversations at schools. In Taiwan, musicians are increasingly using their art to help young people grow in knowledge and pride about their Indigenous heritage. A growing group of Amis and Paiwan artists, spanning genres like electronic and Indie music, sing in their Indigenous languages and host learning spaces where young people can connect (often for the first time) with their cultural and linguistic histories (Huang, 2022). Readers are encouraged to seek out art that connects them to Indigenous perspectives and experiences in their own regions.

14.5.7 Resilience and Beyond

Resilience lenses (discussed further in Chapter 18) are critical in discussion of and engagement with communities facing marginalization. For Indigenous communities in particular, the concept of resilience is sometimes paired with the assertion of a community's continued presence, even in the face of historical and current forces that would hide their existence. Scholars, beginning with Gerald Vizenor, have used the term "survivance" to describe this orientation and phenomenon. Survivance has been referred to as the manifestation of resilience in the face of historical trauma, and includes continual testimony of a community's existence and knowledge, along with the construction of true narratives about history and identity (Wilbur & Gone, 2023).

Meanwhile, decolonizing orientations can benefit practice and scholarship across fields (Banati, 2024). Such perspectives attempt to amplify community sovereignty and capacity and to engage with individuals and collectives on their own terms. For example, decolonizing research in pediatrics may go from asking, "Why does this Pueblo community persistently show poor management of Type 2 diabetes?" to asking, "How do children and families understand their needs and strengths? What would they change about their environments and practices? What do young people here need in order to build their confidence and capacity in shaping their health experience?"

More discussion of research methodologies and advocacy strategies can be found in Chapters 19 and 20.

Reflection Questions

Question 1. Is colonization impacting child development in your community? How?

Question 2. What are two ways that the traumas of colonization may continue long after colonization? What structural factors make this possible?

Question 3. How would your own areas of work and study change with greater prioritization of Indigenous sovereignty?
Question 4. What are two factors or resources that support healthy development of Indigenous children near you?

References

Allen, J., Rasmus, S. M., Fok, C. C. T., Charles, B., Henry, D., & Qungasvik Team. (2018). Multi-level cultural intervention for the prevention of suicide and alcohol use risk with Alaska Native youth: A nonrandomized comparison of treatment intensity. *Prevention Science*, *19*(2), 174–185.

Amnesty International (2024). Indigenous peoples' rights. Amnesty International. https://www.amnesty.org/en/what-we-do/indigenous-peoples/#:~:text=There%20are%20more%20than%205%2C000,speak%20more%20than%204%2C000%20languages.

Banati, P. (2024). Toward a decolonial developmental science in Asia: Exploring adolescent development in communities from the majority world. *Journal of Research on Adolescence*, *34*(2), 513–516.

Bell, S., Deen, J. F., Fuentes, M., Moore, K., Calac, D., Empey, A., Nadeau, K., Oslki, J., Thierry, J., & Weedn, A. (2021). Caring for American Indian and Alaska Native children and adolescents. *Pediatrics*, *147*(4), e2021050498.

Blåhed, H., & San Sebastián, M. (2021). "If the reindeer die, everything dies": The mental health of a Sámi community exposed to a mining project in Swedish Sápmi. *International Journal of Circumpolar Health*, *80*(1), e1935132.

Blume, A. K., Tehee, M., & Galliher, R. V. (2019). Experiences of discrimination and prejudice among American Indian youth: Links to psychosocial functioning. *Handbook of Children and Prejudice: Integrating Research, Practice, and Policy*, 389–404.

Booth, C., Nourian, M. M., Weaver, S., Gull, B., & Kamimura, A. (2017). Policy and social factors influencing diabetes among Pima Indians in Arizona, USA. *Policy*, *7*(3), 35–39.

Brave Heart, Y. H. M. (1998). The return to the sacred path: Healing the historical trauma and historical unresolved grief response among the Lakota through a psychoeducational group intervention. *Smith College Studies in Social Work*, *68*, 280–30

Bruner, M. W., Hillier, S., Baillie, C. P., Lavallee, L. F., Bruner, B. G., Hare, K., Lovelace, R., & Lévesque, L. (2016). Positive youth development in Aboriginal physical activity and sport: A systematic review. *Adolescent Research Review*, *1*, 257–269.

Burke, S., Bouey, J., Madsen, C., Costello, L., & Schmidt, G. (2023). Supporting indigenous kinship caregivers. *Practice*, *35*(4), 317–333.

Cheran, K., Murthy, C., Bornemann, E. A., Kamma, H. K., Alabbas, M., Elashahab, M., Abid, N., Manaye, S., & Venugopal, S. (2023). The growing epidemic of diabetes among the indigenous population of Canada: A systematic review. *Cureus*, *15*(3), e36173. https://doi.org/10.7759/cureus.36173

Crooks, C. V., Chiodo, D., Thomas, D., & Hughes, R. (2010). Strengths-based programming for First Nations youth in schools: Building engagement through healthy relationships and leadership skills. *International Journal of Mental Health and Addiction*, *8*, 160–173.

Eales, L., Gillespie, S., Eckerstorfer, S., Eltag, E. M., & Ferguson, G. M. (2020). Remote acculturation 101: A primer on research, implications, and illustrations from classrooms around the world. *Online Readings in Psychology and Culture, 8*(1), 13.

Empey, A., Garcia, A., & Bell, S. (2021). American Indian/Alaska native child health and poverty. *Academic Pediatrics, 21*(8S), S134–S139. https://doi.org/10.1016/j.acap.2021.07.026

Ettinger, T. (2022). Indigenous cultural considerations during disclosures of child abuse. *SN Social Sciences, 2*(6), 79.

Farrell, J., Burow, P. B., McConnell, K., Bayham, J., Whyte, K., & Koss, G. (2021). Effects of land dispossession and forced migration on Indigenous peoples in North America. *Science, 374*(6567), eabe4943.

Farbotko, C., & Lazrus, H. (2012). The first climate refugees? Contesting global narratives of climate change in Tuvalu. *Global Environmental Change, 22*(2), 382–390. ISSN 0959–3780, https://doi.org/10.1016/j.gloenvcha.2011.11.014.

FLD (2022). HRD Memorial 2021 Report. Frontline Defenders Global analysis 2021. https://www.frontlinedefenders.org/sites/default/files/hrd_memorial_2021_report_final.pdf

Gatwiri, K., McPherson, L., Parmenter, N., Cameron, N., & Rotumah, D. (2021). Indigenous children and young people in residential care: A systematic scoping review. *Trauma, Violence, & Abuse, 22*(4), 829–842.

Gibberd, A. J., Simpson, J. M., & Eades, S. J. (2016). No official identity: A data linkage study of birth registration of Aboriginal children in Western Australia. *Australian and New Zealand Journal of Public Health, 40*(4), 388–394.

Gilmour, B., Alene, K. A., Atalell, K. A., & Clements, A. C. (2023). The prevalence of HIV infection in minority indigenous populations of the South-East Asia and western pacific regions: A systematic review and meta-analysis. *AIDS and Behavior, 27*(7), 2226–2242.

Gone, J. P., Hartmann, W. E., Pomerville, A., Wendt, D. C., Klem, S. H., & Burrage, R. L. (2019). The impact of historical trauma on health outcomes for indigenous populations in the USA and Canada: A systematic review. *American Psychologist, 74*(1), 20.

Hillis, S. D., Blenkinsop, A., Villaveces, A., Annor, F. B., Liburd, L., Massetti, G. M., Demissie, Z., Mercy, J. A.,Nelson, C. A.,Cluver, L., Flaxman, S., Sherr, L., Donnelly, C. A., Ratmann, O., & Unwin, H. J. T. (2021). COVID-19–associated orphanhood and caregiver death in the United States. *Pediatrics, 148*(6), e2021053760.

Huang, K. (2022). 'We are Indigenous people, not primitive people.': The role of popular music in Indigenous language revitalization in Taiwan. *Current Issues in Language Planning, 24*(4), 440–459. https://doi.org/10.1080/14664208.2022.2145540

Jaleel, A., Arlappa, N., Ramakrishna, K. S., Sunu, P. V., Jayalakshmi, G., Neeraja, G., Narasimhulu, D., Kumar, T. S., & Kumar, S. B. (2023). Examining the triple burden of malnutrition: Insights from a community-based comprehensive nutrition survey among indigenous tribal children (0–19 years) in the western ghats hills of India. *Nutrients, 15*(18), 3995. https://doi.org/10.3390/nu15183995

Joseph, G. (2024). The role of sovereignty in Indigenous community-based health interventions: A qualitative metasynthesis. *American Journal of Community Psychology, 73*(1–2), 216–233.

Leckey, R., Schmieder-Gropen, R., Nnebe, C., & Clouthier, M. (2022). Indigenous parents and child welfare: Mistrust, epistemic injustice, and training. *Social & Legal Studies*, *31*(4), 559–579. https://doi.org/10.1177/09646639211041476

Leonard, B., Parker, D. P., & Anderson, T. L. (2020). Land quality, land rights, and indigenous poverty. *Journal of Development Economics*, *143*, 102435.

Lewis, J., Hoover, J., & MacKenzie, D. (2017). Mining and environmental health disparities in Native American communities. *Current Environmental Health Reports*, *4*, 130–141.

Liddell, J. L., Kington, S. G., & McKinley, C. E. (2022). "You got to drive 30 miles to get an apple": Indigenous food sovereignty, food deserts, and changing subsistence practices in the gulf coast. *SN Social Sciences*, *2*(10), 232.

Lima, F., O'Donnell, M., Gibberd, A. J., Falster, K., Banks, E., Jones, J., … Eades, S. (2024). Aboriginal children placed in out-of-home care: Pathways through the child protection system. *Australian Social Work*, *77*(4), 471–485. https://doi.org/10.1080/0312407X.2024.2326505

Love, C. V., Taniguchi, T. E., Williams, M. B., Noonan, C. J., Wetherill, M. S., Salvatore, A. L., Jacob, J., Cannady, T. J., Standridge, J., Spiegel, J., & Jernigan, V. B. B. (2019). Diabetes and obesity associated with poor food environments in American Indian communities: The Tribal Health and Resilience in Vulnerable Environments (THRIVE) Study. *Current Developments in Nutrition*, *3*, 63–68.

Lovett, R., Lee, V., Kukutai, T., Cormack, D., Rainie, S. C., & Walker, J. (2019). Good data practices for Indigenous data sovereignty and governance. In A. Daly, M. Mann, & K. Devitt (Eds.) *Good data* (pp. 26–36). Institute of Network Cultures.

Lucero, J. E., & Roubideaux, Y. (2022). Advancing diabetes prevention and control in American Indians and Alaska Natives. *Annual Review of Public Health*, *43*(1), 461–475.

Mengara D. M. (2019). Colonial intrusion and stages of colonialism in Chinua Achebe's things fall apart. *African Studies Review*, *62*(4), 31–56. https://doi.org/10.1017/asr.2018.85

Menzies, K. (2019). Forcible separation and assimilation as trauma: The historical and socio-political experiences of Australian Aboriginal people. *Social Work & Society*, *17*(1), 1–18.

Mokomane, Z., Enworo, O. C., & Setambule, T. (2021). The role of Indigenous social protection systems in the sustainable development of contemporary African communities. In *Sustainable development in Africa: Fostering sustainability in one of the world's most promising continents* (pp. 75–89). Springer International Publishing.

Monchalin, L., Marques, O., Reasons, C., & Arora, P. (2019). Homicide and Indigenous peoples in North America: A structural analysis. *Aggression and Violent Behavior*, *46*, 212–218.

Morriseau, T. S. (2022). Determinants of wellness: A perspective on diabetes and indigenous health. *Canadian Journal of Diabetes*, *46*(6), 551–552.

Neubacher, C. (n.d.). Three imperatives for ensuring integration of Indigenous youth. *UN Migration*. https://environmentalmigration.iom.int/blogs/three-imperatives-ensuring-integration-indigenous-youth-when-moving-context-climate-change-environmental-degradation-and-disasters

O'Connell, M., Buchwald, D. S., & Duncan, G. E. (2011). Food access and cost in American Indian communities in Washington State. *Journal of the American Dietetic Association*, *111*(9), 1375–1379.

Olson, R., Hackett, J., & DeRoy, S. (2016). Mapping the digital terrain: Towards Indigenous geographic information and spatial data quality indicators for Indigenous knowledge and traditional land-use data collection. *The Cartographic Journal, 53*(4), 348–355.

Peters, E. (2011). Still invisible: Enumeration of Indigenous peoples in census questionnaires internationally. *Aboriginal Policy Studies, 1*(2), 66–100.

Petrov, A. N., Dorough, D. S., Tiwari, S., Welford, M., Golosov, N., Devlin, M., Degai, T., Ksenofontov, S., & DeGroote, J. (2023). Indigenous health-care sovereignty defines resilience to the COVID-19 pandemic. *The Lancet, 401*(10387), 1478–1480.

Ram, A. L., & Shahzar, E. (2024). Why Indigenous communities face climate displacement challenges. *World Economic Forum.* https://www.weforum.org/stories/2024/02/indigenous-challenges-displacement-climate-change/

Richards, T. N., Schwartz, J. A., & Wright, E. (2021). Examining adverse childhood experiences among Native American persons in a nationally representative sample: Differences among racial/ethnic groups and race/ethnicity-sex dyads. *Child Abuse & Neglect, 111*, 104812.

Rosas-Jiménez, C., Tercan, E., Horstick, O., Igboegwu, E., Dambach, P., Louis, V. R., Winkler, V., & Deckert, A. (2022). Prevalence of anemia among Indigenous children in Latin America: A systematic review. *Revista de saude publica, 56*, 99.

Sanchez, J., Maiden, J., Barton, E., Walters, L., Quinn, D., Jones, N., Doyle, A. K., & Lim, D. (2023). Factors that sustain indigenous youth mentoring programs: A qualitative systematic review. *BMC Public Health, 23*(1), 429.

Singer, J., Hoang, H., & Ochiai, C. (2015). Post-displacement community resilience: Considering the contribution of indigenous skills and cultural capital among ethnic minority Vietnamese. *Asia Pacific Viewpoint, 56*(2), 208–222.

Smallwood, R., Woods, C., & Usher, K. (2021). Understanding the impact of historical trauma due to colonization on the health and well-being of indigenous young peoples. A systematic scoping review. *Journal of Transcultural Nursing, 32*(1). https://doi.org/10.1177/1043659620935955

Smylie, J., & Firestone, M. (2015). Back to the basics: Identifying and addressing underlying challenges in achieving high quality and relevant health statistics for indigenous populations in Canada. *Statistical Journal of the IAOS, 31*(1), 67–87.

Taylor, J, Doran, B., Parriman, M., & Yu, E. (2012). Statistics for community governance: The Yawuru Indigenous population survey of Broome.

Uink, B., Bennett, R., Hill, B., van den Berg, C., & Rolfe, J. (2022). Interrogating relationships between student support initiatives and Indigenous student progression. *NCSEHE project final report. National Centre for Student Equity in Higher Education, Curtin University.*

United Nations Office of the High Commissioner for Human Rights (2007). UN declaration on the rights of indigenous peoples. https://www.ohchr.org/en/indigenous-peoples/un-declaration-rights-indigenous-peoples

Walters, K. L., Beltran, R., Huh, D., & Evans-Campbell, T. (2010). Dis-placement and dis-ease: Land, place, and health among American Indians and Alaska Natives. In Burton, L. M., Kemp, S., Leung, M., & Mathews, S., ed. *Communities, neighborhoods, and health: Expanding the boundaries of place* (pp. 163–199). Springer New York.

Whitesell, N. R., Beals, J., Crow, C. B., Mitchell, C. M., & Novins, D. K. (2012). Epidemiology and etiology of substance use among American Indians and Alaska natives: Risk, protection, and implications for prevention. *The American Journal of Drug and Alcohol Abuse*, *38*(5), 376–382. https://doi.org/10.3109/00952990.2012.694527

Wilbur, R. E., & Gone, J. P. (2023). Beyond resilience: A scoping review of Indigenous survivance in the health literature. *Development and Psychopathology*, 35(5), 1–15.

Wilson, D., Mikahere-Hall, A., Jackson, D., Cootes, K., & Sherwood, J. (2021). Aroha and manaakitanga—That's what it is about: Indigenous women, "love," and interpersonal violence. *Journal of Interpersonal Violence*, *36*(19–20), 9808–9837.

World Bank (2023). Indigenous youth train to save the earth by sharing knowledge. https://www.worldbank.org/en/news/feature/2023/08/07/j-venes-ind-genas-se-capacitan-para-salvar-la-tierra-conectando-saberes

15 Exceptional Children

15.1 Introduction

It is expected that adults help to meet children's needs until children can meet these needs on their own. For example, an infant is expected to be dressed by a caregiver, then to begin conducting more and more of these activities independently through toddlerhood and the preschool years, until she is able to dress without help in the early elementary years. Children, of course, show different rates of developing such skills. Some children may never show mastery of these tasks, either independently or supported, and their needs in the long term differ markedly from the needs of their peers in the same communities. These differences may be due to physical disabilities, intellectual impairments, neurodevelopmental disorders, or serious mental health challenges that may constrain their abilities to navigate their environments, form mutual relationships, and engage in age-expected activities.

The term *exceptional children* serves to emphasize that these children's levels of need distinguish them from the rest of their age cohorts (Schwean & Sakloske, 2010). Just as importantly, this term is a reminder of the incredible *potential* of differently developing children and the particular goodness that can come about when adults build communities that amplify these children's dignity and joy.

15.2 Who Are Exceptional Children?

Most people reading this can recall children they have known, cared for, and loved whose needs differ from those of their peers. Figure 15.1 depicts some domains in which a child may show notable difference from their peers. Importantly, many disabilities and conditions affect multiple spheres of functioning at once.

Developmental differences sometimes result from established biological processes (e.g., a single nucleotide polymorphism, an infection), though the ultimate cause of these processes is often unknown. An increasing number of children worldwide experience complex physical, relational, and psychological needs as a result of acute exposure to adversities like armed conflict or family

DOI: 10.4324/9781003488385-18

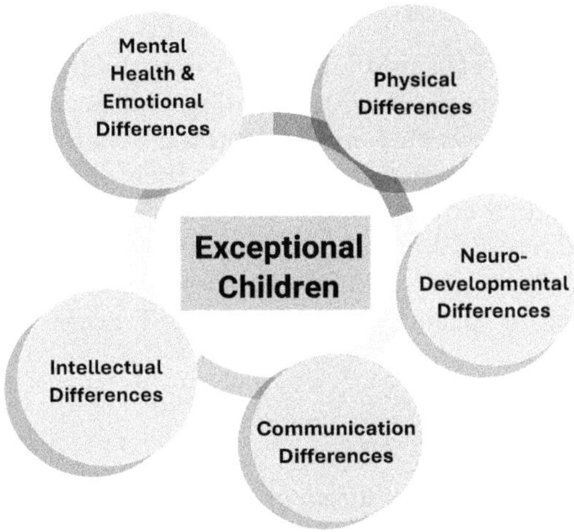

Figure 15.1 Exceptional children.

separation. Still more are impacted by systemic violence, such as the toxin exposure, economic marginalization, and social adversity that, owing to structural racism, disproportionately impact children from minoritized racial and ethnic backgrounds. These exposures can leave children vulnerable to a host of developmental risks and challenges, from asthma to cerebral palsy to maternal and infant mortality (Beech et al., 2021).

15.2.1 *Physical Differences*

Differences in physical development can affect children's mobility and appearance and, as such, are sometimes obvious and visible (e.g., limb differences, or musculoskeletal conditions that require wheelchair use). Other times, these differences can be more subtle to notice (e.g., respiratory conditions and digestive disorders). Unsurprisingly, the way a child navigates a space, from a classroom to a playground, is shaped directly by their physical abilities.

15.2.2 *Neurodevelopmental Differences*

The development of the brain during the prenatal and early childhood periods is incredibly complex, and there are near-infinite ways in which the structures and connectivity of this organ can diverge from expected development. Interruptions of typical neurulation, neural migration, and myelination processes can cause significant disabilities in a developing child. In many cases, as noted above, the root causes of neurodevelopmental differences are unknown. The category of neurodevelopmental disorders is incredibly broad and captures everything from autism to cerebral palsy to numeracy disorders to attention deficit hyperactivity disorder.

15.2.3 *Intellectual Differences*

Due to differences in brain development, some children have substantially more trouble than their peers with retaining and processing information, solving problems, and thinking in the abstract. When a child's intellectual functioning is much lower than expected for their age level, they may have trouble navigating their environments, attaining independence in their activities, and succeeding at school. An estimated 2–3% of a given population is affected by intellectual disabilities. In some cases, these developmental trajectories are tied to specific syndromes (e.g., Trisomy 21 or fetal alcohol spectrum disorder).

15.2.4 *Communication Differences*

Communicating one's needs is a salient developmental task that is actually made up of many sub-tasks, such as learning to produce distinct phonemes, building vocabulary, mastering spoken grammar, mastering writing, and more granular skills, such as self-advocacy or the parsing of pragmatic from semantic meanings. A child may show atypical development in any or all of these skills. Resulting communication disorders are often considered neurodevelopmental disorders and are here given their own section to reflect their unique developmental impacts.

A speech disorder can include challenges with articulation, speech dysfluency (i.e., stutters), and difficulty modulating volume when speaking. Males and monolingual children may be at higher risk for these conditions (Choo et al., 2022). Speech disorders often co-occur with other conditions, such as other neurodevelopmental disorders. Communication is connected to the acquisition of other developmental milestones, such as maintenance of friendships and school success.

15.2.5 *Mental Health and Emotional Differences*

A child's emotional skills, such as self-regulation, empathy, and affective labeling (e.g., knowing whether one is sad, afraid, or angry), are foundational for many other developmental tasks. When these skills are not gained as expected, or are compromised by environmental insults, a child may experience significant developmental disturbance. For example, persistent emotion dysregulation may compromise a child's ability to form stable relationships with others. An inability to enjoy age-expected activities, or high levels of pervasive fears, may lead a child to show behavioral restriction and fail to explore the environment.

15.3 Considerations When Discussing Developmental Differences

In talking about children whose development is following an atypical or unusual path, it is important to remember a few principles. These may help child-serving professionals to consider diverse facets of a child's experience and to attend to the individual in front of them.

15.3.1 Heterogeneity

There is a wide range of functioning in people diagnosed with certain conditions; many people with intellectual disabilities have rich social and occupational lives, for example. Some children who suffer from anxiety are able to thrive academically, while others struggle with attending school or completing homework. Many children who experience spinal cord injuries go on to live independently. A common phrase in developmental and clinical psychology states: "If you have met a person with autism, that means you have met one person with autism." In other words, it is rarely possible to generalize from one person's lived experience to another's, even if both share a diagnostic label.

15.3.2 Chronicity

Frequently, exceptional children will have needs that differ from those of their peers for the rest of their lives. For example, children with significant intellectual disabilities or medical complexities like chronic seizure disorders frequently benefit from coordinated services that span medical, emotional, social and occupational domains (Bigby & Beadle-Brown, 2016; Friedman et al., 2014). In other cases, children's needs differ from those of their peers for a shorter time. When a child breaks her arm, for example, she may need help with tasks like brushing her teeth that she had previously been able to conduct independently. Cancer treatment may last for many months or years and change a child's immune system, but individuals' rates of immune recovery in the years that follow vary substantially (Guilcher et al., 2021). Gastrostomy tubes are placed for long-term (e.g., certain muscular dystrophies) and short-term (e.g., postoperative recovery) purposes alike. In some cases, conditions may fluctuate in severity over time, such as with asthma, depression, or Crohn's disease.

The chronicity of a child's developmental differences may shape the services they receive in several ways. Some support programs consider chronicity a de facto criterion of entry—for example, a school district may offer remote education options only to children who go through a lengthy qualification and evaluation period, and not to children for whom an injury, illness, or recovery period lasts only a few weeks. Caregivers for children whose needs are new or shorter-term may not be familiar with the resources that serve exceptional children, or may not have built skills at changing gastrostomy equipment, administering medication, and connecting with special education services. Conversely, institutional factors like family medical leave policies or insurance premiums may be designed to better support people with shorter-term needs. In other words, the design and delivery of resources to serve exceptional children must be sensitive to varying levels of chronicity and the ways that the duration, permanence, newness, and cyclicality of a child's needs may shape the services they receive and qualify for, as well as their caregivers' experiences providing this type of support.

15.3.3 Disability

Specification of distinct needs need not always be conceptualized as a disability. For example, some children show intellectual capacities that far exceed age-typical levels. In many ways, this difference can support positive development—for example, by opening up opportunities at school and in the community, providing a connection point with adults, supporting the development of good problem-solving skills, and promoting positive self-esteem through competence and the joy of mastery. At the same time, the small body of literature examining children with high intelligence reveals some challenges that can accompany these capacities, such as a fear of underperformance, lower self-worth, and low social acceptance (Cook et al., 2020; Kroesbergen et al., 2016). Additionally, in the face of trauma, children with very high intellectual capacity may face distinct vulnerabilities, such as greater understanding of some of the morally unsettling facets of an experience (Masten, 2025, p. 172). Overall, these children frequently need and deserve resources that differ from those of their peers. Many developmental differences that have been viewed in the past as deficits are increasingly understood to present both distinct support needs and also distinct opportunities. For example, individuals diagnosed with autism spectrum disorder or hearing differences often enjoy high levels of community, belonging, and pride from connections with others who have similar experiences.

Case Study: The Thai Child Development Foundation

The Thai Child Development Foundation (TCDF) is an organization that supports learning and thriving in children with intellectual and developmental disabilities, both through its own specialized Forest School Academy (FSA), and also through collaborations with schools, government agencies, and local leaders across rural Thailand (Thongchan & Gurney, 2021). Some of TCDF's programs include tailored curricula in academics, self-care, communication, and physical health at the FSA; occupational training for older children; home-visiting support; and parent workshops on empowering children with special needs, gender equity, and child safety. Critically, these services are designed for sustainability—for example, they rely on equipping families and communities to meet children's unique needs in the long term through practices like training local women in child development and advocacy. Many children who participate in TCDF's programming return to their local public schools with the support of the organization. As young adults, many enjoy being employed, living independently, and serving their communities through TCDF's sustainable economic initiatives in agriculture, tourism, and hospitality.

15.4 Exceptional Children in Times of Crisis

UNICEF estimates 10% of children worldwide, or roughly 240 million, have a disability. In armed conflicts, children with disabilities face heightened risks (IRRC, 2023), including of human rights violations like sexual violence, use as human shields, and even use as suicide bombers (UNICEF, 2025). A study in West Darfur, Sudan found that children with disabilities fared more poorly than their peers with regard to psychological wellbeing amid protracted conflict (Bakhshi et al., 2018).

A few multisystem factors contribute to the differential vulnerability of exceptional children during crises. First, children may have more difficulty fleeing attacks and reaching safety, as infrastructure damage makes evacuation difficult for those with mobility challenges, and warning systems, like broadcasts or sirens, may be imperceptible to those with vision and hearing impairments. This inability to evacuate can have long-term impacts on physical and mental health and academic outcomes (NCD, 2023). Supply chain issues, destruction of medical facilities, busyness of care providers, and poverty may impede children from accessing essential services and supports. Many experience interruption to education when strained school systems further struggle to serve their special needs. Depending on children's communication abilities and styles, the adults around them may also have trouble grasping how a child's needs are changing in response to the crisis.

Before Russia's 2022 invasion of Ukraine, Ukraine had an estimated 90,000 children living in residential institutions like orphanages—the largest such population in Europe—and nearly half of these children had disabilities. The war separated many of these children from their usual support networks. In fact, families that include a child with disabilities are more likely to be separated during armed conflict, which renders children more vulnerable to future harms (UNICEF, 2022). As a result, many of Ukraine's exceptional children have lost connections to their loved ones in recent years. Furthermore, official evacuation plans often fail to account for individuals with developmental and mobility differences, so children with disabilities frequently face barriers to accessing appropriate shelter, support, and medical resources during and after displacement.

Exceptional children are also particularly vulnerable during extreme weather events. The World Health Organization (WHO) estimates that 35 million people around the world have been displaced because of natural disasters such as floods, earthquakes, hurricanes, or tsunamis. Between 3.5 and 5 million of those displaced in emergency shelters or refugee camps have disabilities, with one third of them being children (WHO, 2011). On the ground, many people with disabilities receive delayed or deficient support with evacuation and provision of basic needs, given that these groups are often overlooked in disaster planning (Harvard, 2023). In addition, severe weather events are contributing to an increase in disability (Kotch et al., 2019). Floods are especially likely to cause injury, disability, and death (Ahmed et al., 2020). Community preparedness is a protective factor from disaster-related injury and impairment, though children and elderly people remain the most vulnerable to harm.

15.5 Promising Approaches

In many cases, a community can reduce the disability that a person experiences by making public spaces more navigable through, for example, wheelchair ramps, sensory-friendly hours in public spaces, or playgrounds that are accessible to all children. Building family agency through workshops, peer mentorship programs, and community liaison services can help adults develop long-term skills to support their exceptional children's unique needs, from medical care to special education systems. Often, children with unique needs benefit when systems of care are built for multisystem coordination across spheres of support. For example, government and non-profit agencies may collaborate to equip therapeutic foster care placements, and school districts may work with healthcare providers to help provide children with assistive communication devices.

It is critical, of course, for crisis response planning to attend to exceptional children's needs, whether in the design of mobile rescue services, temporary housing, emergency healthcare, or daycare spaces in refugee camps. A "universal design approach"—in which accessibility is at the core of planning, rather than added at the end—can improve navigability and usability for all people who enter a space, beyond those with access needs. Finally, exceptional children and the adults who care for them have rich insights about what is helpful to them. As discussed in Chapters 19–21, the voices of people with lived experiences belong at the center of planning for our world's changing needs.

15.6 Conclusion

Exceptional children are particularly vulnerable during and after environmental crises and armed conflicts, given that they may have higher dependence on systems around them, and given that their support needs are not always accounted for in disaster planning. Coordinated, proactive, and multisystem supports (locally, regionally, nationally, and internationally) can help exceptional children to survive and thrive, both during crises and in times of relative stability. Broadly, all children can benefit from the design of structures and spaces that attend to individual developmental differences.

Belief systems around the world emphasize the importance of caring for those with the most vulnerability, and in this light, exceptional children help reveal communities' potential, encouraging adults to work together for the thriving of each individual.

Reflection Questions

Question 1. What are some of the benefits of a lens of "exceptional children" as opposed to simply "children with disabilities"?

Question 2. What have you seen your community doing to help make systems and spaces more navigable for children with developmental differences?

Question 3. How would your community's resources (schools, disaster response, healthcare facilities, etc.) be different if they were designed with the needs of exceptional children in mind?

References

Ahmed, S., Hasan, Md., Z, Pongsiri, M. J., Ahmed, M. W., & Szabo, S. (2020). Effects of extreme weather on injury, disability and death in Bangladesh. *Climate and Development*, *13*(4), 306–317. https://doi.org/10.1080/17565529.2020.1772705

Bakhshi, P., Babulal, G. M., & Trani, J. (2018). Education and disability in a conflict affected context: Are children with disabilities less likely to learn and be protected in Darfur? *World Development*, *106*, 248–259, ISSN 0305-750X. https://doi.org/10.1016/j.worlddev.2018.01.019

Beech, B. M., Ford, C., Thorpe Jr, R. J., Bruce, M. A., & Norris, K. C. (2021). Poverty, racism, and the public health crisis in America. *Frontiers in Public Health*, *9*, 699049.

Bigby, C., & Beadle-Brown, J. (2016). Culture in better group homes for people with intellectual disability at severe levels. *Intellectual and Developmental Disabilities*, *54*(5), 316–331.

Choo, A. L., Smith, S. A., & Li, H. (2022). Prevalence, severity and risk factors for speech disorders in US children: The national survey of children's health. *Journal of Monolingual & Bilingual Speech (JMBS)*, (4)1, 109–126.

Cook, F., Hippmann, D., & Omerovic, E. (2020). The sleep and mental health of gifted children: A prospective, longitudinal, community cohort study. *Gifted and Talented International*, *35*(1), 16–26.

Friedman, S. L., Kalichman, M. A., Council on Children with Disabilities, Norwood Jr, K. W., Adams, R. C., Brei, T., Burke, R. T., Davis, B. E., Houtrow, A., Kuo, D. Z., Levy, S. E., Turchi, R. M., Wiley, S. E. & Murphy, N. A. (2014). Out-of-home placement for children and adolescents with disabilities. *Pediatrics*, *134*(4), 836–846.

Guilcher, G. M., Rivard, L., Huang, J. T., Wright, N. A., Anderson, L., Eissa, H., Pelletier, W., Ramachandran, S., Schechter, T., Shah, A. J., Wong, K. & Chow, E. J. (2021). Immune function in childhood cancer survivors: A Children's oncology group review. *The Lancet Child & Adolescent Health*, *5*(4), 284–294.

Harvard (2023). *Disability in times of climate disaster*. Harvard University Center for the Environment. January 19. https://www.environment.harvard.edu/news/disability-time-climate-disaster

IRRC (2023). At risk and overlooked. Children with disabilities and armed conflict. *International Review of the Red Cross*, *105*(922), 192–216. https://doi.org/10.1017/S181638312200087X

Kotch, L. C., Jill, J., & Rumrill, P. D. (2019). Emerging disabilities that result from or are exacerbated by severe weather events: Implications for rehabilitation counselors. *Rehabilitation Research, Policy and Education. Special Issue on Emerging Disabilities*, *33*(1). https://doi.org/10.1891/2168–6653.33.1.8

Kroesbergen, E. H., van Hooijdonk, M., Van Viersen, S., Middel-Lalleman, M. M., & Reijnders, J. J. (2016). The psychological well-being of early identified gifted children. *Gifted Child Quarterly*, *60*(1), 16–30.

Masten, A. S. (2025). *Ordinary magic: Resilience in development*. Guilford.

National Council on Disabilities (NCD) (2023). The impact of extreme weather events on people with disabilities. May 4. https://www.ncd.gov/assets/uploads/reports/2023/ncd-extreme-weather-2023.pdf

Schwean, V. L., & Saklofske, D. H. (eds.). (2010). *Handbook of psychosocial characteristics of exceptional children*. Kluwer Academic/Plenum Publishers. ISBN 978-1-4419-3309-6.

Thongchan, W. & Gurney, K. (2021). Global Fund for Children. Empowering children with disabilities in Thailand. https://globalfundforchildren.org/story/empowering-children-with-disabilities-in-thailand/

UNICEF (2022). Ukraine ware response: Children with disabilities. June 10. https://www.unicef.org/emergencies/ukraine-war-response-children-disabilities

UNICEF (2025). Protecting children with disabilities during armed conflict. https://www.unicef.org/disabilities/emergencies/armed-conflict#:~:text=Armed%20groups%20have%20been%20known,violence%20soars%20during%20armed%20conflict.

World Health Organization (2011). *World report on disability. 2011*. 24 p. Monography em En | BIGG | ID: biblio–1052751 Geneva, Switzerland.

Part IV

Introduction

Interventions and Solutions

This part of the book highlights approaches, policies, and programs that have the potential to mitigate major developmental risks of the 21st century while promoting children's positive development. The first chapters that follow describe ways of delivering developmental supports to children and their communities. Trauma-informed care (Chapter 16) is one strategy that can inform direct services, as well as the design of systems. The concept of child rights (Chapter 17) may appear abstract at first, but can actually translate into concrete policy design, both within communities and between nations. One such example, discussed in Chapter 17, is UNICEF's Child Friendly Cities Initiative (CFCI). As this book has illustrated so far, a lens of developmental resilience science can help with planning interventions and resources for developing children, and Chapter 18 describes these approaches in more depth.

For adults around the globe to act as an adaptive system, they must maintain awareness and responsiveness to children's changing needs. The book therefore concludes with strategies for listening to children and their communities and responding effectively to what they share. These strategies include ethical, effective research that expands individual and collective agency (Chapter 19); advocacy and activism, including through art and creative expression (Chapters 20 and 21); promoting peace (Chapter 22); and centering young people in ongoing climate justice efforts (Chapter 23).

There is a wide tent for those who hope to support children's futures. A given strategy may resonate with some readers more than with others. All of them can be accessible to people with a wide range of educational backgrounds, disciplines, developmental stages, and governing values; the only requirement is a commitment to work toward a world more honoring for its newest members. As Part IV shows, this work can be hopeful and joyful, even as it is sober-minded. The fruit, of course, makes it all the more worthwhile.

DOI: 10.4324/9781003488385-19

16 Trauma-Informed Care

16.1 Introduction: Principles of Trauma-Informed Care

Public awareness of psychological trauma has grown substantially in the last 60 years, spurred by both clinicians and community advocates, including those associated with women's movements and veterans' movements (Herman, 1992). Once thought of as rare and exceptional, trauma exposure is now understood to be quite common, including among children (Finkelhor et al., 2013). Individual traumas are events or circumstances that are experienced as life-threatening or seriously harmful to one's sense of safety and that have the potential to have lasting adverse impacts on a person's functioning and wellbeing (SAMHSA, 2014). Providers and researchers increasingly acknowledge that trauma does not only result from acute events, but also from chronic circumstances like poverty or the effects of structural racism (McLaughlin et al., 2020). For children, trauma may also take the form of disruption to the caregiving system (e.g., through parental loss or separation), which fundamentally undermines the child's sense of safety (Cohodes et al., 2021; van der Kolk et al., 2019). As discussed elsewhere in this book, scholars and practitioners increasingly acknowledge the impacts of historical and intergenerational trauma on child development, such that even children who are not themselves directly exposed to atrocities like genocide may be affected by them nonetheless, even generations later (Gone et al., 2019; Narayan et al., 2019).

The concept of trauma-informed care (TIC) began to formally coalesce in the 1980s. Unlike many theories of intervention, the core principles of TIC emerged from the observations of clinicians and direct service providers—initially, providers working with adult women who used substances, as well as with individuals experiencing homelessness (Sciolla, 2017). These providers began to share their observations with communities of research and practice. First, they noted that trauma exposure was very common in populations experiencing health needs, approaching 100% in some communities. Second, they observed that systems of care rarely honored the impacts that trauma exposure had on current functioning. Relatedly, people with histories of trauma exposure were often poorly served by healthcare systems; for example, the symptoms they displayed led them to be labeled disruptive in care settings.

DOI: 10.4324/9781003488385-20

Perhaps most pointedly, these clinicians noticed that many practices common in healthcare environments—such as paternalistic healthcare decision-making or assumed comfort with physical touch—resembled events that were traumatizing to care participants. In this way, care environments sometimes acted as sites of retraumatization.

TIC acknowledges the need to consider patients' life experiences in order to deliver effective care. SAMHSA outlines an approach to TIC that incorporates four key elements: (1) realizing the widespread impact of trauma; (2) recognizing how trauma may affect clients, staff, and others in the program, organization, or system; (3) responding by applying knowledge about trauma into practice; and (4) preventing retraumatization (Marsac et al., 2016). The most rudimentary understandings of TIC are *minatory*—that is, providers work to prevent or reduce harm in care settings by, for example, learning to warn patients before they touch them. Just as importantly, though, TIC can be viewed as a *hortatory* ethical framework, one that brings about positive good rather than simply avoiding harm. With this lens, TIC principles and practices can help transform points of care into sites of empowerment that are a part of individuals' and communities' healing journey; that amplify their connection to loved ones and other protective resources; that improve their health literacy and ownership of their own wellbeing practices; and that promote wellness among providers and staff as well (Menschner & Maul, 2016; Raja et al., 2015).

16.2 Trauma-Informed Care for Children Who Are Displaced

Children who flee their homes almost definitionally experience trauma exposure, which can have long-term impacts on health and development. This population's needs present a clear argument for the importance of integrating TIC principles across service sectors, both for individual providers and for systems as a whole.

16.2.1 Emotional and Behavioral Health Conditions Associated with Trauma

Young refugees often suffer from trauma-related sequelae like post-traumatic stress disorder (PTSD), internalizing challenges (anxiety, depression, etc.), and externalizing challenges (hyperactivity, defiance, aggression, etc.; Dangmann, 2022), though these psychological needs often go undetected and untreated (Sanchez-Cao et al., 2012; Spaas et al., 2022). A referral to a therapist who is adept at working with refugee children is optimal. At the same time, forcibly displaced children often have access to high levels of resilience resources that protect their functioning even after significant trauma exposures. Providers serving these children are encouraged to expect both trauma exposure and also resilience.

When families endure displacement, they may experience trauma all along the "Arc of Migration" (Oberg, 2019). This includes trauma from the country of origin (e.g., injuries and loss of loved ones); trauma experienced during migration (e.g., dangerous routes and adversity in refugee camps); and trauma experienced after their arrival in a new country (e.g., exposure to racism or community violence).

Refugee and immigrant children often present with a mixture of symptoms and do not necessarily fulfill a single diagnostic category. For example, a child may present with a mixture of post-traumatic and depressive symptomatology (Fazel & Stein, 2002). For this reason, and due to cultural and individual differences in symptom presentation, broad symptom screeners will sometimes be useful. Of note, it is often more accurate to reference brief measures validated for use in a given cultural community than long measures not yet tested in a family's ethnic or language group (Alemi et al., 2023).

Broadly, trauma screenings with immigrants and refugees are often most effective when they take the form of conversations (rather than forms), when they occur after significant rapport has been built (e.g., well into a visit, or at a follow-up), and when they rely on both cultural humility and competence (e.g., consultations with cultural experts who can provide education on culturally specific signs of traumatic stress; Hodges et al., 2024). Frequently, children and families also benefit from brief psychoeducation, including normalization of the lasting effects of trauma. It is important for care providers to remember that they themselves do not have an inherent right to learn about a person's trauma history.

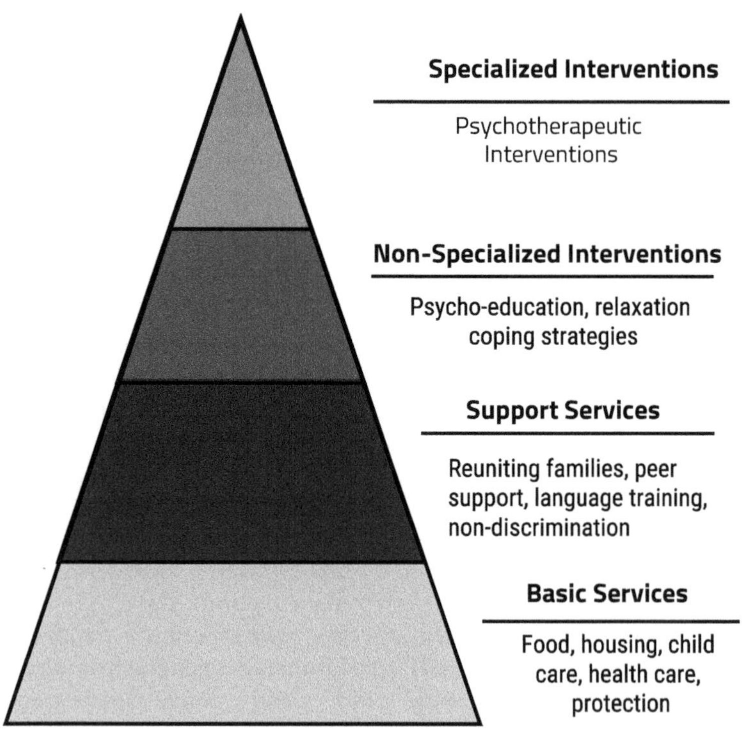

Figure 16.1 Levels of trauma-informed care.

Tiered models can be an important part of TIC for immigrant and refugee children and for others experiencing multisystem stress (Fazel et al., 2014). Figure 16.1 outlines the continuum of care from basic services and security to specialized care for refugee families and their children.

Table 16.1 provides guidance for conducting TIC in the clinical setting with immigrants and refugees, adapted from Miller et al. (2019). Many of these practices generalize well to service with other populations. Providers are encouraged to see all clinical interactions as chances to help build trust with refugee and immigrant clients, support care participants' health literacy, empower families to direct their own healthcare process, and affirm the dignity and agency of care participants, all of which can help to erode some of the effects of trauma (Abdi et al., 2021).

Table 16.1 Trauma-informed care principles with youth who have experienced displacement

Practice a strengths-based approach to care	Children's resilience reflects the functioning of adaptive systems within and around them. Lead social history and/or psychosocial assessment with questions regarding family strengths. ***"Tell me a little bit about yourself. What are some things that you're really proud of?"***
Create an immigrant-friendly healthcare environment	Advocate for safe and inclusive environments, including within your own clinic. **Post welcoming signage in multiple languages. Ensure staff learn norms of body language and communication for the populations they serve.**
Promote trusting relationships within the healthcare environment	Social workers, patient advocates, and support groups can be useful in helping families navigate the new health care system. ***"I know that you have had a difficult journey and now you are entering a new and unfamiliar health system. Would you be interested in talking with our social worker, Fadumo? She helps Somali families connect with new resources."***
Ask for permission to discuss potentially difficult subjects	TIC acknowledges that youth and families can be retraumatized if they are forced to prematurely share information about traumatic events. If there are any signs of fear or anxiety, it is best to follow-up at a different time. ***"I want to make sure that we're giving you the best medical care possible. In order to make sure I understand what you have been through, I would like to ask a few more questions about what has happened on your journey. You don't have to answer, and you can still get care here. Is that okay with you?"***
Recognize the impact of trauma on the developing brain; screen for trauma and associated emotional conditions when appropriate	TIC acknowledges the pervasive impact of trauma, including screening for past experiences of trauma. Mood, anxiety, and behavioral symptoms may reflect traumatic stress. If a family or youth shares stories of trauma, validate their experiences and emotions. ***"These memories sound very frightening. I can imagine that they might make it hard to focus in school or fall asleep at night. Do you notice that at all?"***

(*Continued*)

Table 16.1 (Continued)

Treat trauma-related disorders appropriately	Take time to compassionately discuss with families the relationships between traumatic events and physical/mental health difficulties. In documentation, utilize diagnostic phrasing like *"stress- and trauma-related disorder"* to explain the root causes of symptoms. In the referral and treatment of trauma related mental health disorders, support youth's agency by asking about their treatment preferences. ***"It makes sense that you have trouble feeling safe right now because of what happened to you. Can we think of some strategies together to help you feel safer at school?'"***
Utilize a multi-generational approach to care	Parents, extended family, caregivers, and safe adults outside the family are among the most protective factors for young people's healing after stress and trauma. ***"Who have you relied on or trusted on your journey here?"***
Know your own local resources and make sure they are trustworthy	Partnerships with other individuals and agencies in your area outside of health care can be an invaluable resource for TIC with refugee and immigrant youth. ***"Besides health care, do you have other immediate needs that our team might be able to help you with? Can we refer you to others who may be able to help?"***
Recognize that trauma may not end after migration	Trauma may continue long after migration, including through racism, xenophobia, Islamophobia, and community violence exposure. ***"How is your housing working for you? Does it feel safe and stable?"***
Advocate for your patients in and outside the clinic	Advocacy is a strategy to transform secondary trauma, grief, and anger into action. ***Stay aware of opportunities to use your position and perspectives to advocate for new resources and support for families that have been forcibly displaced.***

Adapted from Miller et al. (2019).

16.3 Effective Treatment Options for Trauma Exposure and PTSD

There are several clinical interventions that are demonstrated to be effective for children and youth experiencing traumatic stress symptoms. Importantly, many are adaptable with regard to their delivery style, setting, and duration. This section presents a few therapies that have shown evidence of effectiveness with refugee youth. Some therapies developed for adults also show preliminary evidence of effectiveness in use with children, including with young refugees and immigrants (e.g., Eye Movement Desensitization and Reprocessing, or EMDR; Ahmad et al., 2007).

16.3.1 Trauma-Focused Cognitive Behavioral Therapy (TF-CBT)

TF-CBT involves a mixture of skill-building (e.g., teaching trauma-sensitive parenting tactics, cognitive reappraisal, and coping skills) and habituation paradigms (e.g., gradual child-led exposure and creation of a trauma narrative), often with a relational lens that works to increase the regulation and support of caregiving relationships (Unterhitzenberger et al., 2015). It has been adapted for use with refugee children, with pilot studies suggesting clinical effectiveness (Chipalo, 2021). For example, a TF-CBT adaptation called My Way or ("Mein Weg" in German) relies on group sessions and incorporates meditation and relaxation practices (Pfeiffer & Goldbeck, 2017). Intervention participants have shown reduced physiological manifestations of stress, startle response, hypervigilance, sleeping and attention problems, and anger dysregulation. Refugee children reported significantly fewer symptoms in the domains of re-experiencing and avoidance, as well as improvements in cognition and mood. Teaching Recovery Techniques (TRT) is another intervention based on TF-CBT in a group setting. This intervention was developed by the Children and War Foundation of Norway. Both PTSD and depression symptoms decreased significantly after TRT (Sarkdadi et al., 2018).

16.3.2 Narrative Exposure Therapy for Children (KIDNET)

KIDNET is a short-term psychotherapeutic approach for the treatment of PTSD in children. It consists of the child and therapist constructing a chronological narrative of the child's exposure to positive and negative life events over the course of 6–10 sessions. Research has demonstrated its success in the treatment of refugee children experiencing PTSD symptoms, with results lasting over a year (Ruf et al., 2010). There is presently a rater-blinded, multi-center, randomized-controlled trial comparing KIDNET to treatment as usual within the German general healthcare system (Wilker et al., 2020).

16.3.3 Trauma Systems Therapy for Refugees (TST-R)

Adapted from Trauma Systems Therapy (TST), TST-R holds that children's trauma-related needs require both individual and environmental intervention, and that the most regulating environments for children exposed to trauma are those that meet physical and emotional safety needs and cultural needs at the same time. In this tiered model, implementers deliver trainings on children's trauma and cultural needs to large numbers of family members or school staff; children participate in non-clinical skills groups at school that deliver social-emotional learning content while supporting acculturative needs; and youth needing more intensive services are referred to individual or family-level therapy. All tiers are co-facilitated by clinicians and cultural brokers, members of children's ethnic or national communities who have expertise navigating the resettlement society. TST-R generates high buy-in from families (Benson et al., 2018; Cardeli et al., 2020). Meanwhile, clinical TST-R therapy corresponds with reductions in trauma and depression symptom domains (Ellis et al., 2013).

16.3.4 Expressive Arts Intervention (EXIT)

Expressive Arts Intervention (EXIT) is based on Intermodal Expressive Arts and uses music education and arts-based therapy to help children access playful or imaginative mental states (Meyer et al., 2017). Results have demonstrated that EXIT helped refugee children with symptoms of trauma and post-traumatic stress symptoms, while improving their sense of safety, calm, connectedness, efficacy, and hope for the future.

16.4 Trauma-Informed Care in the Broader World

TIC has the potential to build point-of-service experiences that are actively healing for people who have experienced adversity. Clearly, this goal is likely to have positive impacts in any place humans are present. Those who serve children have begun to envision the implementation of TIC by foster care providers, and trials have found that adults and children alike benefit from these practices (Lotty et al., 2020). Juvenile detention facilities may also see lower rates of violence when TIC programs are implemented, especially when many individuals participate (Baetz et al., 2021). Some programs for humanitarian settings are already developed with TIC principles in mind (Meštrović, & Bandov, 2024). Schools, of course, are also at the front lines of trauma response, and TIC practices have the potential to improve education and psychosocial outcomes when delivered with regularity and fidelity during the school day (Thomas et al., 2019).

Case Study: Sesame Street Around the World

Sesame Street's global partnerships work to design and deliver programming in humanitarian settings like refugee camps. In addition to delivering early childhood educational content, these programs offer child-friendly language for understanding community challenges, teach coping skills, and provide safety messaging (e.g., body autonomy) that is at the core of TIC (Kohn et al., 2020). One specialized program, WASH UP!, relays messages about using clean water, hand washing with soap, and proper latrine use to children in Ghana, Mali, Niger, Malawi, Zambia, Zimbabwe, Honduras, and Afghanistan (World Vision, 2017). This program has also been expanded to include additional socio-emotional content for Syrian refugee children in Iraq, Jordan, and Lebanon.

16.5 Conclusion

The restoration of safety—physical, social, and emotional—is critical to children's and families' healing after trauma. TIC principles not only help to increase the felt safety of care environments, but also build providers' skills at conducting valid and hospitable assessments, facilitating positive engagement from care participants, and discerning promising paths forward in care. TIC is cost-effective and broadly beneficial to all those who receive care, regardless of trauma exposure, consistent with the principles of universal design (Domino et al., 2005). TIC principles have the potential to support children's wellbeing across a wide range of settings.

Reflection Questions

Question 1. Can you identify an encounter where your words or actions may have unknowingly retraumatized a person you were working with? What about times where your words or actions seemed to help promote agency, empowerment, and safety?

Question 2. In addition to the tools and practices identified in the chapter, are there additional strategies that you have utilized that could be helpful with children exposed to trauma?

Question 3. Consider where you work and learn. How could these systems and spaces become more trauma-informed?

Question 4. Are you aware of trauma-informed care practices that are being implemented with children in your community?

Question 5. What could it look like to use the principles of TIC in your *personal* life?

References

Abdi, S. M., Miller, A. B., Agalab, N. Y., & Ellis, B. H. (2021). Partnering with refugee communities to improve mental health access: Going from "why are they not coming" to "what can I (we) do differently?". *Cultural Diversity and Ethnic Minority Psychology*. https://doi.org/10.1037/CDP0000476

Ahmad, A., Larsson, B., & Sundelin-Wahlsten, V. (2007). EMDR treatment for children with PTSD: Results of a randomized controlled trial. *Nordic Journal of Psychiatry*, *61*(5), 349–354. https://doi.org/10.1080/08039480701643464

Alemi, Q., Panter-Brick, C., Oriya, S., Ahmady, M., Alimi, A. Q., Faiz, H, Haskim, N., Hashemi, S., A., S., Manaly, M., A., & Ventevogel, P. (2023). Afghan mental health and psychosocial well-being: Thematic review of four decades of research and interventions. *BJPsych Open*, *9*(4), e125. https://doi.org/10.1192/bjo.2023.502

Baetz, C. L., Surko, M., Moaveni, M., McNair, F., Bart, A., Workman, S., Tedeschi, F., Guo, F., Quinian C., & Horwitz, S. M. (2021). Impact of a trauma-informed intervention for youth and staff on rates of violence in juvenile detention settings. *Journal of Interpersonal Violence*, *36*(17–18), NP9463–NP9482.

Benson, M. A., Abdi, S. M., Miller, A. B., & Heidi Ellis, B. (2018). Trauma systems therapy for refugee children and families. In N. Morina, & A. Nickerson (Eds.), *Mental health of refugee and conflict-affected populations: Theory, research and clinical practice* (pp. 243–259). Springer International Publishing. https://doi.org/10.1007/978-3-319-97046-2_12

Cardeli, E., Davis, S., Issa, O., & Ellis, B. H. (2020). Trauma Systems Therapy for Refugees (TST-R) in a multi-ethnic refugee population in Maine, USA: Early findings from a programme evaluation project with children and adolescents. *The Lancet Global Health*, *8*, S9. https://doi.org/10.1016/S2214-109X(20)30150-9

Child and Adolescent Trauma Screen (CATS). ISTSS at https://istss.org/clinical-resources/assessing-trauma/child-and-adolescent-trauma-screen-(cats)

Chipalo, E. (2021). Is trauma focused-cognitive behavioral therapy (TF-CBT) effective in reducing trauma symptoms among traumatized refugee children? A systematic review. *Journal of Child & Adolescent Trauma*, *14*(4), 545–558. https://doi.org/10.1007/s40653-021-00370-0

Cohodes, E. M., Kribakaran, S., Odriozola, P., Bakirci, S., McCauley, S., Hodges, H. R., Sisk, L. M., Zacharek, S. J., & Gee, D. G. (2021). Migration-related trauma and mental health among migrant children emigrating from Mexico and Central America to the United States: Effects on developmental neurobiology and implications for policy. *Developmental Psychobiology*, *63*(6), e22158. https://doi.org/10.1002/dev.22158

Dangmann, C. (2022). Good starts: Mental health and resilience in resettled Syrian refuge youth. PhD Dissertation in child and youth participation and competence development, Inland Norway University of Applied Sciences. ISBN printed version: 978–82–8380-323–5.

Derluyn, I., Mels, C., & Broekaert, E. (2009). Mental health problems in separated refugee adolescents. *Journal of Adolescent Health*, *44*, 291–297.

Domino, M., Morrissey, J. P., Nadlicki-Patterson, T., & Chung, S. (2005). Service costs for women with co-occurring disorders and trauma. *Journal of Substance Abuse Treatment*, *28*, 135–143.

Ellis, B. H., Miller, A. B., Abdi, S., Barrett, C., Blood, E. A., & Betancourt, T. S. (2013). Multi-tier mental health program for refugee youth. *Journal of Consulting and Clinical Psychology*, *81*(1), 129. https://doi.org/10.1037/a0029844

Fazel, M., Hoagwood, K., Stephan, S., & Ford, T. (2014). Mental health interventions in schools in high-income countries. *The Lancet Psychiatry*, *1*(5), 377–387. https://doi.org/10.1016/S2215-0366(14)70312-8

Fazel, M., & Stein, A. (2002). The mental health of refugee children. *Archives of Disease in Childhood*, *87*(5), 366–370.

Finkelhor, D., Turner, H. A., Shattuck, A., & Hamby, S. L. (2013). Violence, crime, and abuse exposure in a national sample of children and youth: An update. *JAMA Pediatrics*, *167*(7), 614–621. https://doi.org/10.1001/jamapediatrics.2013.42

Gone, J. P., Hartmann, W. E., Pomerville, A., Wendt, D. C., Klem, S. H., & Burrage, R. L. (2019). The impact of historical trauma on health outcomes for indigenous populations in the USA and Canada: A systematic review. *American Psychologist*, *74*(1), 20. https://doi.org/10.1037/amp0000338

Herman, J. L. (2015). *Trauma and recovery: The aftermath of violence--from domestic abuse to political terror*. Hachette UK.

Hodges, H. R., Wahidy, Z., Bashari, K., & Abdi, S. M. (2024). Cognitive and neuropsychological assessment of Afghan refugee children. *Professional Psychology: Research and Practice*, *55*(6), 537–546. https://doi.org/10.1037/pro0000593

Kohn, S., Foulds, K., Murphy, K. M., & Cole, C. F. (2020). Creating a Sesame Street for the Syrian Response Region. *YC Young Children*, *75*(1), 32–41.

Lotty, M., Dunn-Galvin, A., & Bantry-White, E. (2020). Effectiveness of a trauma-informed care psychoeducational program for foster carers–Evaluation of the Fostering Connections Program. *Child Abuse & Neglect*, *102*, 104390.

Marsac, M. L., Kassam-Adams, N., Hildenbrand, A. K., Nicholls, E., Winston, F. K., Leff, S. S., & Fein, J. (2016). Implementing a trauma-informed approach in pediatric healthcare networks. *JAMA Pediatrics*, *170*, 70–77. https://doi.org/10.1001/jamapediatrics.2015.2206.

McLaughlin, K. A., Colich, N. L., Rodman, A. M., & Weissman, D. G. (2020). Mechanisms linking childhood trauma exposure and psychopathology: A transdiagnostic model of risk and resilience. *BMC Medicine*, *18*(1), 1–11. https://doi.org/10.1186/S12916-020-01561-6

Menschner, C., & Maul, A. (2016). *Issue brief: Key ingredients for successful trauma-informed care implementation*. Center for Health Care Strategies.

Meštrović, T., & Bandov, G. (2024). The interplay of sustainable development goals on education and peace: Enhancing trauma-informed approaches in informal learning environments for displaced and vulnerable populations. *Health Policy, Economics and Sociology*, *8*(2). https://doi.org/10.52340/healthecosoc.2024.08.02.05

Miller, K., Brown, C. R., Shramko, M., & Svetaz, V. (2019). Applying trauma-informed practices to the care of refugee and immigrant youth: 10 clinical pearls. *Children*, *6*, 94. https://doi.org/10.3390/children6080094

Meyer, DeMott, M. A., Jakobsen, M., Wentzel-Larsen, T., & Heir, T. (2017). A controlled early group intervention study for unaccompanied minors-can expressive arts alleviate symptoms of trauma and enhance life satisfaction? *Scandinavian Journal of Psychology*, 58, 510–518.

Narayan, A. J., Ippen, C. G., Harris, W. W., & Lieberman, A. F. (2019). Protective factors that buffer against the intergenerational transmission of trauma from mothers to young children: A replication study of angels in the nursery. *Development and Psychopathology*, *31*(1), 173–187. https://doi.org/10.1017/S0954579418001530

Oberg, C. N. (2019). The arch of migration and the impact on children's health and well-being: Forward to the special issue-children on the move. *Children*, *6*, 100. https://doi.org/10.3390/children6090100

Pfeiffer, E., & Goldbeck, L. (2017). Evaluation of a trauma-focused intervention for unaccompanied young refugees-A pilot study. *Journal of Traumatic Stress*, *30*, 531–536.

Raja, S., Hasnain, M., Hoersch, M., Gove-Yin, S., & Rajagopalan, C. (2015). Trauma informed care in medicine: Current knowledge and future research directions. *Family & Community Health*, *38*(3), 216–226. https://doi.org/10.1097/fch.0000000000000071

Ruf, M., Schauer M., Neuner, F., Catani, C., Schauer, E., & Elbert, T. (2010). Narrative Exposure Therapy for 7- to 16-year-olds: A randomized controlled trial with traumatized refugee children. *Journal of Traumatic Stress*, *23*, 437–445. https://doi.org/10.1002/jts.20548

SAMHSA (2014). SAMHSA's concept of trauma and guidance for a trauma-informed approach SAMHSA's trauma and justice strategic initiative. https://store.samhsa.gov/product/SAMHSA-s-Concept-of-Trauma-and-Guidance-for-a-Trauma-Informed-Approach/SMA14-4884

Sanchez-Cao, E., Kramer, T., & Hodes, M. (2012). Psychological distress and mental health service contact of unaccompanied asylum-seeking children. *Child: Care, Health, and Development*, *39*(5), 651–659.

Sarkdadi, A., Adahl, K., Stenvall, E., Segonja, R., Batti, H., Gavra, P., Fangstrom, K., & Salari, R. (2018). Teaching recovery techniques-evaluation of a group intervention for unaccompanied refugee minors with symptoms of PTSD in Sweden. *European Child & Adolescent Psychiatry*, *27*, 467–479.

Sciolla, A. F. (2017). An overview of trauma-informed care. *Trauma, Resilience, and Health Promotion in LGBT Patients: What Every Healthcare Provider Should Know*, 165–181. https://doi.org/10.1007/978-3-319-54509-7_14

Spaas, C., Verelst, A., Devlieger, I., Aalto, S., Andersen, A. J., Durbeej, N., Hilden, P. K., Kankaanpää, R., Primdahl, N. L., Opaas, M., Osman, F., Peltonen, K., Sarkadi, A., Skovdal, M., Jervelund, S. S., Soye, E., Watters, C., Derluyn, I., Colpin, H., & De Haene, L. (2022). Mental health of refugee and non-refugee migrant young people in European secondary education: The role of family separation, daily material stress and perceived discrimination in resettlement. *Journal of Youth and Adolescence*, *51*(5), 848–870. https://doi.org/10.1007/s10964-021-01515-y

Thomas, M. S., Crosby, S., & Vanderhaar, J. (2019). Trauma-informed practices in schools across two decades: An interdisciplinary review of research. *Review of Research in Education*, *43*(1), 422–452. https://doi.org/10.3102/0091732X18821123

Unterhitzenberger, J., Ebelre-Sejari, R., Rassenhofer, M., Sukale, T., Rosner, T., & Goldbeck, L. (2015). *BMC Psychiatry*, *15*, 260. https://doi.org/10.1186/s12888-015-0645-0

van der Kolk, B., Ford, J. D., & Spinazzola, J. (2019). Comorbidity of developmental trauma disorder (DTD) and post-traumatic stress disorder: Findings from the DTD field trial. *European Journal of Psychotraumatology*, *10*(1). https://doi.org/10.1080/20008198.2018.1562841

Wilker, S., Catani, C., Wittmann, J., Preusse, M., Schmidt, T., May, T., Erti, V., Doering, B., Rosner, R., Zindler, A., & Neuner, F. (2020). The efficacy of Narrative Exposure Therapy for Children (KIDNET) as a treatment for traumatized young refugees versus treatment as usual: Study protocol for a multi-center randomized control trial (YOUTREAT). *Trials*, *21*, 185. https://doi.org/10.1186/s13063-020-4127-4

World Vision. (2017). Sesame Street, World Vision partnership expands to 11 countries with lifesaving hygiene lessons. *World Vision*. https://sesameworkshop.org/about-us/press-room/sesame-street-world-vision-partnership-expands-11-countries-now-reaching/

17 Children's Rights

17.1 Imagining an Equitable World

As conflict, environmental crises, and climate change converge, adults must work with children to reimagine a better world. A child rights lens emerged in response to this need. This chapter presents a brief history of this approach, along with examples of international consensus on this topic and an illustration of a child rights orientation in action: UNICEF's Child-Friendly Cities Initiative (CFCI).

An understanding of health is at the core of a child rights approach. Health is not simply the absence of disease, but is a state of physical, social, and mental wellbeing that includes access to resilience factors, community, and opportunities (WHO, 1946). As has been described throughout this book, factors around a child—economic, social, and environmental—influence both biology and also social, emotional, and spiritual health. Wherever individuals face systematic disadvantage in their experiences of the world, such as social, economic, and environmental adversities, health disparities are likely to emerge (Braveman et. al., 2010). Worldwide, markers like race, ethnicity, income, healthcare access, housing stability, food security, geography, transportation, and the built environment act as social determinants of health, shaping children's likelihood of negative and positive health outcomes alike (Berkman, 2009). Critically, many social determinants of health are associated with health risks because of the ways that they interact with structural inequities. For example, a person's immigrant status influences their risk for mental health challenges due, in large part, to the discriminatory treatment that immigrants may experience during resettlement; the heightened risk of additional adversities that can come from economic vulnerabilities; and challenges accessing resources and supports (Sangalang et al., 2019). Any discussion of child health requires attention to structural disparities in children's experiences of their environments.

Racism is responsible for child health disparities in many communities around the world. Racism is often held to exist on multiple levels, including structural, personally mediated, and internalized (Jones, 2000). In U.S. society, for example, racism has shaped the design of many social systems (e.g., social security, education, banking, housing, healthcare, etc.). These systems confer advantages to White people while generating cumulative (and

DOI: 10.4324/9781003488385-21

often chronic) adverse outcomes for people who are not White; meanwhile, they normalize historical, cultural, institutional, and interpersonal dynamics that perpetuate disadvantages (Bonilla-Silva, 1997). For example, in one large study of children presenting to American emergency rooms, African American, Latine, and American Indian patients received lower triage scores (and therefore waited longer for care) than their White peers with similar injuries or illnesses (Zook et al., 2016). A child rights approach is not complete without a holistic understanding of wellbeing and attention to the many ways that social inequity shapes a child's access to health and developmental resources.

17.2 The Codification of Children's Rights

Most communities have long held that there are appropriate and right ways to treat children. For example, the traditions and sacred texts of Islam emphasize the importance of naming children, treating them fairly, and educating them. A human rights approach references shared understandings of "rights to" and "rights to protection from." These conceptualizations, first, place responsibility on adults to ensure these rights are honored. They also define limits to one party's behavior insofar as the needs of another are impeded. For example, a government's right to pass laws stops short of entitling it to legalize ethnic cleansing, and a parent's right to discipline a child stops short of allowing cruel

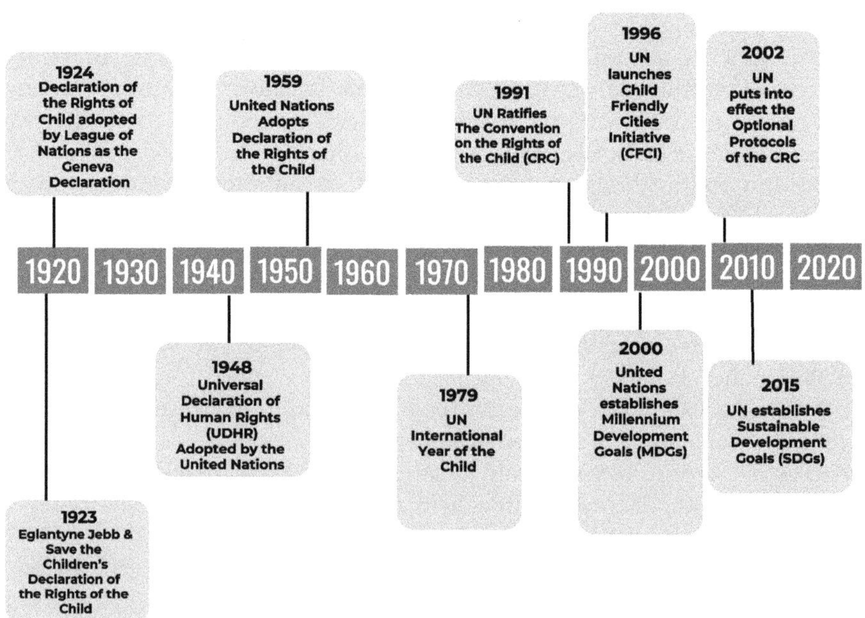

Figure 17.1 Timeline of the international codification of children's rights.

or inhumane treatment. There is not space in this text to describe a detailed history of human rights or child rights. Instead, this section briefly attends to international agreements about child rights over the last century. Figure 17.1 provides a timeline of key events in international children's rights discourse since WWI.

One "ignition moment" in the global movement for child rights is traceable to a British social reformer named Eglantyne Jebb (see case study below). Following WWI's devastating toll on the health and development of children, Jebb presented a brief document to the League of Nations in Geneva that outlined what she viewed as the five core rights of a child. The League adopted this statement, the Declaration on the Rights of the Child, marking the first instance of intergovernmental approval of a human rights document. The five tenets of this Declaration are that children have the right to receive material and spiritual resources required for healthy development; have their needs met in times of adversity; be the first to receive aid during crises; be protected against exploitation and supported in earning a livelihood; and be raised with awareness of how they can contribute to their communities.

Case Study: Eglantyne Jebb

Eglantyne Jebb was raised in a wealthy British family. In the years after World War One, an Allied blockade of Germany and Austria-Hungary blocked humanitarian aid to these countries and led to widespread starvation. After seeing moving photographs of children who were experiencing starvation, Jebb and her colleagues launched a pressure campaign to end the blockade. This campaign involved handing out flyers in London's Trafalgar Square that indicted the British government for their role in this starvation. Jebb was arrested and fined, but her rousing speech in her own defense so moved the judge that he paid her fine himself. She and her colleagues (including her sister, Dorothy) launched a fund to continue these efforts: the Save the Children Fund, which is still in action today. In the years that followed, Save the Children raised awareness and funds to support children caught in the crossfires of global conflict. In 1921, they sent 600 tons of food and medical supplies via cargo ship to Russia. Jebb was known to say, "Every generation of children offers mankind the possibility of rebuilding his ruin of a world" (Save the Children, 2025).

After embracing this Declaration, the League directed all member states to apply these principles toward protecting all children (LeBlanc, 1995). In 1959, the United Nations adopted an expanded version of this document, which also referenced civic, political, economic, social, and cultural rights for all children. However, the Declaration was not supported by an enforceable treaty or international oversight (Mower, 1997).

The International Year of the Child occurred in 1979, when the United Nations and the broader world celebrated and encouraged global efforts to promote the rights of children (Jupp, 1989). In the following years, the UN drafted a Convention that would adapt the principles of the Declaration into a more enforceable international treaty. On November 20, 1989, the General Assembly adopted the UN Convention on the Rights of the Child (CRC), thirty years to the day after adopting the Declaration on the Rights of the Child. In 1990, a sufficient number of member countries ratified the Convention to enshrine it as international law, establishing that governments, institutions, citizens, and families are responsible for safeguarding the rights of children (Goldhagen et al., 2020a; Oberg & Zastrow, 2004). As of 2025, the Convention has been ratified by every country in the world except for the United States; while U.S. effort was instrumental in preparing the Convention, and while the U.S. Ambassador to the UN signed the treaty, the United States has failed to ratify the CRC for decades (Vissing, 2017). The causes of this refusal are complex, but have included U.S. partisanship (i.e., failure to reach a supermajority in the Senate), fears of relinquishing power to another entity like the UN, continued use of life sentences without parole for juveniles (forbidden by Article 37), and a fear of infringing on the rights of families. Of note, the fact that the CRC offers many affirmations of families' rights, and ratifying the treaty does not subject a country to UN enforcement of its laws (but merely requires periodic reports on progress toward goals).

17.3 Guiding Principles of the CRC

The 54 articles of the CRC describe children's civic, political, social, economic, and cultural rights, which are held to be inalienable—that is, they cannot be forfeited, compromised, or lost, regardless of a child's circumstances. At their core, the Articles reflect a commitment to ensuring children's survival and optimal development, promoting their best interests, and respecting children's views (Maurás, 2011). The following section describes these core principles. Of note, **Article 1** defines children as those below the age of 18 years of age, though notions of maturity vary substantially across cultures and domains.

17.3.1 Nondiscrimination

Article 2 of the convention espouses nondiscrimination, establishing that children have a right to be free from disparate treatment based on their own, their family's, or their community's identity, including national origin, heritage, language, religion, political beliefs, income, disability, and other markers. Other articles similarly emphasize states' responsibilities in promoting equity, including through delivering education that prepares children to exercise tolerance for those who differ from them. Many nations and their institutions fail to protect children from discrimination. For example, children who have been through forced displacement often face xenophobia in their resettlement societies, and they may also have more difficulty accessing resources (Klein & von dem Knesebeck, 2018). Children and youth with minoritized sexual or gender identities are often subject to interpersonal discrimination and may also face higher barriers to accessing mental health care (Bhugra et al., 2022).

17.3.2 The Best Interest of the Child

Article 3 establishes that individuals and systems with authority over children must act in the best interest of the child and that children's needs are to be considered in all decisions that affect them (Goldhagen et al., 2015). Many other articles in this document reflect this principle by enshrining children's right to, say, contact with family members under most circumstances; freedom from economic exploitation; and protection from neglectful or abusive caregiving. These articles also offer a developmentally sensitive framing of children's autonomy—namely, that children's capacities to act in their own best interest evolve over time.

17.3.3 Survival and Optimal Development

Article 6 establishes that states and state institutions are responsible for ensuring children's access to resources for survival, health, and development, including shelter, nutritious food, clothing, and quality medical care. The CRC relies on an expansive version of health that includes optimal physical, emotional, social, and cognitive development (WHO, 1946). Among the articles supporting this principle are those establishing a child's rights to be free from dangers, including those related to abuse, armed conflict, and unsafe labor. Articles also support children's rights to access positive resources for their development, such as free primary school, family connections, and adequate sanitation. Many other articles safeguard children's cultural and emotional development, including their rights to a name, to beliefs, and to opportunities to learn the language of their culture.

Case Study: Period Poverty and Menstrual Justice

Around the world, the simple fact of menstruation is a major driver of gender inequity in education, with many girls and young women lacking menstrual supplies, adequate sanitation, and social support to allow them to attend school during their periods. A group of high school students and their teacher started The Pad Project in 2013. In addition to providing menstrual health education and hygiene products, this organization has also helped distribute machines that manufacture inexpensive sanitary products within communities (The Pad Project, 2025). Meanwhile, Huru International partners with community organizations across East Africa to distribute reusable hygiene products, spark conversations about sexual and financial health, and even deliver high-quality menstrual education to boys, which helps reduce stigma against their female classmates and friends (Huru International, 2025). One prominent figure in menstrual justice is Arunachalam Muruganantham, who was saddened to learn about the shame and discomfort his wife, Shanthi, faced during her period, given that the family could not afford menstrual products. In response, he spent several years developing materials and manufacturing processes that could produce sanitary pads for a very low cost, even testing his own designs using a fake uterus filled with animal blood. His persistence bore fruit. Since the early 2000s, communities across India and other nations have used Mr. Muruganantham's machine to produce inexpensive period products. All in all, grassroots efforts like this have already helped to save millions of school and work days for girls and women worldwide.

17.3.4 Respect for the Child's Views

Article 12 outlines the importance of listening to the opinions of children who can form their own views and considering them in proportion to a child's age and maturity. This and other articles enshrine children's rights to participate in all levels of society, including arts and culture. For example, **Article 15** states that children and youth have the right to assemble peacefully, **Article 16** describes the right to private communication, and **Article 17** supports children's rights to seek information. Some of the ways in which adults can honor these rights are by supporting children's access to digital technologies in helpful and developmentally appropriate ways (see Chapter 13). Adults also respect these rights by honoring children's informed assent to healthcare and social services where possible and by ensuring that children can safely give testimonies during court proceedings, for example (Bensted et al., 2015).

17.3.5 Child Rights and Child Vulnerabilities

These four principles are at the core of all articles of the CRC. Critically, all rights are understood to be both interconnected—informing one another—and indivisible, meaning that all are equal in importance. As such, the CRC can inform holistic approaches to children's wellbeing in diverse cultural communities and contexts.

A number of the rights outlined in the CRC are especially pertinent when children are facing marginalization or contexts that could harm their wellbeing. **Article 23**, for example, states that children with disabilities are entitled to resources that optimize their development, health, quality of life, and participation in their communities (see Chapter 15). **Article 8** safeguards a child's right to an identity, including nationality, which is a rebuke of cultural genocide (see Chapter 11). Relatedly, **Article 30** states that countries must respect a child's ethnicity, religion, and language, a principle especially relevant to children from minoritized ethnic and religious groups, including Indigenous communities (see Chapter 14). Similarly, several articles are relevant to children experiencing forced displacement (see Chapter 9). **Article 22** asserts that refugee children must receive humanitarian assistance and protection throughout their journey. **Articles 9 and 10** demand that children are protected from family separation, and that efforts are made to quickly reunite families. Other articles establish children's rights to protection from crimes against humanity (see Chapter 11). For example, **Articles 34–38** focus on protections from sexual exploitation, labor exploitation, slavery, torture, and armed conflict. All readers of this text are encouraged to explore the United Nations Convention on the Rights of the Child in more detail.

In the years after the CRC was ratified, many policy makers and advocates for child rights noted that two particular issues could benefit from additional clarity and strength, and two additional protocols were adopted. First, in 2000, the UN passed the Optional Protocol on the Involvement of Children in Armed Conflict (Coomaraswamy, 2010), which has been ratified by 173 countries (including the United States). This protocol asserts that children under 18 will not be drafted into a nation's army, that those who enlist prior to age 18 will not be directly involved in armed combat before 18, and that non-state armed forces (e.g., militias) cannot recruit children for any purpose. The second measure, the Optional Protocol on the Sale of Children, Child Pornography and Child Prostitution, arose out of growing concerns around child sexual trafficking and the availability of child abuse imagery online (UNHCR, 2000). This protocol has been ratified by 178 member nations.

17.4 Child-Friendly Cities

In 1996, UNICEF launched a new initiative to translate the UN Convention on the Rights of the Child into actionable interventions at the local level. The Child-Friendly Cities Initiative (CFCI) works with local governments and communities to design infrastructure, governance, and resources that can optimize children's wellbeing and healthy development (Goldhagen et al., 2020b). The CFCI process also involves carefully attending to children's own voices and working to integrate these opinions into governmental decisions and public programming. In 2018, over 40 countries and over 3,000 cities were engaged in the CFCI (UNICEF, 2018). Table 17.1 highlights the five goals that underpin the CFCI (Goldhagen et al., 2020b), along with examples (UNICEF, 2025).

To establish a Child-Friendly City, municipalities partner with UNICEF to conduct needs assessments, develop action plans, implement these plans, and evaluate the fruits of these efforts, involving children at each step of the way (UNICEF, 2025). Communities may choose to address issues as diverse as emergency preparedness, education, gender equity, water access,

Table 17.1 UNICEF child-friendly cities initiative: goals and examples

Goal	*Definition*	*Examples*
Safety and Inclusion	All children are treated with fairness and respect by their communities and local authorities	- Community- and school-based workshops address digital safety - Meet-up groups connect families that are facing social isolation
Equitable Social Services	All children have access to excellent services and supports	- Service access processes are audited from a perspective of refugee needs - Women facing structural adversity receive prenatal healthcare, nutrition, and occupational support
Safe Living Environment	All children have safe, enriching, and clean environments	- Road crossings, signage, and street lighting are redesigned from a perspective of child safety - Public WiFi zones and sports centers help protect youth from gang activity
Play and Leisure	All children enjoy abundant rest and play	- City spaces are repurposed for play areas - Children partner with contractors in designing wheelchair-accessible playgrounds
Child and Youth Participation	All children's voices and priorities are considered in public decisions, including design of policies and programs	- Youth boards shape services for other children experiencing housing loss - Children work with local leaders to build maps of community resources that support education, play, and celebration

environmental justice, or healthcare, to name a few (UNICEF, 2024). Out of the 3,000 cities involved in the CFCI worldwide, two are in the United States (Houston and Minneapolis; Oberg, 2024).

17.5 Conclusion

A child rights approach has the potential to focus global attention on the most important issues affecting children's safety, wellbeing, and development. The UN's Convention on the Rights of the Child has helped to establish consensus across international communities on indivisible, inalienable, and interconnected rights to which children are entitled. While enforcement of documents like the CRC is limited, there are examples of successful structures that support communities in reaching these goals for children. One example is the CFCI, which helps equip the design of public services, spaces, and programs that promote healthy development. This initiative benefits from flexibility and responsiveness at the local level, along with commitment to centering children's voices at each level of planning and implementation. Generations of children can benefit from internationally supported and locally implemented initiatives to protect children's rights.

Reflection Questions

Question 1. The UN Convention on the Rights of the Child is sometimes criticized for having limited enforcement mechanisms (i.e., countries that ratify it agree to have their progress monitored and to receive recommendations from an international committee, but a country may or may not investigate or prosecute violations). Can you think of any ways that it can still be beneficial to children?

Question 2. Referencing the CRC, describe an issue in your community from a child rights perspective.

Question 3. If your community was engaged in the Child-Friendly Cities Initiative, what projects would you expect it to take on?

References

Bensted, R., Hargreaves, D. S., Lombard, J., Viner, R. M. (2015). Comparison of healthcare priorities in childhood and early/late adolescence: Analysis of cross-sectional data from eight countries in the Council of Europe Child-friendly healthcare survey. *Child: Care, Health and Development*, *41*, 160–165.

Berkman, L. F. (2009). Social epidemiology: Social determinants of health in the United States: Are we losing ground? *Annual Review of Public Health*, *30*, 27–41.

Bhugra, D., Killaspy, H., Kar, A., Levin, S., Chumakov, E., Rogoza, D., Bagga, H., Owino – Wamari. Y., Everall, I.,Bishop A., Javate, J., Westmore, I., Ahuja, A., Torales, J., Rubin, H., Castaldelli-Maia, J., Ng, R., Nakajima, G. A., Levounis, P., & Ventriglio, A. (2022). IRP commission: Sexual minorities and mental health: Global perspectives. *International Review of Psychiatry*, 34(3-4), 171–199.

Bonilla-Silva, E. (1997). Rethinking racism: Toward a structural interpretation. *American Sociological Review*, *62*(3), 465–480.

Braveman, P. A., Cubbin, C., Egerter, S., Williams, D. R., & Pamuk, E. (2010). Socioeconomic disparities in health in the United States-what patterns tell us. *American Journal of Public Health*, *100*(1), S186–S196.

Coomaraswamy, R. (2010). The Optional protocol to the convention on the rights of the child on the involvement of children in armed conflict – towards universal ratification. *The International Journal of Children's Rights*, *18*(4), 535–549. https://doi.org/10.1163/157181810X527978

Goldhagen J., Clarke A., Dixon P., Guerreiro, A. I., Lansdown, G., & Vaghri, A. (2020a). Thirtieth anniversary of the UN Convention on the Rights of the Child: Advancing a child rights-based approach to child health and well-being. *BMJ Paediatrics Open*, *4*, e000589. https://doi.org/10.1136/bmj po-2019–000589

Goldhagen, J., Mercer, R., & Webb, E. (2015). Toward a child rights theory in pediatric bioethics. In M. Montello F. Miller, & J. Lantos (Eds.), *Perspectives in biology and medicine* (3rd ed.). Summer 2015.

Goldhagen, J. L., Shenoda, S., Oberg, C. N., Mercer, R., Kadir, A., Raman, S., Waterston, T., & Spencer, R. J. (2020b). Rights, justice, and equity: A global agenda for child health and wellbeing. *Lancet Child/Adolescent*, *4*(1), 80–90. https://doi.org/10.1016/S2352-4642(19)30346-3

Huru International. (2025). https://www.huruinternational.org/

Jones, C. PP. (2000). Levels of racism—A theoretic framework and a gardener's tale. *American Journal of Public Health*, *90*, 1212–1215.

Jupp, M. (1989). The international year of the child: Ten years later. *Proceedings of the Academy of Political Science* (pp. 31–44). https://doi.org/10.2307/1173949

Klein. J., & von dem Knesebeck, O. (2018). Inequalities in health care utilization among migrants and non-migrants in Germany: A systematic review. *International Journal of Health Sciences, 17*, 160.

LeBlanc (1995). *The convention on the rights of the child—United Nations lawmaking on human rights* (p. xv). University of Nebraska Press.

Maurás, M. (2011). Public policies and child rights: Entering the third decade of the convention on the rights of the child. *The ANNALS of the American Academy of Political and Social Science*, *633*(1), 52–65. https://doi.org/10.1177/0002716210382993

Mower, A. G. (1997). *The convention on the rights of the child—international law support for children* (p. 11). Greenwood Press.

Oberg, C. N. (2024). The child friendly cities initiative-minneapolis model. *Maternal and Child Health Journal*, February. https://doi.org/10.1007/s10995-024-03921-7

Oberg, C. N., & Zastrow, C. (2004). Pediatrics and social policy—advocating for children's rights. *Current Problems in Pediatric and Adolescent Health Care*, *34*(8), 286–308.

The Pad Project. (2025). https://thepadproject.org/who-we-are/

Sangalang, C. C., Becerra, D., Mitchell, F. M., Lechuga-Peña, S., Lopez, K., & Kim, I. (2019). Trauma, post-migration stress, and mental health: A comparative analysis of refugees and immigrants in the United States. *Journal of Immigrant and Minority Health*, *21*, 909–919.

Save the Children. (2025). Meet Eglantyne Jebb - Founder of Save the Children. *Save the Children.* https://www.savethechildren.org/us/about-us/why-save-the-children/eglantyne-jebb

UNHCR (2000). Optional protocol to the convention on the rights of the child on the sale of children, child prostitution and child pornography. May 25. https://www.ohchr.org/en/instruments-mechanisms/instruments/optional-protocol-convention-rights-child-sale-children-child

UNICEF (2018). UNICEF child friendly cities and communities handbook. April. https://www.childfriendlycities.org/media/2251/file/CFCI%20Handbook%20-%20EN.pdf

UNICEF (2024). https://www.unicef.org/eap/what-we-do

UNICEF. (2025). Child-friendly cities initiative. https://www.childfriendlycities.org/

Vissing, Y. (2017). Children rights in the United States: 25 years later and counting, Chapter 6. In T. Liefaard, & J. Slotj-Nielsen (Eds.), *The United Nations convention on the rights of the child-taking stock after 25 years and looking ahead* (pp. 73–100). ISBN: 978-90-04-29504-9. https://doi.org/10.1163/9789004295056_007

WHO (1946). Preamble to the constitution of the world health organization as adopted by the international health conference, New York, 19–22 June 1946; signed on 22 July 1946 by the representatives of 61 States (Official Records of the World Health Organization, no. 2, p. 100) and entered into force on 7 April 1948.

Zook, H. G., Kharbanda, A. B., Flood, A., Harmon, B., Puumala, S. E., & Payne, N. R. (2016). Racial differences in pediatric emergency department triage scores. *The Journal of emergency medicine*, *50*(5), 720–727.

18 Developmental Resilience Science and Resilience-Informed Systems

18.1 Introduction

To study—and, most especially, to invest in—child development amid the risks of the present century requires the use of dual lenses: sobriety and hope. The field of developmental resilience science (DRS) aims to integrate these two lenses, offering accounts of the potential (and even tendency) of complex systems, from individual biology to large cultural communities, to adapt successfully to serious threats to their functioning and survival (Masten et al., 2021). Part II described many of the factors that have been found to be associated with resilient outcomes in children exposed to various developmental risks. These resilience factors, from stable caregiving to cultural pride to involvement in well-functioning schools, are implicated in key developmental processes, including in children's adaptation to risk. This chapter explores in more depth the resilience frameworks that drive research and practice today. Finally, it presents theoretical and practical guidance for designing systems, policies, and practices in ways that promote resilient child development amid 21st-century risks.

18.2 Resilience in the Developing Child

Making judgments about the quality and success of adaptation in light of risk requires some understanding of normative or typical functioning. These judgments reflect a child's attainment of competence markers, or "milestones," behaviors and capacities that indicate development is proceeding as expected (Obradović et al., 2006). Competence markers are the observable fruits of multiple aggregated capacities that reveal the health of coordinated systems within a person. For example, when a baby takes her first steps unassisted, adults around her can conclude that she has developed musculature in her upper and lower body to keep her balanced while she walks; that she has absorbed sufficient nutrients to fuel this exertion; that social and non-social motivational systems are active; and that she has learned enough visuospatial perception to orient herself to her surroundings. When a middle school child has had a mutual and respectful friendship with a classmate for a whole

DOI: 10.4324/9781003488385-22

year, we can conclude that both children have levels of social motivation, communication skills, and emotion regulation capacities that approximate or exceed their community's expectations of youth in this developmental stage.

Since well before the middle of the 20th century, researchers and practitioners have understood that serious enough insults to a developing system can damage the system's functioning. Readers may recall studies of children who, lacking a nurturing and responsive caregiver, show disorganized attachment styles that can interfere with emotion regulation processes (Girme et al., 2021; Śliwerski et al., 2020), of child abuse increasing the risk of depression later in life, or of exposure to harsh discipline interfering with social processing patterns to increase the frequency of interpersonal conflict (Godleski & Ostrov, 2020; Martinelli et al., 2018). It is the presence of developmental competence in people exposed to significant risks that signals a resilient outcome.

Frequently, discussion of resilience is impeded by the popular and historic belief that resilience is an individual trait, comparable to "grit" or "toughness." Understandably, many people resist the implication that it is the job of a person (especially a child) exposed to risk to supply the internal resources required to overcome this challenge. (Even worse, perhaps, is the implication that those who struggle to adapt successfully to adversity have flaws at the level of their character.) Such trait-like understandings of resilience run counter to the current scientific understandings of the phenomenon. According to DRS frameworks, resilience is an outcome of (rather than an input to) adaptive processes. Far from being an individual accomplishment, it results from the interaction of resources at each level of a person's ecology. Some trait-level resources within a person are associated with positive outcomes after adversity, such as a sense of agency, optimism, and cognitive skills (Masten & Barnes, 2018). However, these typically act through mediation or moderation processes rather than direct causal processes. In fact, it is said that as a child's exposure to adversity increases, individual traits matter less and less to outcomes, their contributions eclipsed by the adaptive and supportive capacity of the systems around the person (Ungar et al., 2013). In the torn economic and social fabric that accompanies armed conflict, even a four-year-old who has remarkable cognitive skills is unlikely to meet core developmental competencies in the absence of ecological resilience factors like responsive caregiving, household organization, nutrition infrastructure, and environmental safety.

Indeed, developmental resilience processes frequently occur without the knowledge of the individuals they benefit. A twelve-year-old facing housing loss may not be aware that his involvement in organized sports through school is helping to physiologically regulate his diurnal rhythms and maintain his sense of efficacy and belonging amid chaotic housing transitions. A family whose nation is at war may not be attuned to the fact that continued revenue from the nation's core exports is keeping food prices stable in their local market, or that social and political movements in the past century have led their country's leaders to prioritize keeping schools open rather than redirecting children to labor.

Attending to the factors that protect and promote wellbeing amid threats as serious as climate change, genocide, and forced displacement may initially appear naïve or escapist. How could school engagement or hopefulness matter for people whose community is threatened by famine? Are resilience researchers simply avoiding the discomfort of attending to the horror of human rights violations?

18.3 Developmental Resilience Science (DRS)

In contrast, resilience science is a sober study of risk that takes seriously the ways that adversity threatens children. First, conducting resilience research requires making accurate, granular assessments of the nature and extent of threats. For example, how exactly does abuse versus neglect in infancy threaten social processing? How are the impacts of caloric deprivation magnified by the presence of household disorganization (Laude, 1999)? How does prolonged separation from a caregiver cause damage to the neural circuitry of emotion regulation in toddlerhood versus early childhood (Cohodes et al., 2021)? It is no coincidence that the fields of DRS and developmental psychopathology have always had a strong influence on one another, as methods of assessing risk and its potential impact are shared across these disciplines. Additionally, as discussed below, resilience-informed interventions are concerned with ending and preventing threats so that adaptive systems can engage to the fullest extent (Sanson et al., 2022).

DRS has indeed produced remarkable stories of hope, of course. Even amid some of the worst threats imaginable to child development, the majority of youth go on to function at or above average levels. Research on individuals and school communities exposed to serious threats has found that within a few years, *90%* of youth may be functioning at or above the levels expected for non-exposed samples (Betancourt et al., 2013; Lai et al., 2019). Across fields as diverse as ecology, economics, and human development, positive adaptation appears to be the normative reaction of systems exposed to threat. These efforts at adaptation are most likely to be successful, of course, when threats have ceased and necessary resources are reintroduced.

That is to say, rather than naïve optimism, DRS can be said to reflect *realism*. The story told by DRS—that adversity is not ultimately expected to fundamentally limit the trajectory of human development in people whose exposome includes species-typical resilience factors—appears, from decades of research, to be true. It is also a story that resonates with its most important listeners: the children whose development is threatened by past, present, and looming threats, along with the adults who care for them. A thriving family life continues to matter to Somali refugee families, even while exposure to ongoing racism, xenophobia, and economic marginalization continues (Betancourt et al., 2015). Parents facing displacement from their home have dreams for their children that do not merely amount to the avoidance of mental illness or poverty but also include happiness and friendship. In fact, experts recommend that those designing and delivering services for communities facing marginalization and risk use language and frameworks that emphasize the potential of individuals and systems to adapt positively rather than simply their likelihood of being damaged (Abdi, 2018).

Case Study: Appalachian Children Coalition

Many children growing up in the Appalachian region of the Eastern United States face complex social challenges like intergenerational poverty, environmental damage related to industry, difficulties related to family members' substance use, and disparities in healthcare access (Hash et al., 2024). Resilience science emphasizes that as children face poverty and challenging environmental conditions, strong networks within communities help them to access support and resources (Raniga & Mthembu, 2016). The Appalachian Children Coalition (ACC) works to connect people who serve children in Appalachia, whether they are caregivers, educators, or clinicians, in order to support a culture of resource-sharing and collaboration. Their work involves developing and distributing best-practices guidance on young people's use of digital media and substances; supporting staff retention among youth mental health providers; and helping equip schools to deliver primary care. The ACC's methods and goals closely reflect those of DRS (ACC, 2025; Masten & Hodges, 2025).

18.4 Principles of Resilience-Informed Systems

This section describes some of the characteristics of systems that are designed to promote resilient outcomes for children exposed to significant stress and adversity. Resilience processes are frequently conserved across domains, so many of the approaches outlined here are likely to be meaningful to structures as diverse as families, classrooms, healthcare systems, and lawmaking bodies (Masten et al., 2021). Readers are encouraged to consider how their existing work already entails engagement in the activities below and whether there may be additional opportunities to deepen the resilience-promoting capacities of their systems. Table 18.1 provides a list of the principles of resilience-informed systems discussed in this chapter.

Table 18.1 Principles of resilience-informed systems

- Adding protective and promotive factors
- Amplifying connections to resources
- Fueling adaptive systems
- Appreciating physiological processes
- Supporting emotion regulation
- Encouraging nurturing relationships
- Building supportive communities
- Reducing risk

18.4.1 Adding Protective and Promotive Factors

When children are exposed to developmental risks and adversity, there are usually extensive resources around them that initiate and maintain positive adaptation. These include promotive factors—resources associated with more favorable outcomes under high and low levels of stress alike—along with protective factors, whose importance is clearest when vulnerability and stress levels are high. Resilience-informed systems equip children with these promotive and protective factors, both by ensuring that these resources exist in the child's environment and also by facilitating the child's access to them (Jabr & Cahan, 2014; Nakkash et al., 2012).

Promotive factors can be thought of as "universal developmental resources." They are often so central to the fabric of communities that it is easy to forget they are implicated in children's positive adaptation. Some promotive factors are material. For example, nutritional food is critical to physical and cognitive development, and infrastructures like balanced school lunch programs make macronutrients and calories available to large groups of children each day (Vernarelli & O'Brien, 2017). Unsurprisingly, family financial stability is associated with mental health benefits (Shangani et al., 2017; Zimmerman et al., 2021).

Many promotive factors are social and interpersonal. Within the home, children whose caregiving environments are marked by sensitivity, warmth, and nurture show lower rates of mental health difficulties and higher levels of social competence (DePasquale & Gunnar, 2020). Social connections, including connection with religious communities, are broadly associated with longer life spans and higher levels of subjective well-being (Diener et al., 2018; McGinnis, 2016). Community centers and gathering places like parks can provide safe opportunities for building within- and inter-generational relationships and transmitting community culture (Betancourt et al., 2015). A sense of belonging at school is associated with higher levels of prosocial behaviors and lower levels of unhealthy behaviors (Allen et al., 2016). It also appears broadly associated with lower rates of depression and higher rates of self-efficacy in Somali refugee youth with high and low levels of reported trauma exposure alike (Kia-Keating & Ellis, 2007).

Many promotive factors serve protective roles when they are accessed under stressful circumstances. Stable childcare, whether center-based or informal, is a helpful resource for all families. For families with lower incomes, it can help caregivers to maintain employment and work sufficient hours, buffering against the risks of more severe poverty (Brady, 2016; Scarborough et al., 2021). Sleep, critical for all children, serves an adaptive purpose under conditions of higher stress, supporting the rebuilding of cellular and neural structures weakened by stress (Caldwell et al., 2020). Similarly, religious practice is broadly associated with wellbeing, but may take on new importance for people exposed to higher levels of adversity (Diener et al., 2018; Duggan et al., 2016).

Protective factors may be present in a community or individual at all times, but they are mobilized under conditions of adversity or risk, much like airbags and seatbelts matter for outcomes when an accident has occurred. Emergency rooms are an obvious infrastructural example, as are resources for people experiencing economic adversity, like food shelves and unemployment resources. There is a growing movement to prepare medical, behavioral, and infrastructural workforces to respond to natural disasters and terrorist attacks. Such a group of people can mobilize rapidly to set up communication networks, mobile medical units, gathering places, reunification processes, and shelter systems after a crisis (Masten & Motti-Stefanidi, 2020). Redesigning and equipping existing systems to maintain function during crises is a critical part of community resilience. For example, schools that had prepared for the possibility of remote learning before the COVID-19 pandemic were better equipped to ensure quality education after the crisis began (Diliberti et al., 2020). Other community-level protective factors include mental health systems designed to support people in crisis (Hogan & Goldman, 2021). International systems like peacekeeping interventions, human rights legislation, and food programs can also act as protective factors for communities facing adversity (Oberg et al., 2022).

Within individuals, broad protective factors include conflict resolution and problem-solving skills (Abraham & Sher, 2019). Youth who have experienced trauma may rely on collective or individual practices of meaning-making and coping to mourn and heal (Hosseini & Punzi, 2023; Johnson, 2010). A tendency toward active and positive rather than passive or negative coping is also associated broadly with adaptive outcomes (Cardoso, 2018). Some protective factors are specific to certain types of risk. For example, strong racial and ethnic identity can buffer against some of the effects of racial and ethnic discrimination (Chavez-Dueñas et al., 2019; Jones & Neblett, 2016).

18.4.2 Amplifying Connection to Resources

For a system to be resilience-informed, members must be aware of the promotive and protective resources contained within the system and, simultaneously, aware of the barriers and facilitators children may face to accessing these resources. The benefits of even the best online learning materials and virtual healthcare platforms depend on children's access to reliable internet (Afzal et al., 2022). School lunch programs only help children who can get to school (Vernarelli & O'Brien, 2017). Delivering nutritious food and water to children affected by armed conflict, land productivity decline, or economic collapse depends on the integrity of transportation infrastructures. In fact, living close to a road is already predictive of a child's nutritional diversity and dietary resilience, an association that will likely grow as climate change drives further declines in land productivity and water access (Galway et al., 2018; Ickowitz et al., 2014).

Resilience-informed systems are characterized by *curiosity* and *humility*, reflecting awareness of the adaptive resources they offer to children while never assuming these resources are reaching the children who need them. Barriers and facilitators to accessing resources may include practical, social, cultural, and structural factors, from transportation to religious beliefs (Abdi, 2018).

18.4.3 *Fueling Adaptive Systems*

Many of the assets described above can be described as *simple resources*: Their direct impacts, however critical, are usually limited in time and scope, and each asset serves a small number of functions for a child. Providing appropriate footwear to a child in a refugee camp may allow her to safely play with others outdoors and attend school (supporting her cognitive, social, physical, and identity development), and these activities may allow her caregivers time to engage in work, build friendships, or seek healthcare (which indirectly benefits the child through improved household functioning and caregiver well-being). The impact of these simple resources cannot be overstated. However, the shoes will only ever be shoes; their *direct* benefit to the child is limited in time (i.e., only while she is wearing them) and scope (i.e., serving simply to cover her feet).

Frequently, an influx of or connection to new resources is sufficient to help a child enter a resilient developmental path after adversity. However, the most sustainable and promising resilience-promoting interventions frequently invest in the health and availability of powerful *adaptive systems* around a child. Adaptive systems have the capacity to respond with situation-specific support as a person's or community's needs evolve. The following pages describe examples of these adaptive systems.

18.4.4 *Appreciating Physiological Processes*

Many biological processes serve a regulatory function. The sympathetic and parasympathetic nervous systems coordinate a person's activation and deactivation in accordance with situational needs. When functioning as expected, the hypothalamic-pituitary-adrenal (HPA) axis can titrate hormones to help a person respond dynamically to stressors and opportunities in the environment (Karin et al., 2020). Elaborate hormonal feedback loops guide moment-by-moment changes in cortisol levels. Metabolic processes plumb each bite of food for the nutrients needed in the body at a given time, with enzyme levels changing according to the organism's prior nutrient intake (Martínez-Gómez & Roberts, 2022). Healthy sleep appears to support cardiac responses to stress (Lü et al., 2018). Investing in a developing child's physical health is likely to support adaptation to changing circumstances for decades to come.

18.4.5 *Supporting Emotion Regulation*

Closely intertwined with physiological processes is a child's emotion regulation capacity. Emotion regulation is not a single system but includes biological circuits (such as the HPA axis and dopaminergic motivational systems; Baik, 2020; Karin et al., 2020), social practices (such as support-seeking; Garcia et al., 2020; Oppedal & Idsoe, 2015), and cognitive or behavioral skills (such as meaning-making, re-appraisal, or an orientation toward the future; Hosseini &

Punzi, 2023; Metzger et al., 2021). When young people are able to access these internal or external resources successfully, they can be buffered against many of the impacts of stress (Graham et al., 2015). Critically, each system that supports emotion regulation acts dynamically to promote goal-congruent behavior. A student benefits from accessing enthusiasm and energy during recess to connect with peers on the playground, reducing his sensation-seeking urges during math class (while maintaining enough energy to focus), and then calming down further when it is time to go to sleep. Similarly, it can be beneficial for a person to access negative emotionality to garner motivation to solve a problem, and then wholly experience positive emotions when the goal is met. The capacity to access and leverage emotions in service of goals helps a young person to benefit from their changing environment.

18.4.6 Encouraging Nurturing Relationships

It is unsurprising that positive social engagement is predictive of developmental competence for those exposed to a wide range of stressors (Feldman, 2021): Successfully connecting with others also guarantees ongoing connection to ever-evolving, situationally tailored support. In early life, caregiving relationships are the most important social adaptive systems. Sensitive caregivers are able to offer social stimulation when a child is alert and eager, feed her when she is hungry, clean her when she is dirty, and facilitate down-regulation when the child needs to sleep (DePasquale et al., 2019; Masten & Palmer, 2019). Additionally, developmental sensitivity to a child's needs can inform, say, whether a caregiver provides physical co-regulation to a young child who is distressed or scaffolds an older child in using his own emotion regulation strategies (Bernier et al., 2010; Borelli et al., 2021). When families have faced high levels of adversity, responsive parenting can buffer young children from developing behavioral and emotional difficulties (Greene et al., 2020).

As children grow, relationships outside of the home increasingly serve as adaptive systems as well (Mahon & Yarcheski, 2017). Friendships with peers can support goals as diverse as self-esteem development, hope for the future, help-seeking skills, and mood regulation (Costello et al., 2023). Under challenging circumstances like forced displacement, connections with peers can help youth cope with discrimination and access practical resources (Oppedal & Idsoe, 2015).

18.4.7 Building Social Structures

Resilience-informed international aid systems may intervene in a crisis to meet practical needs of an affected group while mobilizing local sociocultural resources in support of long-term, sustainable flourishing (Panter-Brick, 2023). Of course, these structures must tailor responses to the needs of each crisis, adapting approaches to within-country cultural differences, partnering with the appropriate individuals and organizations in each region, and adding, withdrawing, or changing supports as conditions change. For example, a famine relief program must consider dietary needs and preferences of each ethnic and religious group in a region, social norms around support-seeking, and the ideal balances between direct nutritional aid and support of food infrastructure at a given time.

In addition to providing psychosocial and spiritual benefits, religious and cultural organizations can promote civic engagement, physical health, and mental health (Coombs et al., 2022; Onyishi et al., 2022; Oskooii & Dana, 2018). Ethnic and religious peers in one's community can support needs as diverse as meaning-making during times of adversity, celebration during noteworthy milestones, identity development, and protection from some of the psychological harm of discrimination (Ip et al., 2023). Amplifying connections to these adaptive social structures through neighborhood cohesion, school belonging, religious involvement, or family cohesion connects children to responsive resources for the long term (Allen et al., 2016; Hobfoll, 2012).

18.4.8 Promoting Risk Reduction

As described, positive adaptation is, by and large, a common outcome in individuals and communities exposed to risks, due to the abundance of promotive and protective resources and the affected party's connection to other adaptive systems. However, the adaptive capacity of a system is not infinite and can be depleted as a result of chronic or severe stress. This is true, of course, of everything from the immune system to the global economy. Therefore, resilience-informed systems are also concerned with reducing the risks to which each child, family, and community is exposed. When risks are reduced, resources in the community and family can be used to promote flourishing rather than simply survival (Kilburn et al., 2017).

Fortunately, an abundance of research and common-sense wisdom can guide risk reduction efforts, from the individual to the chronosystem. Eliminating childhood adversity, particularly family–level adversity, would result in a 30% decrease in the lifetime incidence of mental health conditions around the world (Kessler et al., 2010), in part through easing the burden on adaptive systems. Ending practices of residential discrimination and reducing neighborhood violence will protect mental health among young people exposed to forced displacement and allow community-level adaptive systems to support development in the long term (e.g., Gillespie et al., 2020). Reducing young people's exposure to interpersonal discrimination can also protect their biological and social regulatory systems from strain (Njoroge et al., 2021; Samari et al., 2018; Siddiqi et al., 2017). Finally, as described throughout this book, climate change and armed conflict pose multisystem threats to child development. A resilience-informed global strategy for the 21st century entails ending reliance on fossil fuels and mobilizing community-led efforts toward peacebuilding and sustainable development.

Another pernicious risk begs mention: the separation of children from the systems that help them adapt after adversity. Forced displacement can abruptly compromise a child's connections to friendships and relationships within their cultural communities (Hodges & Abdi, 2023). The long-term risk profiles of children exposed to adversity differ substantially depending on their access to stable caregivers (Cohodes et al., 2021). A resilience-informed immigration policy suite, for example, prioritizes keeping families and communities together so that children can benefit from the relational assets and adaptive systems known to support their development. A resilience-informed economic system amplifies (rather than restricts) access to quality education, which is itself an adaptive system, equipping students to meet a society's changing needs.

18.4.9 Cultural Responsiveness

While there is striking cross-cultural similarity in resilience processes, there are also distinctive features observed in each community (Durbrow et al., 2016; Suárez-Orozco et al., 2018). While a strong sense of individual mastery is associated with more positive outcomes in some communities, those from collectivist or interdependent communities may benefit more from the tendency to attribute their successes to collaboration with others (Hobfoll et al., 2002). Particular beliefs (such as a faith that God keeps promises) may facilitate positive adaptation within a given culture (Pieloch et al., 2016). Resilience-informed systems frequently promote a person's connection to culturally conferred protective factors. For immigrant and refugee adolescents, contact with the heritage culture from afar through family, media, clubs, and events can support the development of a healthy, integrated identity (Gillespie et al., 2024). Programs that support young people's mental health should attend to relational dynamics within the patients' communities, asking who should be in the room when interventions are delivered, which leaders' endorsements and support can best support treatment delivery, and which interpersonal processes can best be leveraged to promote long-term positive outcomes (Goodkind et al., 2010; Rose-Clarke et al., 2020).

18.4.10 Leveraging Sensitive Periods

Many types of threat and deprivation impact young children with particular acuity, threatening developmental processes as they unfold and potentially cascading into other domains of functioning. However, there is also evidence that children's heightened sensitivity to negative events in their environment may correspond and coincide with heightened sensitivity to *positive* events and resources (Belsky & Pluess, 2009; Pluess & Belsky,

2013). Infancy and early childhood are examples of these "vantage sensitivity" periods, but they are not the only ones: A renewal of social and neural plasticity in adolescence can both amplify the impact of positive resources and also allow for recalibration of adaptive systems (DePasquale et al., 2019; Gee, 2022).

Resilience-informed systems can use knowledge of developmental science to plan the timing of interventions and supports. Supporting prenatal and perinatal access to nutrition and socioeconomic resources can reduce the impact of family stress on infant brain development, as both infant and parental sensitivity to the environment are heightened during this period (Nolvi et al., 2023). Interventions that support parenting sensitivity and environmental stability may have particularly strong effects for toddlers and early elementary-aged children, as this is a period in which children form the foundations of co-regulation and safety learning (Cohodes et al., 2023; Paley & Hajal, 2022). In addition to promoting an attitude of hopefulness in the context of mounting global risks, this perspective of vantage sensitivity or "positive vulnerability" is a powerful motivator for the urgent introduction of supports and reduction of risks early in the lifespan.

18.5 Resilience-Informed Systems in the 21st Century

It should be fairly clear from the previous section that most of the assets associated with positive development among children exposed to adversity are not unusual resources. Rather, they are very common; some are species-expected (such as functional metabolic systems and attachment relationships), and many are so mundane as to be passed over in accounts of overcoming (such as a responsive landlord, a childcare center, a predictable bus route, or a stable group of childhood friends). The term "ordinary magic" describes a contradiction at the core of resilience science: that positive adaptation after adversity is itself noteworthy, but there is rarely anything noteworthy or attention-grabbing about the assets and processes that support these outcomes (Masten, 2001).

It is fitting that the concept of ordinary magic emerged in scholarship right at the beginning of this tumultuous century. In the face of the multisystem risks to child development described throughout this book, it is reassuring to recall that resilient outcomes largely depend not on children's own "grit" or "toughness," nor on resources that are already rare (and increasingly scarce), but predominantly on the "stuff" of ordinary lives: relationships, ritual, community, hope, meaning-making.

In a resilience-informed system, every adult is aware of the roles they can play in promoting children's positive development after adversity. To illustrate the diversity of these roles, and to encourage readers to identify the parts they play in supporting children's resilience, this chapter closes with a few examples of the fruits a resilience lens can bear in various social systems.

In a Resilience-Informed City:

- New road-building projects ask how, with the least disturbance to environments and communities, resources and humans can flow between neighborhoods.
- Continuing education is available and affordable, allowing adults to build skills that meet their family's needs and the city's needs in a changing world.
- Youth can access easy on-ramps to activism, leadership, and civic engagement, which amplifies their agency and also drives need-informed policies and solutions.
- Drainage, communications, transit, and other infrastructure systems are built to account for natural disasters, droughts, and floods. Preparedness plans (ambulance re-routes, post-disaster information relays, etc.) allow operations to resume quickly after crises.

In a Resilience-Informed School System:

- Social and emotional learning curricula help children to learn the emotion regulation skills that will help them adapt to changing circumstances for their whole lives (Mahoney et al., 2018; Seff et al., 2024; Shi et al., 2022).
- The adults who drive school buses are supported with competitive salaries in their critical role of granting children access to the resilience caravan of the school community.
- Support staff like crossing guards, cafeteria workers, and custodians are trained to intervene in bullying. They are also supported in identifying children who may need mental health support.
- Clubs, staff, and curricula reflect the cultural and social identities of students. Children can connect positively with co-ethnic peers and leaders and access culturally specific protective resources.

Healthcare organizations, economies, immigration structures, and countless other systems similarly stand to benefit from applying resilience lenses. The resulting designs can reduce the risks to which children are exposed, increase access to critical resources, magnify the adaptive capacity of surrounding systems, engage responsively with culture and context, and tailor approaches developmentally.

Of note, the field of DRS is changing as the century progresses. Some changes are readily apparent, such as the field's increased reliance on multi-system modeling tactics, emphasis on multinational collaboration, and new focus on climate processes (Hasselman, 2023; Sanson et al., 2022). Other changes are on the horizon. For example, resilience science may begin soon to incorporate more methods from prevention science, asking how assets and adaptive systems may be acting to prevent the onset of risks. One other area of future growth in DRS is in the study of forcibly displaced children and youth; it is estimated that the field is at least four decades behind with regard to this population (Jafari et al., 2022). As the scale and complexity of immigration stories grow around the world, resilience scientists can help communities and interventionists prepare and respond in ways that support positive development. The field of DRS is itself, ideally, an adaptive system, taking in the evolving needs of the world's children as the century progresses and, in turn, changing its own goals and methods.

Reflection Questions

Question 1. According to DRS frameworks, resilience is an outcome of adaptive processes at diverse levels of a person's ecology. What have been some of the most important resources, internal or external, in your own adaptation to stress? Your community's adaptation?

Question 2. What roles can adults like you play in promoting children's positive development after adversity?

Question 3. How is your community already exhibiting principles of resilience-informed systems? How can it improve in this regard?

References

Abdi, S. M. (2018). *Mental health of migrant children.* August 28. Oxford Research Encyclopedia of Global Public Health. https://doi.org/10.1093/acrefore/9780190632366.013.12

Abraham, Z. K., & Sher, L. (2019). Adolescent suicide as a global public health issue. *International Journal of Adolescent Medicine and Health, 31*(4). https://doi.org/10.1515/ijamh-2017-0036

Afzal, A., Firdousi, S. F., Waqar, A., & Awais, M. (2022). The influence of internet penetration on poverty and income inequality. *Sage Open, 12*(3), 21582440221116104. https://doi.org/10.1177/21582440221116104

Allen, K., Kern, M. L., Vella-Brodrick, D., Hattie, J., & Waters, L. (2016). What schools need to know about fostering school belonging: A meta-analysis. *Educational Psychology Review, 30*(1), 1–34. https://doi.org/10.1007/S10648-016-9389-8

Appalachian Children Coalition (2025). https://www.appchildren.org/about

Baik, J.-H. (2020). Stress and the dopaminergic reward system. *Experimental & Molecular Medicine, 52*(12), 1879–1890. https://doi.org/10.1038/s12276-020-00532-4

Belsky, J., & Pluess, M. (2009). Beyond diathesis stress: Differential susceptibility to environmental influences. *Psychological Bulletin, 135*(6), 885–908. https://doi.org/10.1037/a0017376

Bernier, A., Carlson, S. M., & Whipple, N. (2010). From external regulation to self-regulation: Early parenting precursors of young children's executive functioning. *Child Development, 81*(1), 326–339.

Betancourt, T. S., Abdi, S., Ito, B. S., Lilienthal, G. M., Agalab, N., & Ellis, H. (2015). We left one war and came to another: Resource loss, acculturative stress, and caregiver–child relationships in Somali refugee families. *Cultural Diversity and Ethnic Minority Psychology, 21*(1), 114. https://doi.org/10.1037/a0037538

Betancourt, T. S., McBain, R., Newnham, E. A., & Brennan, R. T. (2013). Trajectories of internalizing problems in war-affected Sierra Leonean youth: Examining conflict and postconflict factors. *Child Development*, *84*(2), 455–470. https://doi.org/10.1111/j.1467-8624.2012.01861.x

Borelli, J. L., Lai, J., Smiley, P. A., Kerr, M. L., Buttitta, K., Hecht, H. K., & Rasmussen, H. F. (2021). Higher maternal reflective functioning is associated with toddlers' adaptive emotion regulation. *Infant Mental Health Journal*, *42*(4), 473–487. https://doi.org/10.1002/imhj.21904

Brady, M. (2016). Gluing, catching and connecting: How informal childcare strengthens single mothers' employment trajectories *Work, Employment and Society*. *30*(5), 821–837. https://doi.org/10.1177/0950017016630259

Caldwell, B. A., Ordway, M. R., Sadler, L. S., & Redeker, N. S. (2020). Parent perspectives on sleep and sleep habits among young children living with economic adversity. *Journal of Pediatric Health Care*, *34*(1), 10–22. https://doi.org/10.1016/j.pedhc.2019.06.006

Cardoso, J. B. (2018). Running to stand still: Trauma symptoms, coping strategies, and substance use behaviors in unaccompanied migrant youth. *Children and Youth Services Review*, *92*, 143–152. https://doi.org/10.1016/j.childyouth.2018.04.018

Chavez-Dueñas, N. Y., Adames, H. Y., Perez-Chavez, J. G., & Salas, S. P. (2019). Healing ethno-racial trauma in Latinx immigrant communities: Cultivating hope, resistance, and action. *American Psychologist*, *74*(1), 49–62. https://doi.org/10.1037/amp0000289

Cohodes, E. M., Kribakaran, S., Odriozola, P., Bakirci, S., McCauley, S., Hodges, H. R., Sisk, L. M., Zacharek, S. J., & Gee, D. G. (2021). Migration-related trauma and mental health among migrant children emigrating from Mexico and Central America to the United States: Effects on developmental neurobiology and implications for policy. *Developmental Psychobiology*, *63*(6), e22158. https://doi.org/10.1002/dev.22158

Cohodes, E. M., Sisk, L. M., Keding, T. J., Mandell, J. D., Notti, M. E., & Gee, D. G. (2023). Characterizing experiential elements of early-life stress to inform resilience: Buffering effects of controllability and predictability and the importance of their timing. *Development and Psychopathology*, 1–14. https://doi.org/10.1017/S0954579423000822

Coombs, A., Joshua, A., Flowers, M., Wisdom, J., Crayton, L. S., Frazier, K., & Hankerson, S. H. (2022). Mental health perspectives among Black Americans receiving services from a church-affiliated mental health clinic. *Psychiatric Services*, *73*(1), 77–82. https://doi.org/10.1176/appi.ps.202000766

Costello, M. A., Allen, J. P., Womack, S. R., Loeb, E. L., Stern, J. A., & Pettit, C. (2023). Characterizing emotional support development: From adolescent best friendships to young adult romantic relationships. *Journal of Research on Adolescence*, *33*(2), 389–403. https://doi.org/10.1111/jora.12809

DePasquale, C. E., Donzella, B., & Gunnar, M. R. (2019). Pubertal recalibration of cortisol reactivity following early life stress: A cross-sectional analysis. *Journal of Child Psychology and Psychiatry*, *60*(5), 566–575. https://doi.org/10.1111/jcpp.12992

DePasquale, C. E., & Gunnar, M. R. (2020). Parental sensitivity and nurturance. *The Future of Children*, *30*(2), 53–70.

Diener, E., Lucas, R. E., & Oishi, S. (2018). Advances and open questions in the science of subjective well-being. *Collabra: Psychology*, *4*(1), 15. https://doi.org/10.1525/collabra.115

Diliberti, M., Schwartz, H., Hamilton, L., & Kaufman, J. (2020). Prepared for a pandemic? How schools' preparedness related to their remote instruction during COVID-19. *Prepared for a Pandemic? How Schools' Preparedness Related to Their Remote Instruction During COVID-19*. https://doi.org/10.7249/RRA168-3

Duggan, C., Wilson, C., DiPonio, L., Trumpower, B., & Meade, M. A. (2016). Resilience and happiness after spinal cord injury: A qualitative study. *Topics in Spinal Cord Injury Rehabilitation*, *22*(2), 99–110. https://doi.org/10.1310/sci2202-99

Durbrow, E. H., Pen, L. F., Masten, A., Sesma, A., & Williamson, I. (2016). Mothers' conceptions of child competence in contexts of poverty: The Philippines, St Vincent, and the United States. *International Journal of Behavioral Development*, *25*(5), 438–443. https://doi.org/10.1080/016502501316934860

Feldman, R. (2021). Social behavior as a transdiagnostic marker of resilience. *Annual Review of Clinical Psychology*, *17*(1), 153–180. https://doi.org/10.1146/annurev-clinpsy-081219-102046

Galway, L. P., Acharya, Y., & Jones, A. D. (2018). Deforestation and child diet diversity: A geospatial analysis of 15 Sub-Saharan African countries. *Health & Place*, *51*, 78–88. https://doi.org/10.1016/j.healthplace.2018.03.002

Garcia, J., Vargas, N., Clark, J. L., Magaña Álvarez, M., Nelons, D. A., & Parker, R. G. (2020). Social isolation and connectedness as determinants of well-being: Global evidence mapping focused on LGBTQ youth. *Global Public Health*, *15*(4), 497–519. https://doi.org/10.1080/17441692.2019.1682028

Gee, D. G. (2022). When do sensitive periods emerge later in development? *Trends in Cognitive Sciences*, *26*(2), 97–98. https://doi.org/10.1016/j.tics.2021.12.001

Gillespie, S., Cardeli, E., Sideridis, G., Issa, O., & Ellis, B. H. (2020). Residential mobility, mental health, and community violence exposure among Somali refugees and immigrants in North America. *Health & Place*, *65*. https://doi.org/10.1016/j.healthplace.2020.102419

Gillespie, S., Hodges, H. R., Abdi, K., Gibson, H., Harnack, L., & Ferguson, G. M. (2024). Remote enculturation among Black immigrant adolescents in the United States. *Journal of Applied Developmental Psychology*, *91*, 101627. https://doi.org/10.1016/j.appdev.2023.101627

Girme, Y. U., Jones, R. E., Fleck, C., Simpson, J. A., & Overall, N. C. (2021). Infants' attachment insecurity predicts attachment-relevant emotion regulation strategies in adulthood. *Emotion*, *21*(2), 260–272. https://doi.org/10.1037/emo0000721

Godleski, S. A., & Ostrov, J. M. (2020). Parental influences on child report of relational attribution biases during early childhood. *Journal of Experimental Child Psychology*, *192*, 104775. https://doi.org/10.1016/j.jecp.2019.104775

Goodkind, J. R., LaNoue, M. D., & Milford, J. (2010). Adaptation and implementation of cognitive behavioral intervention for trauma in schools with American Indian youth. *Journal of Clinical Child and Adolescent Psychology: The Official Journal for the Society of Clinical Child and Adolescent Psychology, American Psychological Association, Division 53*, *39*(6), 858–872. https://doi.org/10.1080/15374416.2010.517166

Graham, J. R., Calloway, A., & Roemer, L. (2015). The buffering effects of emotion regulation in the relationship between experiences of racism and anxiety in a black American sample. *Cognitive Therapy and Research*, *39*(5), 553–563. https://doi.org/10.1007/s10608-015-9682-8

Greene, C. A., McCarthy, K. J., Estabrook, R., Wakschlag, L. S., & Briggs-Gowan, M. J. (2020). Responsive parenting buffers the impact of maternal PTSD on young children. *Parenting*, *20*(2), 141–165. https://doi.org/10.1080/15295192.2019.1707623

Hash, K. M., Schreurs, B. G., Tolley, S. M., & Fiske, A. (2024). Health disparities in appalachian and other rural communities. *The International Journal of Aging and Human Development*, *98*(1), 56–68.

Hasselman, F. (2023). Understanding the complexity of individual developmental pathways: A primer on metaphors, models, and methods to study resilience in development. *Development and Psychopathology*, *35*(5), 2186–2198. https://doi.org/10.1017/S0954579423001281

Hobfoll, S. E. (2012). Conservation of resources and disaster in cultural context: The caravans and passageways for resources. *Psychiatry: Interpersonal and Biological Processes*, *75*(3), 227–232. https://doi.org/10.1521/psyc.2012.75.3.227

Hobfoll, S. E., Jackson, A., Hobfoll, I., Pierce, C. A., & Young, S. (2002). The impact of communal-mastery versus self-mastery on emotional outcomes during stressful conditions: A prospective study of native American women. *American Journal of Community Psychology 2002 30:6*, *30*(6), 853–871. https://doi.org/10.1023/A:1020209220214

Hodges, H., & Abdi, S. (2024). *Forced displacement. Encyclopedia of Adolescence* (2nd ed., Vol. 2, pp. 112–127). https://doi.org/10.1016/B978-0-323-96023-6.00018-X

Hogan, M. F., & Goldman, M. L. (2021). New opportunities to improve mental health crisis systems. *Psychiatric Services*, *72*(2), 169–173. https://doi.org/10.1176/appi.ps.202000114

Hosseini, M., & Punzi, E. (2023). "Through my poems, I wanted a sense of recognition": Afghan unaccompanied refugee minors' experiences of poetic writing, migration, and resettlement. *Journal of Poetry Therapy*, *36*(2), 131–143. https://doi.org/10.1080/08893675.2022.2147033

Ickowitz, A., Powell, B., Salim, M. A., & Sunderland, T. C. H. (2014). Dietary quality and tree cover in Africa. *Global Environmental Change*, *24*, 287–294. https://doi.org/10.1016/j.gloenvcha.2013.12.001

Ip, K. I., Wen, W., Sim, L., Chen, S., & Kim, S. Y. (2023). Associations of household and neighborhood contexts and hair cortisol among adolescents from low-income Mexican immigrant families [PDF]. *Minnesota Population Center Working Paper Series*. https://doi.org/10.18128/MPC2023-01

Jabr, D., & Cahan, S. (2014). Schooling effects on cognitive development in a difficult environment: The case of refugee camps in the West Bank. *International Studies in Sociology of Education*, *24*(2), 165–188. https://doi.org/10.1080/09620214.2014.900949

Jafari, H., Kassan, A., Reay, G., & Climie, E. A. (2022). Resilience in refugee children and youth: A critical literature review. *Canadian Psychology / Psychologie Canadienne*, *63*(4), 678–694. https://doi.org/10.1037/cap0000320

Johnson, C. M. (2010). African-American teen girls grieve the loss of friends to homicide: Meaning making and resilience. *OMEGA - Journal of Death and Dying*, *61*(2), 121–143. https://doi.org/10.2190/OM.61.2.c

Jones, S. C. T., & Neblett, E. W. (2016). *Racial-ethnic protective factors and mechanisms in psychosocial prevention and intervention programs for black youth*. https://doi.org/10.1007/s10567-016-0201-6

Karin, O., Raz, M., Tendler, A., Bar, A., Korem Kohanim, Y., Milo, T., & Alon, U. (2020). A new model for the HPA axis explains dysregulation of stress hormones on the timescale of weeks. *Molecular Systems Biology*, *16*(7), e9510. https://doi.org/10.15252/msb.20209510

Kessler, R. C., McLaughlin, K. A., Green, J. G., Gruber, M. J., Sampson, N. A., Zaslavsky, A. M., Aguilar-Gaxiola, S., Alhamzawi, A. O., Alonso, J., Angermeyer, M., Benjet, C., Bromet, E., Chatterji, S., Girolamo, G. de, Demyttenaere, K., Fayyad, J., Florescu, S., Gal, G., Gureje, O., Haro, J. M., Hu, C,... Williams, D. R. (2010). Childhood adversities and adult psychopathology in the WHO World Mental Health Surveys. *The British Journal of Psychiatry*, *197*(5), 378–385. https://doi.org/10.1192/bjp.bp.110.080499.

Kia-Keating, M., & Ellis, B. H. (2007). Belonging and connection to school in resettlement: Young refugees, school belonging, and psychosocial adjustment. *Clinical Child Psychology and Psychiatry*, *12*(1), 29–43. https://doi.org/10.1177/1359104507071052

Kilburn, K., Handa, S., Angeles, G., Mvula, P., & Tsoka, M. (2017). Short-term impacts of an unconditional cash transfer program on child schooling: Experimental evidence from Malawi. *Economics of Education Review*, *59*, 63–80. https://doi.org/10.1016/j.econedurev.2017.06.002

Lai, B. S., Esnard, A.-M., Wyczalkowski, C., Savage, R., & Shah, H. (2019). Trajectories of school recovery after a natural disaster: Risk and protective factors. *Risk, Hazards & Crisis in Public Policy*, *10*(1), 32–51. https://doi.org/10.1002/rhc3.12158

Laude, M. (1999). Assessment of nutritional status, cognitive development, and mother-child interaction in Central American refugee children. *Revista Panamericana de Salud Pública*, *6*(3), 164–171. https://doi.org/10.1590/S1020-49891999000800003

Lü, W., Hughes, B. M., Howard, S., & James, J. E. (2018). Sleep restriction undermines cardiovascular adaptation during stress, contingent on emotional stability. *Biological Psychology*, *132*, 125–132. https://doi.org/10.1016/j.biopsycho.2017.11.013

Mahon, N. E., & Yarcheski, A. (2017). Parent and friend social support and adolescent hope. *Clinical Nursing Research*, *26*(2), 224–240. https://doi.org/10.1177/1054773815619881

Mahoney, J. L., Durlak, J. A., & Weissberg, R. P. (2018). An update on social and emotional learning outcome research. *Phi Delta Kappan*, *100*(4), 18–23. https://doi.org/10.1177/0031721718815668

Martinelli, A., Ackermann, K., Bernhard, A., Freitag, C. M., & Schwenck, C. (2018). Hostile attribution bias and aggression in children and adolescents: A systematic literature review on the influence of aggression subtype and gender. *Aggression and Violent Behavior*, *39*, 25–32. https://doi.org/10.1016/j.avb.2018.01.005

Martínez-Gómez, M. G., & Roberts, B. M. (2022). Metabolic adaptations to weight loss: A brief review. *The Journal of Strength & Conditioning Research*, *36*(10), 2970. https://doi.org/10.1519/JSC.0000000000003991

Masten, A. S. (2001). Ordinary magic. Resilience processes in development. *The American Psychologist*, *56*(3), 227–238. https://doi.org/10.1037//0003-066x.56.3.227

Masten, A. S., & Barnes, A. J. (2018). Resilience in children: Developmental perspectives. *Children*, *5*(7), Article 7. https://doi.org/10.3390/children5070098

Masten, A. S., & Hodges, H. R. (2025). Ordinary magic: Promoting resilience in children and their support systems. *Appalachian Children Coalition, Newsletter.*

Masten, A. S., Lucke, C. M., Nelson, K. M., & Stallworthy, I. C. (2021). Resilience in development and psychopathology: Multisystem perspectives. *Annual Review*

Review of Clinical Psychology, *17*(1), 521–549. https://doi.org/10.1146/annurev-clinpsy-081219-120307

Masten, A. S., & Motti-Stefanidi, F. (2020). Multisystem resilience for children and youth in disaster: Reflections in the context of COVID-19. *Adversity and Resilience Science*, *1*(2), 95–106. https://doi.org/10.1007/s42844-020-00010-w

Masten, A. S., & Palmer, A. R. (2019). Parenting to promote resilience in children. In *Handbook of parenting: The practice of parenting* (vol. 5, 3rd ed., pp. 156–188). Routledge/Taylor & Francis Group. https://doi.org/10.4324/9780429401695-6

McGinnis, J. M. (2016). Income, life expectancy, and community health: Underscoring the opportunity. *JAMA*, *315*(16), 1709–1710. https://doi.org/10.1001/JAMA.2016.4729

Metzger, I. W., Anderson, R. E., Are, F., & Ritchwood, T. (2021). Healing interpersonal and racial trauma: Integrating Racial socialization into trauma-focused cognitive behavioral therapy for African American youth. *Child Maltreatment*, *26*(1), 17–27. https://doi.org/10.1177/1077559520921457

Nakkash, R. T., Alaouie, H., Haddad, P., El Hajj, T., Salem, H., Mahfoud, Z., & Afifi, R. A. (2012). Process evaluation of a community-based mental health promotion intervention for refugee children. *Health Education Research*, *27*(4), 595–607. https://doi.org/10.1093/her/cyr062

Njoroge, W. F. M., Forkpa, M., & Bath, E. (2021). Impact of racial discrimination on the mental health of minoritized youth. *Current Psychiatry Reports*, *23*(12), 81. https://doi.org/10.1007/s11920-021-01297-x

Nolvi, S., Merz, E. C., Kataja, E.-L., & Parsons, C. E. (2023). Prenatal stress and the developing brain: Postnatal environments promoting resilience. *Biological Psychiatry*, *93*(10), 942–952. https://doi.org/10.1016/j.biopsych.2022.11.023

Oberg, C., Hodges, H. R., & Masten, A. S. (2022). Conflict, war, and famine in childhood. In *The Wiley-Blackwell handbook of childhood social development* (pp. 189–205). John Wiley & Sons, Ltd. https://doi.org/10.1002/9781119679028.ch10

Obradović, J., van Dulmen, M. H. M., Yates, T. M., Carlson, E. A., & Egeland, B. (2006). Developmental assessment of competence from early childhood to middle adolescence. *Journal of Adolescence*, *29*(6), 857–889. https://doi.org/10.1016/j.adolescence.2006.04.009

Onyishi, C. N., Eseadi, C., Ilechukwu, L. C., Okoro, K. N., Okolie, C. N., Egbule, E., & Asogwa, E. (2022). Potential influences of religiosity and religious coping strategies on people with diabetes. *World Journal of Clinical Cases*, *10*(25), 8816–8826. https://doi.org/10.12998/wjcc.v10.i25.8816

Oppedal, B., & Idsoe, T. (2015). The role of social support in the acculturation and mental health of unaccompanied minor asylum seekers. *Scandinavian Journal of Psychology*, *56*(2), 203–211. https://doi.org/10.1111/sjop.12194

Oskooii, K. A. R., & Dana, K. (2018). Muslims in Great Britain: The impact of mosque attendance on political behaviour and civic engagement. *Journal of Ethnic and Migration Studies*, *44*(9), 1479–1505. https://doi.org/10.1080/1369183X.2017.1330652

Paley, B., & Hajal, N. J. (2022). Conceptualizing emotion regulation and coregulation as family-level phenomena. *Clinical Child and Family Psychology Review*, *25*(1), 19–43. https://doi.org/10.1007/s10567-022-00378-4

Panter-Brick, C. (2023). Pathways to resilience and pathways to flourishing: Examining the added-value of multisystem research and intervention in contexts of war and forced displacement. *Development and Psychopathology*, *35*(5), 2214–2225. https://doi.org/10.1017/S095457942300113X

Pieloch, K. A., McCullough, M. B., & Marks, A. K. (2016). Resilience of children with refugee statuses: A research review. *Canadian Psychology / Psychologie Canadienne, 57*(4), 330–339. https://doi.org/10.1037/cap0000073

Pluess, M., & Belsky, J. (2013). Vantage sensitivity: Individual differences in response to positive experiences. *Psychological Bulletin, 139*(4), 901–916. https://doi.org/10.1037/a0030196

Raniga, T., and Mthembu, M. (2016). Family resilience in low income communities: A case study of an informal settlement in KwaZulu-Natal, South Africa. *International Journal of Social Welfare, 26*, 1369–6866. https://doi.org/10.1111/ijsw.12243

Rose-Clarke, K., Pradhan, I., Shrestha, P., B. K., P., Magar, J., Luitel, N. P., Devakumar, D., Rafaeli, A. K., Clougherty, K., Kohrt, B. A., Jordans, M. J. D., & Verdeli, H. (2020). Culturally and developmentally adapting group interpersonal therapy for adolescents with depression in rural Nepal. *BMC Psychology, 8*(1), Article 1. https://doi.org/10.1186/s40359-020-00452-y

Samari, G., Alcalá, H. E., & Sharif, M. Z. (2018). Islamophobia, health, and public health: A systematic literature review. *American Journal of Public Health, 108*(6), e1–e9. https://doi.org/10.2105/AJPH.2018.304402

Sanson, A. V., Malca, K. P., Hoorn, J. V., & Burke, S. (2022). Children and climate change. *Elements in Child Development*. https://doi.org/10.1017/9781009118705

Scarborough, W. J., Collins, C., Ruppanner, L., & Landivar, L. C. (2021). Head start and families' recovery from economic recession: Policy recommendations for COVID-19. *Family Relations, 70*(1), 26–42. https://doi.org/10.1111/FARE.12519

Seff, I., Stark, L., Ali, A., Sarraf, D., Hassan, W., & Allaf, C. (2024). Supporting social emotional learning and wellbeing of displaced adolescents from the middle east: A pilot evaluation of the 'forward with peers' intervention. *BMC Psychiatry, 24*(1), 176. https://doi.org/10.1186/s12888-024-05544-2

Shangani, S., Operario, D., Genberg, B., Kirwa, K., Midoun, M., Atwoli, L., Ayuku, D., Galárraga, O., & Braitstein, P. (2017). Unconditional government cash transfers in support of orphaned and vulnerable adolescents in western Kenya: Is there an association with psychological wellbeing? *PLOS ONE, 12*(5), e0178076. https://doi.org/10.1371/journal.pone.0178076

Shi, J., Cheung, A. C. K., & Ni, A. (2022). The effectiveness of promoting alternative thinking strategies program: A meta-analysis. *Frontiers in Psychology, 13*. https://doi.org/10.3389/fpsyg.2022.1030572

Siddiqi, A., Shahidi, F. V., Ramraj, C., & Williams, D. R. (2017). Associations between race, discrimination and risk for chronic disease in a population-based sample from Canada. *Social Science & Medicine, 194*, 135–141. https://doi.org/10.1016/j.socscimed.2017.10.009

Śliwerski, A., Kossakowska, K., Jarecka, K., Świtalska, J., & Bielawska-Batorowicz, E. (2020). The effect of maternal depression on infant attachment: A systematic review. *International Journal of Environmental Research and Public Health, 17*(8), Article 8. https://doi.org/10.3390/ijerph17082675

Suárez-Orozco, C., Motti-Stefanidi, F., Marks, A., & Katsiaficas, D. (2018). An integrative risk and resilience model for understanding the adaptation of immigrant-origin children and youth. *American Psychologist, 73*(6), 781–796. https://doi.org/10.1037/AMP0000265

Ungar, M., Ghazinour, M., & Richter, J. (2013). Annual research review: What is resilience within the social ecology of human development? *Journal of Child Psychology and Psychiatry, 54*(4), 348–366. https://doi.org/10.1111/jcpp.12025

Vernarelli, J. A., & O'Brien, B. (2017). A vote for school lunches: School lunches provide superior nutrient quality than lunches obtained from other sources in a nationally representative sample of US children. *Nutrients 2017, 9*(9), 924. https://doi.org/10.3390/NU9090924

Zimmerman, A., Garman, E., Avendano-Pabon, M., Araya, R., Evans-Lacko, S., McDaid, D., Park, A.-L., Hessel, P., Diaz, Y., Matijasevich, A., Ziebold, C., Bauer, A., Paula, C. S., & Lund, C. (2021). The impact of cash transfers on mental health in children and young people in low-income and middle-income countries: A systematic review and meta-analysis. *BMJ Global Health, 6*(4), e004661. https://doi.org/10.1136/bmjgh-2020-004661

19 Bearing Witness Through Research

19.1 Introduction

A just future will be one in which the world attends and responds to children's voices for change. In the meantime, given that most societies are built to honor adults' voices over children's, adults can use their privileged positions to magnify the stories of young people. In essence, they can tell the truth. This and the following chapters describe a few ways that adults may be equipped to tell the truth about children's needs, children's rights, and children's potential in the world, through a wide range of professional and public-facing activities. Of course, this list is certainly incomplete; there are as many ways and as many reasons to bear witness as there are people in this world.

Many people reading this will find that their "first language" for witnessing is *research*. In fields as diverse as pediatrics, clinical psychology, urban planning, and economics, professionals synthesize and present stories of human development. These findings spread in print journals, classrooms, the internet, social media, word of mouth, diverse policy and practice channels, and between members of participant communities. Research teams describe the challenges children face, the impacts of these risks, the factors that confer protections, and the effects of interventions.

19.2 Research Strategies

This chapter describes ways in which, when conducted with integrity and excellence, and when communicated thoughtfully through the proper channels, research findings may equip child-friendly actions among caregivers, practitioners, and policy makers. It additionally describes some of the features of research that can help make a difference for child development in the 21st century.

19.2.1 Child-Focused Community Engagement

To tell the truth about children, one must hear from them. Most often, this means going where children are and listening. It is often very difficult for a

DOI: 10.4324/9781003488385-23

university-based researcher to ethically and accurately depict the lived experience of children facing marginalization. This is due, in part, to the process of acculturating to academia (which can involve, among other things, learning to attend to empirical epistemologies above other ways of knowing, as well as an emphasis on products over process) and to the sometimes steep power differentials between researchers and participants. Even when researchers are members of the communities they study, these power differentials can persist, impeding participants' trust in the research process and their belief that findings will benefit their communities. Further, many universities and other research bodies have poor reputations within communities for engaging in exploitative or "helicopter" research, extracting data without committing to sustainable partnerships—or, worse, benefitting from findings at the expense of participants (Hodges et al., 2024).

Community-engaged research emerges as an antidote to these harms and, even more, out of a positive vision for what knowledge co-creation can be: by and for the people most directly involved; part of the engines of structural justice; a tool for social healing; and honoring to local priorities and ways of knowing. There are many iterations of community engagement in research, and readers may be familiar with terms like community-based participatory research (CBPR), participatory action research (PAR), and action research, though the lines between these orientations are sometimes unclear. A few core tenets of community engagement are listed below:

- Research occurring as much as possible in community-run spaces
- Power-sharing between researchers and communities
- Partnerships that promote lasting, sustainable, positive effects within communities
- Capacity-building within communities
- Reliance on long-term partnerships
- Deference to community partners around methods, pacing, and even research questions
- Dedication to the creation of new knowledge useful to communities (rather than extraction of knowledge)

Community engagement exists on a spectrum. One team may simply rely on local organizations to recruit participants in the ways they see fit while another may also use a community advisory board to give feedback on planned questionnaires and methods. Some research teams function in the context of long-term, sustainable research partnerships. While a "gold standard" for community-engaged research is, arguably, a fully community-led study (where, for example, researchers are invited to join a research effort that is ongoing in a community), any study can be improved through power-sharing with community partners. The benefits are likely to include more positive participant experiences, more accurate representation of a community, more representative samples, a greater understanding of constructs in question, more impactful dissemination efforts, and long-term relationships (Foster et al., 2024).

One developmental resilience science team spent years running a research lab inside a homeless shelter. This team's continual presence in this setting, combined with the mutual respect they enjoyed with shelter staff and residents, resulted in a suite of research findings (and even new research questions) on children and families' resilience amid the multisystem stressors of housing loss (Distefano et al., 2021). For example, in partnering with families facing homelessness and the staff that served them, researchers learned of the importance of sleep routines amid the stress of housing loss and began to develop new research protocols and interventions to reflect this family-voiced need (Labella et al., 2017).

In all of this, it is important to remember that children are likely to be themselves key partners in child-focused research. They are, for one thing, natural researchers, often possessing abundant questions and a drive to answer them (Yardley, 2014). Researchers who make space for children to share their questions and participate in knowledge co-creation frequently find eager collaborators with creative methodological ideas and even nuanced interpretations of findings. Those who host colloquia, conferences, and other gatherings of knowledge-producers may be surprised by the fruits that can come from inviting children as honored guests and fellow knowledge-seekers.

19.2.2 Courage and Creativity

As noted throughout this book, many of the issues most relevant to child development in the 21st century foreclose the possibility of simple, lab-based research protocols. It is hard to imagine how the traditional model of university-based research could meaningfully document, for example, the developmental impacts of a disease outbreak in a refugee camp, or the ways that camp structures and social efforts may slow the disease. Even a skilled field researcher cannot arrange ethics board approval, travel arrangements, and a trained team in time to study the immediate impact of a wildfire on children's mental health. These questions may be asked inside a laboratory, but they can rarely (and only partially) be answered there.

To conduct research with children amid the challenges of the century requires flexibility, proactivity, and, for many researchers, a departure from the methods and orientations in which they were trained. For example, some teams have succeeded in measuring long-term changes in physiological stress among young Syrian refugees, including in response to psychosocial support interventions. In one study, local hairdressers were hired to offer participants a free professional haircut and, with participants' permission, collected a sample of hair, which was then analyzed for cortisol concentrations (Dajani et al., 2018). This protocol succeeded in large part due to its low invasiveness and minimal burden to participants. Many scholars, including some from the teams described in this section, have argued for the development of novel research orientations and methodologies that are suited for use in humanitarian, conflict, and post-disaster settings (Panter-Brick, 2023). Such frameworks would not merely be a way of extracting data, but would flow from long-term, interdisciplinary, equitable partnerships that go beyond addressing crises and work sustainably towards community goals.

Research teams hoping to learn about child development amid acute and chronic stressors and strains often benefit from technologies like cellphone surveys or wearable physiology tools. For example, cellphone location data has been used to assess the extent of a community's return to normal movement after a natural disaster and to track the possible spread of pathogens during epidemics (Yabe et al., 2022). Ecological momentary analysis has been used to non-invasively assess the impact of witnessing violence and substance use on young people's social and health behavior (Russel & Gajos, 2020), and these methods may be useful for measuring the impact of some other chronic or frequent stressors on children, such as the death of livestock during droughts or exposure to political extremist rhetoric. Some researchers have already begun to demonstrate the feasibility of using wearable data collection devices such as heart rate monitors, proximity sensors, or electroencephalography (EEG) headbands in settings like rural villages in Malawi or emergency shelters (Leonard et al., 2018; Neto et al., 2021). New partnerships—such as with federal emergency management teams, military groups, and local communities—may allow researchers to proactively plan for data collection before, during, and after a crisis (Morton & Levy, 2011). Propensity score matching and natural experiments also have the potential to support ethical data collection in light of disasters.

19.2.3 Texture

Just as many people have a "first language," many researchers have a "home field" methodology (e.g., magnetic resonance imaging or school-based action research) and theoretical approach (e.g., family systems, global pediatrics, or general strain theory). As previously described, the challenges and opportunities faced by children in the 21st century are often complex and rarely intelligible through one lens alone. To design interventions for malnutrition during a drought, one may find oneself consulting with local and global experts in agriculture, education, transportation, economics, pediatrics and public health.

A transdisciplinary team science approach can help scholars to leverage the diverse skill sets and interpretive instincts of researchers, practitioners, and community members (Ferguson et al., 2019; Stokols et al., 2008). In one study on refugee health, for example, scholars from developmental psychology, nutrition, and advertising came together with community liaisons and youth advisors to design research protocols that would capture multiple facets of young people's health decision-making, from cultural identity to media literacy (Hodges et al., 2024). A person engaged in team science approaches has access to methodological skills through colleagues that they may not have been able to develop on their own; a diverse suite of cultural and theoretical interpretive lenses; and wider dissemination networks for findings.

Arguably, some of the most impactful research findings emerge with one clear narrative. Readers or listeners may walk away grasping a simple truth, such as, "Exposure to racism impacts child development by eroding self-esteem, relationships, and social trust," or, "Healthy sleep is especially critical—but especially vulnerable—in high-stress environments." However, many people find that the essence and import of research findings emerge most clearly when multiple "doors" are available through which one can access them. Mixed methods research can open such doors. In these projects, a chorus of testimonies emerges around a given topic, including (but not limited to) descriptive statistics, graphical depictions of structural models, excerpts from focus group interviews, and community-generated interpretive summaries of research findings. Frequently, the "whole" generated from the presence of multiple methodological lenses is greater than the sum of its parts. For example, a study that reports on the fluctuations in the diurnal cortisol patterns of preschool-aged children in a refugee camp offers a more complete picture of physiological stress and buffering experiences when it includes caregiver accounts of children's morning routines, day-to-day activities, sleep environments, and co-regulation opportunities. It has been said that quantitative methods can help to identify the relationships that exist between variables, while qualitative methods are often necessary for describing the *how* or the *why* of these relationships. Other uses of mixed methods can include using one method to flesh out another (e.g., recording focus group participants reacting to and interpreting survey findings); using one method as a springboard (e.g., growing curious about a phenomenon based on a case study and seeking to grasp it quantitatively); or using one method to identify nuances in findings from another method (e.g., collecting caregivers' narratives about their children alongside survey data on the same topics; Jones & Sumner, 2009).

In addition to adding richness to the findings it produces, mixed methods approaches may improve the accuracy and applicability of research. For example, a team may engage with community members to better appreciate the meaning of constructs (e.g., a study on housing instability may also include textured testimonies from youth about the meaning of "safety" or "home"; Foster et al., 2024). One ethical benefit of this approach is that it allows participants to represent themselves and the constructs of relevance to the audience directly (Hodges et al., 2024). Centering participant voices in this way has the potential to mitigate some of the toxic social effects of poverty and marginalization, which are often defined by the experience of being overlooked, discounted, or not listened to (Jones & Sumner, 2009). In fact, mixed methods research may help to support dignifying and flexible knowledge generation processes in high-intensity or unpredictable environments (Hansen et al., 2016).

From an impact perspective, too, mixed methods arguably increase the chances that each member of the audience may find a "door" through which to enter into the research emotionally and motivationally. At times, a statistic may move a reader to change their mind or take new actions to protect and promote the wellbeing of children. Ninety percent of migrant mothers arriving in the United States from Central and South America reported fearing for their children's lives during the journey (Ornelas & Perreira, 2011). One in thirty U.S. children experiences a bomb or attack threat against their school in a given year (Finkelhor et al., 2013).

Other times, it is the "zoomed in" testimony of a single speaker. Baby Constantin, at four months old, was the youngest child separated from his family at the U.S. border in 2019. His father had sold two pigs and a cow to pay for his emergency C-section in a hospital (Dickerson & Heisler, 2019). Perhaps it is the picture that Fayette S. took of a hallway fire extinguisher in 2016 and the way she described what it meant to have a mentor through the Saving Lives, Inspiring Youth project in Chicago: "a safety support in a time of need" (2016).

19.2.4 Implementation-Informed Dissemination

Regardless of the methods chosen for research, teams are wise to invest in thoughtful dissemination plans. Findings have the greatest impact when they are conveyed in ways that are intelligible, actionable, and compelling. Multi-pronged dissemination strategies are often advisable. For example, findings about parenting practices that support children's wellbeing during residential instability can be distributed directly to community parents, shelter staff, and childcare workers; to clinicians who work with families under stress; to academic audiences who study child development and parenting; and to policy personnel who are equipped to direct funding and public attention toward parenting and housing supports. One clear benefit of this approach is its potential to support the development of children in the here and now. Translational researchers have identified a 17-year "bench to bedside" lag time, such that the average basic research finding takes many years to influence practice and lived experiences (Morris et al., 2011). Of course, children and families exposed to the highest levels of risk and marginalization may benefit from these findings at an even slower rate. Targeted dissemination directly to caregivers and practitioners accelerates the rate at which critical research findings can promote the wellbeing of rapidly developing children.

Broadly speaking, dissemination plans should reflect a goal of capacity-building—that is, how can these findings be leveraged to improve the ability of individuals and systems to meet the needs of children? One assumption that may prove useful in research and practice is the compassionate belief that most individuals and most systems are operating at or above their current capacity to serve; therefore, expanding the ceiling of their functioning (through resources, knowledge, or refinement of operations) is necessary to increase their usefulness to children. Implementation science efforts can accompany basic science and intervention research, identifying ways in which practices and knowledge can gain traction in communities and be maximally leveraged for change (Aboud et al., 2018). For example, an implementation science inquiry (with a capacity-building goal) may ask:

- *What cultural and practical barriers can contribute to the success of an early childhood intervention when it is translated from an urban setting to a rural one?*
- *What training and monitoring components are most important to assuring the fidelity of a brief psychological intervention in transit camps?*
- *What administrative changes can increase the bandwidth of pediatric intensive care nurses so that they are better able to attend to patients' medication side effects?*

Children's rapid development and high dependence on the systems around them make child-focused research especially well-suited for implementation science methods (Wakschlag et al., 2022; Williams & Beidas, 2019). Even small improvements in caregiving skills, institutional capacity, or attitudes toward a practice may bear great amounts of fruit across time and domains for growing children and the adults who care for them.

19.2.5 Policy-Targeted

Some of the risks faced by children occur in the privacy of homes, such as domestic violence and exposure to environmental toxins. However, in all of these cases, children's "exposome" is shaped directly and indirectly by community resources, laws, health campaigns, education, and other forces in the public sphere. For this reason, research that gains the ear and the credence of policy makers may have large impacts on large numbers of children. Those who hope for their research agendas to support many children's development may benefit from building partnerships with leaders in local, national, and global policy spheres and, in doing so, generate and communicate knowledge that can be reflected in new resources, calls for funding, and legal codes.

Child-focused research can be especially impactful when researchers consider framings that speak to economic and political needs in their contexts. Return-on-investment analyses are one such example, as in an experimental study in India that showed how the economic benefits of adding one staff member to public early childhood classrooms outweighed the costs (Ganimian et al., 2024). Another research team identified child trauma and low levels of social support as major root causes behind radicalization and openness to extremist violence (Ellis et al., 2021). This finding, directed through the appropriate policy channels, has begun to help shape U.S. responses to domestic terrorism risks, ensuring that a focus on early life trauma and social connectedness can be centered in prevention programs.

In Minneapolis, Minnesota, on the eve of the city's billion-dollar investment in a new sports stadium, economic researchers conducted a comparative analysis of returns on infrastructural investments from taxpayers and donors (Rolnick & Grunewald, 2003). They found that in contrast to contributions to sports stadiums—on which taxpayers may or may not eventually "break even," seeing a dollar returned to them for every dollar they have invested in the project—each dollar invested in high-quality early childhood education infrastructure was likely to yield high dividends to the average taxpayer and donor down the line. Specifically, each member of the public who contributed a dollar to these infrastructure efforts through taxes could expect to see at least $7.16 return to their pockets over the coming decades, via greater school achievement and retention, decreases in welfare payments, decreases in crime, and greater social security benefits from a higher-earning workforce. Other analyses have found that the dividends from each dollar of such an investment can amount to $13 (Grunewald & Rolnick, 2007). While the ethical arguments for investing in child-friendly policies, practices, and resources often ring out clear as a bell, they may find new (and newly enthusiastic) spokespeople and allies when their economic and civic benefits are made clear.

19.2.6 Resilience-Grounded

When conducting research with groups that are facing marginalization, it is considered best practice to use lenses of resilience and positive adaptation (Abdi, 2018). That is to say, while it is critical to document the mechanisms and impacts of risk, it is just as important to identify strengths and resources present in communities that help to protect children and promote their wellbeing. As a methodology and a theoretical lens, resilience science has several advantages. First, this lens is likely to help teams accurately describe the social, emotional, and environmental landscapes of growing children. After all, a scholar would be remiss in trying to convey the impacts of armed conflict on children's physical health without discussing the ways that adults in a community work together to maintain children's nutrition status; the persistence of religious and cultural rituals even amid danger; and the role of schools in supporting cognitive and social development. Scholars who learn the "short list"—resources and assets associated with positive adaptation to adversity around the globe—have at hand a set of factors to evaluate as covariates, mechanisms, and outcomes (Masten et al., 2021). Second, communities are likely to engage more eagerly with resilience research than with risk research, as these framings frequently resonate more powerfully with participants' self-concepts and beliefs about their children. Such studies may therefore generate more representative samples and invite more avid, equitable community partnerships (Foster et al., 2024; Hodges et al., 2024). Chapter 18 further described the science of resilience, along with some ways in which this science can be applied in support of child rights.

Case Study: The "Bright Spots" Model

One resilience-based research methodology that is likely relevant to a wide range of disciplines is the "bright spots" or "positive deviance" model. In this approach, researchers consider a community where exposure to a given set of risk factors is very high, and where associated adverse outcomes are expected to be high—for example, a neighborhood known to have high levels of air pollution or lead paint, a school district whose graduates rarely attend college, or a conflict-affected area where access to clean drinking water is interrupted. Next, rather than focusing on the most severely impacted children (e.g., those with chronic asthma, who drop out of school the earliest, or who have the most serious water-borne diseases), researchers identify the children who show the *lowest* levels of expected adverse outcomes, deviating from the expected dose-response curves (Marsh et al., 2004). From there, patterns can emerge that point to resilience mechanisms. For example, perhaps children in conflict zones who have lower levels of water-borne diseases are those whose families happen to draw water upstream from other houses or whose parents cook all vegetables thoroughly. Bright spots approaches are often appealing to communities, as they promise to identify strengths. They also tend to generate solutions that are sustainable, affordable, and culturally appropriate, as, by definition, the assets and mechanisms these studies uncover are those that are already present in the community.

19.3 Conclusion: Baby Steps into a Wide Tent

Reading these proposed qualities of impactful child-friendly research may seem daunting to students, junior scholars, and seasoned academics alike. Many academic fields encourage high levels of specialization, and it is all too common for a person's interdisciplinarity to decrease over time as they progress through a career. Meanwhile, it is often hard to envision how existing research engines could be infused with new resilience perspectives, community engagement, and economic or political relevance. However, each facet of effective child-friendly research described above exists on a spectrum, and even initial efforts toward these goals may help to make a research project more ethical, accurate, incisive, and just. For example, a researcher interested in bearing witness to child rights through research may reflect on questions like:

- *Can a pair of fresh eyes read through my manuscript to see whether there are opportunities to use strengths-based framing rather than deficit framing?*
- *Are there actions that a caregiver or practitioner could take based on these findings to support a child's development in the next six months? How could these findings reach them?*

- *Does my institution offer training on community engagement, mixed methods research, implementation science, or writing policy briefs?*
- *Are there people in my community who care about the same goals but use different methods or skill sets?*

The potential fruits of child-friendly research agendas include a generation of researchers who have become sensitive to the particularities of children's lives; a generation of children who know that their voices matter; and a suite of creative solutions to the needs facing real children and their communities today.

Research, of course, is only one way to bear witness to the experiences of children in our world, and it is a fairly recent human invention as a modality of truth-telling. More ancient and universal is creative expression. In fact, some of the most powerfully communicated research findings have a "ring" of art to them; they may speak to the core of one's motivational systems, convey sorrow, ignite hope, or confer a sense of connectedness to others. The next chapter discusses the roles of art and other forms of communication in promoting child rights.

Reflection Questions

Question 1. What factors can make community-engaged research harder to conduct? What about research during humanitarian crises?

Question 2. In your own field of study/work, what would happen if children's voices were more closely incorporated into research and practice?

References

Abdi, S. M. (2018). Mental health of migrant children. In *Oxford research encyclopedia of global public health* (pp. 1–19) (publichealth.oxfordre.com). USA: Oxford University Press. https://doi.org/10.1093/acrefore/9780190632366.013.12

Aboud, F. E., Yousafzai, A. K., & Nores, M. (2018). State of the science on implementation research in early child development and future directions. *Annals of the New York Academy of Sciences*, *1419*(1), 264–271.

Dajani, R., Hadfield, K., van Uum, S., Greff, M., & Panter-Brick, C. (2018). Hair cortisol concentrations in war-affected adolescents: A prospective intervention trial. *Psychoneuroendocrinology*, *89*, 138–146.

Dickerson, C., & Heisler, T. (2019). The youngest child separated from his family at the border was 4 months old. *The New York Times*, June 16, https://www.nytimes.com/2019/06/16/us/baby-constantine-romania-migrants.html.

Distefano, R., Grenell, A., Palmer, A. R., Houlihan, K., Masten, A. S., & Carlson, S. M. (2021). Self-regulation as promotive for academic achievement in young children across risk contexts. *Cognitive Development*, *58*, 101050. https://doi.org/10.1016/j.cogdev.2021.101050

Foster, J. C., Hodges, H. R., Beloborodova, A., Cohodes, E. M., Phillips, M. Q., Anderson, E., Fagbenro, B., & Gee, D. G. (2024). Integrating developmental neuroscience with community-engaged approaches to address mental health outcomes for housing-insecure youth: Implications for research, practice, and policy. *Developmental Cognitive Neuroscience*, 101399. https://doi.org/10.1016/j.dcn.2024.101399

Ellis, B. H., Sideridis, G., Miller, A. B., Abdi, S. M., & Winer, J. P. (2021). Trauma, trust in government, and social connection: How social context shapes attitudes related to the use of ideologically or politically motivated violence. *Studies in Conflict & Terrorism*, *44*(12), 1050–1067.

Ferguson, G. M., Fiese, B. H., Nelson, M. R., & Meeks Gardner, J. M. (2019). Transdisciplinary team science for global health: Case study of the JUS Media? Programme. *American Psychologist*, *74*(6), 725.

Finkelhor, D., Turner, H. A., Shattuck, A., & Hamby, S. L. (2013). Violence, crime, and abuse exposure in a national sample of children and youth: An update. *JAMA pPediatrics*, *167*(7), 614–621.

Ganimian, A. J., Muralidharan, K., & Walters, C. R. (2024). Augmenting state capacity for child development: Experimental evidence from India. *Journal of Political Economy*, *132*(5), 1565–1602.

Hansen, M., O'Brien, K., Meckler, G., Chang, A. M., & Guise, J. M. (2016). Understanding the value of mixed methods research: The children's safety initiative-emergency medical services. *Emergency Medicine Journal*, *33*(7), 489–494.

Hodges, H. R., Gillespie, S., Cherubini, F. D. S., Ibrahim, S. A., Gibson, H., Ali Daad, A. M., Davis, S. L., Abdi, S. M., Senesathith, V., Food, C. Ferguson, G. M., and Food, Culture, & Health Study Team. (2024). Ethical applications of digital community-based research with Black immigrant and refugee youth and families. *American Psychologist*, *79*(1), 9.

Grunewald, R., & Rolnick, A. (2007). A productive investment: Early child development. In Mary Eming Young and Linda M. Richardson (Eds), *Early Child Development: From Measurement to Action. A Priority for Growth and Equity*, 17–32. Washington DC: World Bank

Jones, N., & Sumner, A. (2009). Does mixed methods research matter to understanding childhood well-being? *Social Indicators Research*, *90*, 33–50.

Labella, M. H., Kalstabbakken, A., Johnson, J., Leppa, J., Robinson, N., Masten, A. S., & Barnes, A. J. (2017). Promoting resilience by improving children's sleep: Feasibility among families living in supportive housing. *Progress in Community Health Partnerships: Research, Education, and Action*, *11*(3), 285–293.

Leonard, N. R., Casarjian, B., Fletcher, R. R., Prata, C., Sherpa, D., Kelemen, A., Rajam, S., Salaam, R., Cleland, C. M., & Gwadz, M. V. (2018). Theoretically-based emotion regulation strategies using a mobile app and wearable sensor among homeless adolescent mothers: Acceptability and feasibility study. *JMIR Pediatrics and Parenting*, *1*(1), e9037.

Marsh, D. R., Schroeder, D. G., Dearden, K. A., Sternin, J., & Sternin, M. (2004). The power of positive deviance. *BMJ*, *329*(7475), 1177–1179.

Masten, A. S., Lucke, C. M., Nelson, K. M., & Stallworthy, I. C. (2021). Resilience in development and psychopathology: Multisystem perspectives. *Annual Review of Clinical Psychology*, *17*(1), 521–549.

Morris, Z. S., Wooding, S., & Grant, J. (2011). The answer is 17 years, what is the question: Understanding time lags in translational research. *Journal of the Royal Society of Medicine*, *104*(12), 510–520.

Morton, M., & Levy, J. L. (2011). Challenges in disaster data collection during recent disasters. *Prehospital and Disaster Medicine*, *26*(3), 196–201.

Neto, O. L., Haenni, S., Phuka, J., Ozella, L., Paolotti, D., Cattuto, C., Robles, D., & Lichand, G. (2021). Combining wearable devices and mobile surveys to study child and youth development in Malawi: Implementation study of a multimodal approach. *JMIR Public Health and Surveillance*, *7*(3), e23154.

Ornelas, I. J., & Perreira, K. M. (2011). The role of migration in the development of depressive symptoms among Latino immigrant parents in the USA. *Social Science & Medicine*, *73*(8), 1169–1177.

Panter-Brick, C. (2023). Pathways to resilience and pathways to flourishing: Examining the added-value of multisystem research and intervention in contexts of war and forced displacement. *Development and Psychopathology*, *35*(5), 2214–2225.

Rolnick, A., & Grunewald, R. (2003). Early childhood development: Economic development with a high public return. *The Region*, *17*(4), 6–12.

Russell, M. A., & Gajos, J. M. (2020). Annual research review: Ecological momentary assessment studies in child psychology and psychiatry. *Journal of Child Psychology and Psychiatry*, *61*(3), 376–394.

S., F. (2016). Nicholson photo voice. Saving Lives, Inspiring Youth. https://savinglivesinspiringyouth.weebly.com/nicholson-photovoice.html

Stokols, D., Hall, K. L., Taylor, B. K., & Moser, R. P. (2008). The science of team science: Overview of the field and introduction to the supplement. *American Journal of Preventive Medicine*, *35*(2), S77–S89.

Wakschlag, L. S., Finlay-Jones, A. L., MacNeill, L. A., Kaat, A. J., Brown, C. H., Davis, M. M., Franklin, P., Berkel, C., Krogh-Jespersen, S. & Smith, J. D. (2022). Don't get lost in translation: Integrating developmental and implementation sciences to accelerate real-world impact on children's development, health, and wellbeing. *Frontiers in Public Health*, *10*, 827412.

Williams, N. J., & Beidas, R. S. (2019). Annual research review: The state of implementation science in child psychology and psychiatry: A review and suggestions to advance the field. *Journal of Child Psychology and Psychiatry*, *60*(4), 430–450.

Yabe, T., Jones, N. K., Rao, P. S. C., Gonzalez, M. C., & Ukkusuri, S. V. (2022). Mobile phone location data for disasters: A review from natural hazards and epidemics. *Computers, Environment and Urban Systems*, *94*, 101777.

Yardley, A. (2014). Children describing the world: Mixed-method research by child practitioners developing an intergenerational dialogue. *Educational & Child Psychology*, *31*(1), 48–62.

20 Advocacy through the Lens of Creative Expression

20.1 Introduction

This chapter describes opportunities to bear witness to children's needs, rights, and potential in order to bring about change in the broader world. Advocacy here is understood broadly; as one definition states, it is "the pursuit of influencing outcomes" (Wolfenberger, 1971), or the process of helping to move a community from "what is" to "what should be." Those who engage in advocacy, whether in public or private settings, are attempting to shape policies and practices that impact people's lived experiences, often with attention to a particular domain or issue. Whether one is making a speech at a capitol building in his capacity as a pediatrician or engaging a friend in an earnest conversation about community needs, advocates for children are concerned with shaping ideas, values, and priorities (Cohen et al., 2001). Scholars note that effective advocacy for child rights often invites involvement from people across sectors and systems; ignites passion; is grounded in accurate understandings of an issue and what works to address it; and attends to "upstream" factors shaping children's strengths and vulnerabilities (Cascardi et al., 2015; Devakumar et al., 2016).

20.2 Advocacy Modalities

When readers think of the term "advocacy," it may be easiest to envision the work that occurs in the macrosphere, including through national and international legal codes or public policies. Often, the fruits of these efforts are implemented at an institutional or organizational level, such as through mandated reporting requirements in a healthcare setting or a school's efforts to combat xenophobia in the community. Arguably, any individual who works to change a child's experience for the better and shape the way that others treat them—whether these people are parents, relatives, teachers, therapists, health care providers, social workers, religious leaders, or other community members—comprise the largest group of child advocates in the world. Children, too, advocate for their own needs each day, in public and

DOI: 10.4324/9781003488385-24

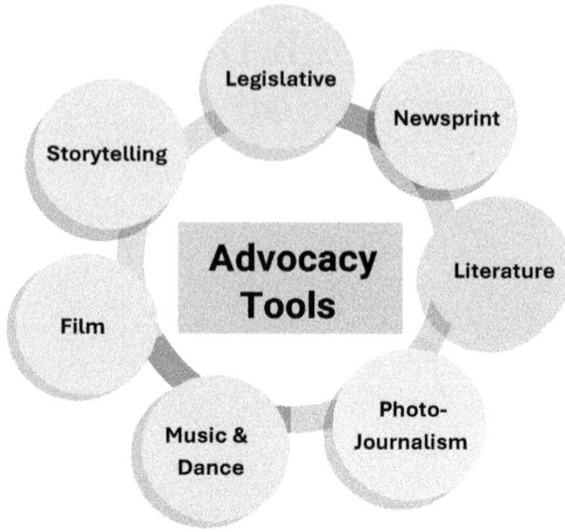

Figure 20.1 Modalities of advocacy and creative expression.

in private, using tools as complex as class-action lawsuits and as simple as crying. This section describes some of the diverse forms of advocacy that can benefit children's development, whether by awakening an audience to injustices that children face, fostering a sense of connectedness and obligation to a new group of children, growing hopefulness about the world that is possible for children, or igniting motivation to act. Figure 20.1 shows some of the diverse forms of child advocacy.

20.2.1 Legislative Advocacy

Efforts to change public policy and law in favor of children's rights, whether at the local, state, national, or international level, requires commitment of like-minded individuals willing to lead a movement toward change and, often, substantial public support. One example of health advocacy that has had many successes in the last century is the anti-tobacco movement. By the 1960s, there was mounting public awareness that use of tobacco products increased the risks of lung cancer, heart disease, stroke, and death. Evidence also accumulated that passive or secondhand cigarette exposure put children at a greater risk of asthma, bronchitis, and respiratory infections. Around the world, many communities advocated for protecting children and adults alike from the effects of tobacco, using tools like research papers, issue briefs, legal testimonies, and political campaigns. Increasingly, states and countries passed age restrictions on tobacco purchases, along with limits on smoking in shared and public spaces. Taxes on cigarettes have been found to be particularly protective of children's smoke exposure (Hawkins et al., 2012). Meanwhile, surveys have found that public opinion in many communities overwhelmingly supports children's rights to smoke-free environments, and even among caregivers who smoke, it is increasingly uncommon for them to do so among children (Semple et al., 2025; Tattan-Birch & Javis, 2022).

An additional example concerns changes in the resources available to children with disabilities. Throughout much of the 20th century, children in the United States who developed differently were frequently placed in institutions, separated from their families and communities. Many underwent procedures like sterilizations and lobotomies. In 1936, a small group of parents in Washington state formed the Children's Benevolent League to advocate for their own and other exceptional children. In its current form, as the Arc of the United States, this organization has been instrumental in bringing about changes in the treatment of children with special needs in domains as diverse as early childhood education, infant screenings, housing, and healthcare access, as well as changes in environmental policies like those impacting lead exposure (The Arc, 2025). In the 1970s, the Arc also played a role in establishing children's rights to a free and appropriate education in public schools, regardless of ability or disability status, in the "least restrictive environment." Today, while there are gaps in implementation, U.S. children with special needs attend schools in their own communities, where they receive education and resources that help them reach their potential.

20.2.2 News Media

There is a long history of writers using newspapers, pamphlets, and similar media to raise awareness about issues affecting children. In the 1870s, *New York Times* coverage of what is widely considered the first child abuse case (concerning a girl named Mary Ellen Wilson) galvanized public outrage over children's vulnerabilities to maltreatment and led to the creation of the first child protection agencies. The 19th and early 20th centuries saw a proliferation of lurid "temperance literature." In addition to sensationalist novellas, these pamphlets offered (purportedly true) anecdotes about families harmed by a person's drinking, with the purpose of depicting the evils brought into society by the availability of alcohol (Leonard & Jacob, 1988). These pamphlets are considered one of the first venues for describing violence against women and children and, arguably, brought stories of domestic violence and child abuse into the public eye.

In the modern day, print and digital news sources continue to draw attention to issues affecting children and other vulnerable groups and offer child rights advocates opportunities to share their perspectives. In addition, social media increasingly plays a role in young people's activism, making it possible for "citizen journalists" to share their lived experiences with people who might not otherwise have access to their voices (Karki, 2024).

Case Study: Shyam Sunder Paliwal

A laborer in the marble industry since age 11, Shyam Sunder Paliwal was raised in the shadow of the mining projects that tore up his district of Rajsamand, India. His love for his community led him to seek and earn election as his village's sarpanch (president or decision-maker) in 2005. When his daughter, Kiran, died of dehydration during a devastating drought the following year, Mr. Paliwal created a model of reform that merges ecological restoration and gender equity efforts, now adopted by over 150 villages worldwide beyond his own community of Piplantri (Mission Sustainability, n.d.; Rawal, 2022). In a state known for high rates of female infanticide, Mr. Paliwal has helped to shift the attitudes of his community toward celebration of girls. He now plants 111 trees whenever a baby girl is born in his village, and the town opens a bank account in the new child's name, contingent on the family's promises to educate her and to abstain from facilitating her marriage before age 18. Piplantri now has a suite of sustainable agriculture and economic efforts as well, including aloe and bamboo farming, and is self-sufficient with regard to electrical power. Groundwater has risen by three inches since Mr. Paliwal's reform efforts, and there have been no serious droughts. Town dumps once full of mining waste are now full of plants.

Mr. Paliwal is considered the founder of eco-feminism for his efforts to address the ways that gender inequity interacts with climate change and environmental degradation to harm individuals and communities.

20.2.3 *Creative Forms*

Given its aim of shifting people's motivations, attention, values, and priorities, it is unsurprising that successful advocacy relies on effective communication that broadens awareness and imagination while motivating new actions. One of the most ancient and effective ways to communicate about lived experience and change people's minds is through art.

20.2.3.1 Literature

Authors of fiction and nonfiction alike often play a role in educating readers about the impacts of past adversity on the lives of children and families while spurring action in the present. These works, of course, may have intended audiences across the lifespan. In 1988, Emily Style coined the concept of "windows" and "mirrors" in describing literature, noting that "mirror" texts reflect a reader's identity and lived experience, while "window" texts let readers glimpse other perspectives (Style, 1988). In 1990, Dr. Rudine Sims Bishop expanded this concept to include "sliding doors," texts that build readers' abilities to imaginatively "step into" another world for themselves (Bishop, 1990).

Many writers use literature to describe collective and individual experiences of adversity and resilience in their own communities. Chinua Achebe was a Nigerian writer whose work deals extensively with colonialism, cultural sovereignty, and collective resilience. One section of his writing (reproduced below from *Anthills of the Savannah* [1987]) comments on storytelling itself as a cultural protective factor.

> "...[I]t is only the story that can continue beyond the war and the warrior. It is the story that outlives the sound of war-drums and the exploits of brave fighters. It is the story... that saves our progeny from blundering like blind beggars into the spikes of the cactus fence. The story is our escort; without it, we are blind. Does the blind man own his escort? No, neither do we the story; rather it is the story that owns us and directs us."
>
> Chinua Achebe, Anthills of the Savannah (1987)

Many books intended for adolescents or adults deal with themes that include children's adversity and resilience. As such, these books—important stories in their own rights—can expose readers to perspectives of children and families exposed to oppression and trauma. Toni Morrison's 1987 *Beloved* was inspired by the true story of Margaret Garner, a U.S. woman born into slavery who was tried for killing her young daughter rather than let her daughter become enslaved again. *Persepolis* (2000–2003), Marjane Satrapi's autobiographical graphic novels, document the author's experiences growing up in Iran during the political violence of the 1980s. Louise Erdrich's 2012 coming-of-age novel, *The Round House,* depicts ways that historical trauma and social inequity act alongside communities' protective mechanisms to shape development for a group of American Indian children. The book also addresses themes around the complexities of prosecuting crimes committed on tribal or reservation land. These and countless other stories can act as "mirrors," "windows," and "sliding doors" to readers, all of which may equip their motivation and capacity to protect children in the here and now.

Of course, not all literature that has the potential to support child advocacy focuses on atrocities. Some engages readers' hopefulness or depicts positive imagined futures. For example, Afro-Futurist writers like Deji Olukotun may use the style of science fiction to help expand readers' imagination of what it may feel like to live in an African continent leading the world in science and economic growth.

Many authors of children's literature have worked to describe the adversities facing today's children in developmentally appropriate ways. Malala Yousafzai's *Malala's Magic Pencil* (2017) describes the activist's journey, including the assassination attempt she suffered, in child-friendly terms. *La Luna Mango* (2019) by Diane de Anda depicts parental deportation from the perspective of a young girl. Armed conflict is represented in literature for children and adolescents, including *The Red Pencil* by Andrea Davis Pinkney (2015) and *A Long Walk to Water* (2010) by Linda Sue Park, both of which are about Sudanese children affected by war and forced displacement. Other books help children learn about climate justice and environmental degradation, like *The Lonely Polar Bear* (2020) by Khoa Le, and *Hoot* (2002) by Carl Hiaasen. *One Plastic Bag* by Miranda Paul (2015) tells the true story of Isatou Ceesay, a Gambian environmental activist and community leader. All of these books may serve to foster children's empathy for those affected by adversities, process their own experiences of adversity, envision stories of hope and resilience in the world around them, and learn the roles they can play in building a better world themselves.

One powerful example of advocacy through child-facing literature is *Every Child a Song: A Celebration of Children's Rights* (2019) by Nicola Davies (Figure 20.2). This book provides an introduction to the concept of children's rights and, specifically, the UN Convention on the Rights of the Child (CRC), using the metaphor of music to describe the urgency of children's survival, development, and thriving:

> When you were born a song began
> Sometimes it didn't sound much like a song.
> Sometimes, no one could hear it.
> But it was there in every heartbeat, every breath; tiny, fragile and unique.
> A melody the world had never heard before.
> It needed love to help it grow, to keep it sheltered and protected.
> Nourished, cherished, celebrated.
> It needed naming and belonging, a home to call its own,
> arms to hold it safe in warmth and welcome.

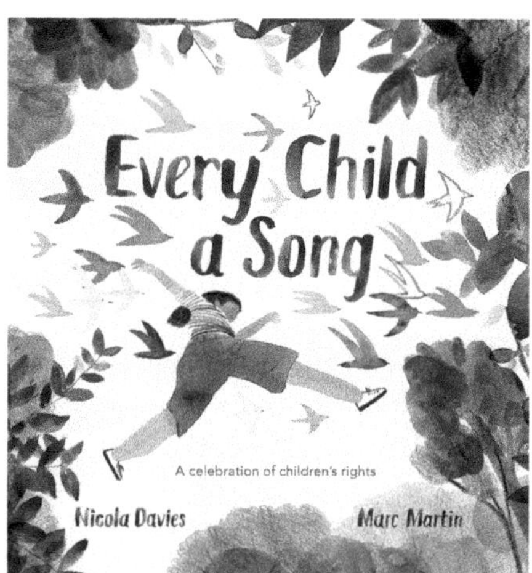

Figure 20.2 Cover of Every Child a Song: A Celebration of Children's Rights, by Nicola Davies.

20.2.3.2 Photography

Some of the most impactful visual images in the child rights movement in the last century have been journalistic photographs. An 1890 photojournalistic collection by Jacob Riis called *How the Other Half Lives*, though rife with racial and ethnic stereotypes, raised widespread awareness about the conditions of people in U.S. immigrant communities living in poverty. Through images, Riis argued that residential instability and poor housing conditions, rather than "weak moral standards" of tenants of overcrowded apartment buildings, were responsible for adverse social and health outcomes among economically marginalized families in New York City. This catalogue helped inspire a set of housing and labor reforms that improved the lives of children.

Lewis Wicks Hines, a sociologist and photographer working at the turn of the century, shone a light on the dangers of child labor in the United States. At the time, child labor was often viewed as a normative trajectory. His photographs are credited with inspiring the first child labor laws in the United States. Figure 20.3 juxtaposes the small stature of the children with the huge mechanical loom they are working. The boys' bare feet emphasizes their vulnerability.

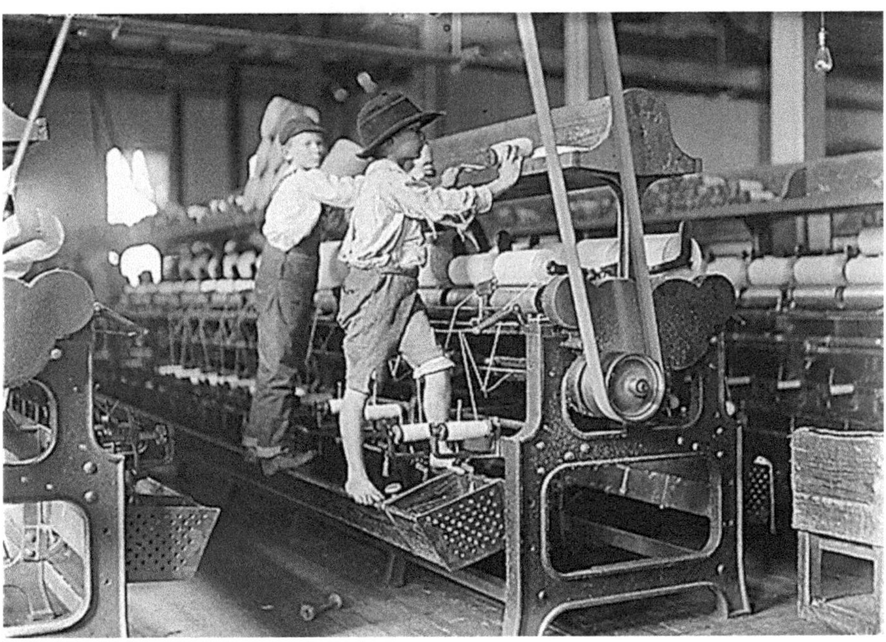

Figure 20.3 Child Labor in Industrial Age.

Case Study: Dorthea Lange

Originally trained as a teacher, Dorothea Lange operated a portrait studio in San Francisco from 1919 to 1940. In 1929, she took her equipment outside the studio to begin photographing people in their daily contexts, including those affected by the Great Depression. Between 1935 and 1939, Lange conducted several documentary photojournalism trips for the Farm Security Administration. One of her pieces from this era, *Migrant Mother,* depicts the farmworker Florence Owens Thompson as she holds her three young children (Figure 20.4). This photograph draws viewers' attention to the individuals in the midst of a national economic crisis. Later, Lange documented Japanese American internment camps in the 1940s, often with particular attention to children and families. Her photographs are notable for their attention to relationships and the empathy that they engender for the people they depict.

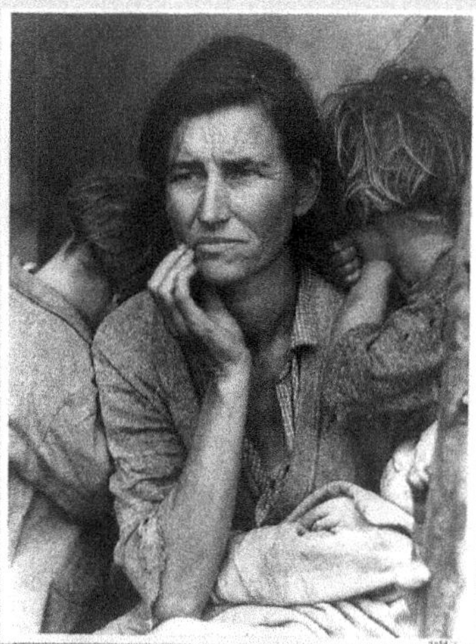

Figure 20.4 Dorthea Lange's *Migrant Mother.*

Some of the most iconic photographs of the 20th century had relevance to children's rights: images of the desegregation of U.S. schools, of the brutal effects of racist violence against children like Emmett Till, of children burned by napalm in the Vietnam War. A 1971 photo by W. Eugene Smith shows an intimate moment in which a mother bathes her daughter, whose musculoskeletal development was affected by mercury poisoning from a local factory's runoff. In an early success for the environmental movement, this photo and others in its series helped galvanize public efforts to hold a corporation financially accountable for the deaths of nearly 2,000 people in Minamata, Japan. This photograph, its title, and its subject are rarely reproduced today in deference to the preference of the family depicted in the image.

Sebastião Salgado of Brazil trained as an economist and went on to become a photographer. He is known for his beautiful, straightforward photos of children and families experiencing poverty and other forms of adversity. In 1984, Salgado undertook a fifteen-month project of photographing the Sahel region of Africa amid a drought. He later photographed conditions of famine and malnutrition in Chad, Ethiopia, Maki, and Sudan, along with people who worked in coffee farming and production.

The photograph *Afghan Girl* (McCurry, 1984) became an emblem of Afghanistan's refugee crisis, depicting 12-year-old Sharbat Gula, who was displaced to Pakistan. (Notably, this photograph was published without Gula's consent.) More recently, in 2015, many members of a Syrian refugee family drowned during an attempted passage of the Mediterranean Sea. Among the victims was two-year-old Alan Kurdi (Shenu). Turkish journalist Nilüfer Demir took a photograph of this child's body that rapidly galvanized international support for those impacted by the Syrian refugee crisis. Yazan al-Kafarneh, a ten-year-old Palestinian boy with cerebral palsy who was photographed during and after his 2024 death by starvation in a Gaza hospital, gave a face to the humanitarian disaster of the Israel-Hamas war.

Today, in the 21st century, photojournalism is an immediate and impactful form of advocacy. As this form of artistic expression continues to grow, both the photographer and intended audience must navigate the emotional drive to action that these images elicit while ethically considering the role of consent from the subject, especially in the case of children experiencing acute adversity.

20.2.3.3 Other Visual Arts

Drawing, painting and other visual arts can play a large role in galvanizing responses to children's needs. Ai Weiwei created *Remembering* (2009) using 9,000 school backpacks to represent the children's lives lost during the 2008 earthquake in Sichuan, China. His work hoped to raise awareness and accountability about corruption in China's construction industry that led to the building shortcuts that rendered school structures so vulnerable to the earthquake. Titus Kaphar, an American artist, created a sort of a modern *pieta* with a Black mother and her baby, though the child exists only as a hole in the canvas of the painting (Figure 20.5). The intent of this work, *Contour of Loss* (2020), was to capture the absence of children and the loved ones who remain following environmental violence like that caused by structural racism.

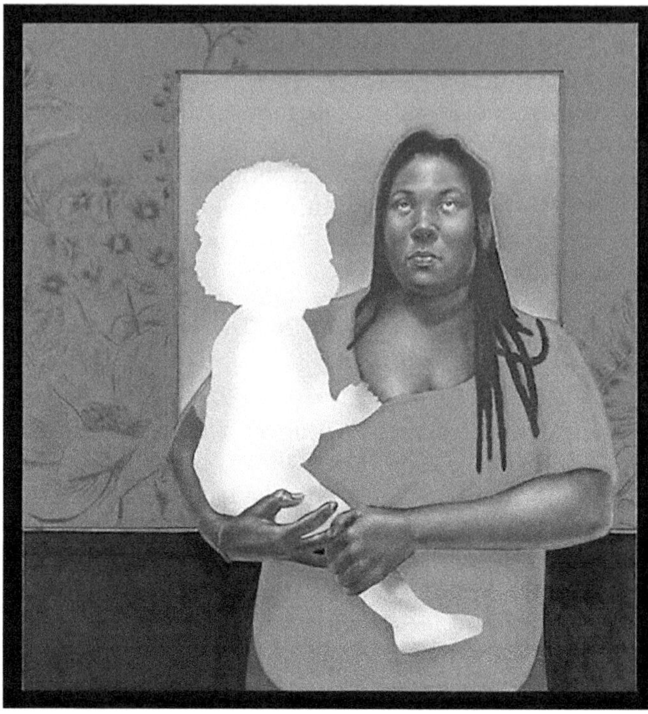

Figure 20.5 Titus Kaphar's *Contour of Loss.*

20.2.3.4 Film and Video

Film is frequently thought of as simply a format for entertainment, yet many readers are aware of its tremendous potential to inform and motivate action. Today's films include full-length movies, biopics, documentaries, shorts, public service announcements (PSAs), and commercials, as well as videos shared through social media. All have the power to be advocacy tools. Davis Guggenheim's 2006 documentary, *An Inconvenient Truth*, represented an early effort to raise international awareness about climate change. In particular, this film appealed to young people as agents of change in addressing climate crises.

Some of the most effective films about children's development amid adversity rely centrally on the voices of the children themselves. *Born into Brothels* (2004; directed by Anan Briski and Ross Kauffman) depicts the lives of children of sex workers in Kolkata, India. This film rested on photography classes for children; youth were provided with cameras and used them to document their daily lives. The film won a 2004 Oscar for best documentary amongst other numerous film awards. Opira Bosco Okot, a filmmaker and a refugee from South Sudan, has used film to advocate for supports for refugees and to raise awareness about the intersections of climate degradation and forced displacement. His advocacy efforts include reforestation projects, educating refugee children to be protectors of their environments, and promoting relationships between refugee communities and members of resettlement societies (Okot, 2022).

20.2.3.5 Music and Dance

A chapter on creative expression would be woefully incomplete without a section on music, as challenging as it is to summarize the advocacy power of music in such a short few paragraphs. Readers in the United States may be familiar with Woody Guthrie's folk music about the challenges of daily life during the Great Depression, or Billie Holliday's famous recording of "Strange Fruit," a song by Abel Meeropol about the murder of Black Americans by mob violence. From James Weldon Johnson's 1900 "Lift Every Voice and Sing" (Howard Gospel Choir, 2024) to Floyd Red Crow Westerman's "Wounded Knee" (1993), music has often encapsulated the striving of marginalized groups for freedom and thriving.

Many readers will be familiar with the use of music therapy on an individual level to help individual children heal after difficult experiences. There are examples, too, of communities creating music together to tell their stories and rebuild collective identity and agency after adversity. Sierra Leone's 10-year civil war ended in 2002 and made over two million people refugees, at least half of whom were children. Many children and youth were forcibly conscripted into the conflict. An organization called Plan International worked with young men and boys in conflict-affected communities there to support meaning-making and community reintegration after the war. Noting that American rap music was a favorite art form for many of these youth and their friends, this organization established a rap collective. Respect Rappers included many youth who had been forced into combat roles. Through street performances and education, they told stories from their own experiences, spread messages of peace, and helped shape cultures of hope and accountability as communities came back together after the war (Plan International, 2008).

Closely connected to music, dance exists in every culture. The Sankofa Center for African Dance and Culture draws community audiences using traditional Ghanaian art forms of drumming and dance-drama, using these gatherings to provide education and advocacy around HIV/AIDS (The Communication Initiative, 2011). Oxfam has brought together women with artificial pregnancy bellies to breakdance and initiate flash mobs in public spaces to raise awareness of maternal and infant mortality risks in low-resource settings (Barberton, 2009). Likely originating in Zimbabwean communities, the Toyi-Toyi dance was eventually used in South Africa to protest nonviolently against apartheid and intimate security forces during demonstrations (Ethnomusicology Explained!, 2015).

20.2.4 *Listening*

The act of witnessing, of course, is not only about the speaker but also the one who receives. Even as adults build their ability to speak about children's needs and rights, they can simultaneously seek out, attend to, and be changed by the voices of young people.

The structures and endorsement of adults often helps to elevate young people's perspectives. In these authors' local setting of the Twin Cities, NorthPoint Health and Wellness Center in North Minneapolis recently created a Youth Poet Laureate program as a way to showcase the resilience of young clinic users. A 2019 collection of creative writing by Somali American youth living in the Twin Cities, *Crossroads*, reflects young people's stories of intergenerational trauma, racism, and injustice, but also of hope and belonging (Hassan, 2019). Youth-centered art shows, theater programs, and other creative venues abound in most cities and towns. Readers are encouraged to seek out these opportunities to hear children's perspectives. The United Nations itself holds an International Child's Arts Competition, an annual event that encourages children to create with any materials available in their surroundings. One associated project, for example, was to design a UN stamp on the theme, "We Can End Poverty" (United Nations, 2007).

Researchers, too, have a role to play in elevating children's voices. A few teams of researchers have documented young Afghan refugees' use of poetry to document their experiences, encouraging those who serve youth affected by displacement to attend to these forms of expression (Hosseini & Punzi, 2023; Olszewska, 2007). Children themselves may participate as creative researcher-witnesses through community-engaged research methods like photovoice or walking surveys. Occasionally, academic conferences invite children and youth to attend and represent their generation, participating in panels or co-interpretation events (Yardley, 2014).

20.3 Conclusion

For advocacy to be sustainable, effective, and inclusive, it must invite wide and diverse participation. Creative expression is a large part of this, engaging a wide range of emotions (hope, anger, sadness, excitement, etc.) and connecting participants more deeply to the world's children.

The burden of truth-telling includes sober-minded honesty about the mounting crises described in this book, the vulnerability of children, and the recalcitrant responses too often seen in world leaders. However, it is essential to tell the truth about child development, including by bearing witness to children's potential and to the resilience already shown by young people and their communities worldwide—that is, an account not only of what is worth fighting *against,* but also of what is worth fighting *for*. Spending time with children in real life is one of the most reliable ways to become grounded once again in realistic hope.

Reflection Questions

Question 1. What do you think makes advocacy efforts effective?
Question 2. Has art ever changed the way you thought or acted?
Question 3. Think about a child rights issue that matters to you. Can you envision what legal or political advocacy could look like in your community? How could this benefit from creative expression?

References

Achebe, C. (1987). *Anthills of the Savannah.* Heinemann.
Barberton, Z. [Zan Barberton]. (2009). *Groove your Bump* [Video]. Vimeo, October 11. https://vimeo.com/7011683
Bishop, R. S. (1990). Mirrors, windows, and sliding glass doors. *Perspectives: Choosing and Using Books in the Classroom. Perspectives: Choosing and Using Books for the Classroom*, 6(3), ix–xi.
Cascardi, M., Brown, C., Shpiegel, S., & Alvarez, A. (2015). Where have we been and where are we going? A conceptual framework for child advocacy. *Sage Open*, *5*(1), 2158244015576763.
Cohen, D., de la Vega, R., & Watson, G. (2001). *Advocacy for social justice: A global action and reflection guide.* Kumarian Press.
Davies, N. (2019). *Every child a song: A celebration of children's rights.* Wren & Rook.
de Anda, D. (2019). *La luna mango.* Albert Whitman & Company.
Devakumar, D., Spencer, N., & Waterston, T. (2016). The role of advocacy in promoting better child health. *Archives of Disease in Childhood*, *101*(7), 596–599.
Ethnomusicology Explained! [Ethnomusicology Explained!]. (2015). Toyi-Toyi revolution: The rhythm of South African protest. [Video]. YouTube, November 2. https://www.youtube.com/watch?v=XPuQBqNhH1M
Hassan, M. A. (Ed.). (2019). *Crossroads: An anthology of resilience & hope by young Somali writers.* Minnesota Humanities Center.
Hawkins, S. S., Chandra, A., & Berkman, L. (2012). The impact of tobacco control policies on disparities in children's secondhand smoke exposure: A comparison of methods. *Maternal and Child Health Journal*, *16*, 70–77.
Hiaasen, C. (2002). *Hoot.* Alfred A. Knopf.
Hosseini, M., & Punzi, E. (2023). "Through my poems, I wanted a sense of recognition": Afghan unaccompanied refugee minors' experiences of poetic writing, migration, and resettlement. *Journal of Poetry Therapy*, *36*(2), 131–143.
Howard Gospel Choir. [Howardgospelchoir]. (2024). *Howard Gospel Choir - "Lift Every Voice and Sing"* [Video]. YouTube, November 10. https://www.youtube.com/watch?v=huXrTXnl2aY
Kaphar, T. (2020). *Contour of loss.* [Oil on canvas.] *The Met.* https://www.metmuseum.org/art/collection/search/848286
Karki, T. (2024). Role of social media in facilitating social justice movements and advocacy in the field of social work. *Current Trends in Information Technology*, *13*(13), 1–7.
Le, K. (2020). *The lonely polar bear.* Happy Fox Books.

Leonard, K. E., & Jacob, T. (1988). Alcohol, alcoholism and family violence. In Hasselt, V. B., Morrison, R. L., Bellack, A. S. & Hersen, M. (Eds.) *Handbook of Family Violence*, Chapter 16, 383–406.

McCurry, S. (1984). *Afghan girl.* [Photograph.] *The Guardian.* https://en.wikipedia.org/wiki/Afghan_Girl

Mission Sustainability (n.d.). Shri Shyam Sunder Paliwal: The man behind the Piplantri model. *Mission Sustainability.* https://missionsustainability.org/blog/shyam-sunder-paliwal/

Okot, O. B. (2022). As a refugee, I have seen the impact of the climate crisis up close. *UNHCR.* https://www.unhcr.org/us/news/stories/refugee-i-have-seen-impacts-climate-crisis-close

Olszewska, Z. (2007). "A desolate voice": Poetry and identity among young Afghan refugees in Iran. *Iranian Studies, 40*(2), 203–224.

Park, L. S. (2010). *A long walk to water.* Clarion Books.

Paul, M. (2015). *One plastic bag.* Millbrook Press.

Pinkney, A. D. (2015). *The red pencil.* Little, Brown Books for Young Readers.

Plan International. [Plan International.] (2008). *Children on the Frontline: Sierra Leone 1* [Video]. YouTube, February 19. https://www.youtube.com/watch?v=RAFV2utYmkQ

Rawal, U. D. (2022). Daughter, water & trees: How this mantra made Piplantri a model village of India. *30 Stades.* https://30stades.com/2022/01/10/girl-child-birth-trees-plantation-piplantri-shyam-sundar-paliwal-rajasthan-environment-conservation/

Semple, S., Tigova, O., Howell, R., Davie, E., Gorini, G., Turner, S. W., Vardavas, E., Clancy, C, Peruga, A., Fernández, E., & O'Donnell, R. (2025). Protecting children from second-hand tobacco smoke in the home: The need for a new approach. *Tobacco Control.*

Style, E. (1988). Curriculum As window and mirror. *Listening for All Voices*, Oak Knoll School monograph.

Tattan-Birch, H., & Jarvis, M. J. (2022). Children's exposure to second-hand smoke 10 years on from smoke-free legislation in England: Cotinine data from the Health Survey for England 1998–2018. *The Lancet Regional Health–Europe, 15.*

The Arc (2025). *Our history.* https://thearc.org/about-us/history/

The Communication Initiative (2011). Sankofa Center for African Dance and Culture. The Communication Initiative. https://global.comminit.com/content/sankofa-center-african-dance-and-culture

United Nations (2007). 'We Can End Poverty' exhibit on show at United Nations. Meetings Coverage and Press Release. https://press.un.org/en/2007/note6110.doc.htm

Weiwei, A. (2009). *Remembering.* [Backpacks and building.] Artsy. https://www.artsy.net/article/joanne-artman-gallery-art-society-ai-weiwei

Westerman, F. R. C. (1993). Wounded Knee [Song]. *The Land Is Your Mother.* Hen House Studios.

Wolfenberger, W. (1971). Joint commission on mental health of children and US department of education, health, education, and welfare. *Child Advocacy Perspectives.*

Yardley, A. (2014). Children describing the world: Mixed-method research by child practitioners developing an intergenerational dialogue. *Educational & Child Psychology, 31*(1), 48–62.

Yousafzai, M. (2017). *Malala's Magic Pencil.* Little, Brown Books for Young Readers.

21 Protest and Youth Voices

21.1 Introduction

This chapter focuses on peaceful protest, an extension of advocacy, as a way to bring about positive change for children. Closely related is adults' obligation to listen to youth's voices when they speak on behalf of themselves and other young people about their lived experiences and ask adults for better treatment. A perusal of international law will find that the word "protest" is not necessarily included in human rights documents. However, international human rights law safeguards the right to peaceful assembly and the expression of one's views in public, including through actions like demonstrations, strikes, rallies, sit-ins, vigils, and of course, cultural and religious celebrations, provided that these activities are peaceful (Wall, 2023). The United Nations ratified the Universal Declaration of Human Rights (UDHR) in 1948, and affirmed the rights to freedom of opinion and freedom of expression in Article 19 and the rights to peacefully assemble in Article 20 (UDHR, 2024). These rights extend to the digital space and entitle people to seek, receive, and share information through media. The United Nations International Covenant on Civil and Political Rights (ICCPR) also protects freedom of assembly and peaceful expression of views. Many regional treaties and national constitutions have similar provisions. Civil disobedience — the refusal to follow unjust laws — is also widely protected.

21.2 Principles of Protest

Protest depends on leveraging one's sources of power, which can be understood in various ways. First, and most obviously, power can be political, enacted through voting, speaking to representatives, or taking actions that shape news coverage of important issues. Power is also economic, and many people choose to use their money or their buying power in ways that motivate corporations or legislative bodies to make desired changes. Another form of power is physical. In the context of nonviolent protest activities, physical power does not involve using force to harm other people, but rather using one's own body and the space it takes up as a form of power. Examples include sit-ins, lie-ins, and marches that

DOI: 10.4324/9781003488385-25

alter the flow of others' daily activities. Additionally, power is relational, social, and communicative. People employing this type of power in protest may use the roles that they have as communicators through face-to-face interpersonal conversations, through their platforms as leaders, through social media, or through other types of social interactions to steer others' attention and motivation toward addressing a certain issue. This type of power overlaps particularly strongly with advocacy work (see Chapter 20).

Many people justifiably stand out as individual icons of protest throughout history, such as Rosa Parks, the "Tank Man" of Tiananmen Square, and Thích Quảng Đức, the Buddhist monk who set himself on fire in 1963 to protest the Vietnamese government's treatment of other Buddhists. Notably, political, economic, physical, and social power can all be magnified when they are used collectively. One person's economic boycott of a brand that uses child labor (or, relatedly, a "buycott," where people agree to purchase only ethically sourced goods) is much less powerful than a widespread shift in consumer behaviors. Indeed, there is precedent for large swaths of consumers successfully incentivizing manufacturers to eliminate child labor in the supply chain by "voting with their wallets" (Brantley, 2025).

Scholars in the fields of protest and activism often note that the type of power used in protest and the type of power against which people protest are very different from one another (Pansardi & Bindi, 2021). Frequently, the term "power-*over*" is used to describe unjust or imbalanced use of power, where one party's power comes at the expense of another's agency, freedom, and thriving—for example, when armed militia groups intimidate children from attending school, or when corporate policies interfere with the enactment of parental leave policies. Power-over is the ability to coerce another. Conversely, "power-*to*" is present when a person or a group exerts their agency to bring about a desired outcome. This has often been equated with *ability*. "Power-*with*" has great relevance to protest, resulting as it does from the collaborative and collective intentions and actions of multiple individuals and groups. For example, these three types of power are present in the protest of Rosa Parks. Laws and norms of racial segregation, along with cultural mores and the wills of individual actors, exerted *power-over* by determining the mobility of Black Americans and their access to resources in their communities. Parks showed *power-to* by exercising her ability to choose where to sit on the bus on December 1st, 1955 in Montgomery, Alabama. Beyond Parks' own agency, this protest was made possible by *power-with*, the support and connectedness of multiple parties working together for change, as her bus ride was planned and supported through networks like the National Association for the Advancement of Colored People (NAACP), the American Civil Liberties Union (ACLU), the Student Nonviolent Coordinating Committee (SNCC), and the Southern Christian Leadership Conferences (SCLC) led by the Reverend Dr. Martin Luther King Jr.

Protest is most likely to be successful when it begins with clear identification of the *power-over* dynamics at play in maintaining unjust conditions (e.g., appreciating the role of a small number of corporations in exacerbating climate change and identifying ways that economic forces shape the politics of climate justice); when protest participants are attuned to their own *power-to* (e.g., believing that their agency as consumers has a meaningful impact on corporate activities, and having ways to meet their needs without relying on these corporations); and when participants coordinate and sustain their activities using *power-with* (e.g., sharing creative workarounds to avoid reliance on polluting corporations, coordinating boycotts and buycotts that increase in size, supporting one another practically and emotionally, and informing one another about political candidates' climate track records). The co-existence of these three types of power alongside one another is what makes it possible for protest to be effective and ethical. That is to say, a group of protesters need not necessarily amass coercive *power-over* to cow corporate leaders into submission; rather, their power exists on different axes, from a combination of *power-to* and *power-with*. In this way, even individuals and groups with substantially lower levels of resources and social capital have succeeded in bringing about changes in spheres of greater capital and influence.

Related to *power-with* and *power-to* is the concept of community partnership. Waves of protest activities often have one overarching goal, such as bringing about an end to violence in a region or divesting money from corporations that are harming people. However, the articulation of these goals and the approaches toward meeting them may look different in each pocket of a protesting community. Networks and coalitions can allow many diverse voices to converge around a particular issue while maintaining communities' sovereignty to choose and design sustainable and feasible protest options for themselves.

Protest is often risky, as those with *power-over* rarely want to part with it, and disruptions to the status quo are threatening to anyone—perpetrators and bystanders alike—who benefit from it. People marching may encounter tear gas or officers in riot gear. A shopkeeper who puts up a sign voicing support for a marginalized group may lose some business. Preparing for risk helps to make protest possible. Additionally, thoughtful protest activities often account for positionality, as risk is not distributed uniformly across a network of advocates or protesters. For example, if a big box store is revealed to use child labor in its clothing products, many customers living in poverty may want to boycott this chain but be unable to, as their families depend on these affordable brands. The burden of boycotting/buycotting may fall more on those with somewhat more flexibility in their spending. Relatedly, the risk of protesting against unjust immigration practices (e.g., family separation at the southern U.S. border) may be highest for those who are themselves undocumented, and so those with more secure legal status may have special roles to play in protest activities.

Finally, protest is often fueled by testimonies and stories. As described in Chapters 19 and 20, accounts of one's own or someone else's lived experiences can help new people connect with causes and movements (amplifying *power-with*) and build individuals' motivation to act (adding to their *power-to*).

21.3 Peaceful Protests Prior to the 21st Century

Readers may feel discouraged and powerless amid mounting global crises like armed conflict, food shortages, environmental disasters, and the existential threat of climate change. The next two sections of this chapter describe successful protests prior to the year 2000 and in the years since then.

21.3.1 Mahatma Gandhi and the Dandi Salt March

Mohandas Karamchand "Mahatma" Gandhi (1869–1948) was raised in India under British colonial rule. Initially educated as a lawyer, he dedicated much of his life to peaceful, non-violent protest. In addition to helping to lead campaigns to support the rights of women and members of the "untouchable" castes, Gandhi is credited as one of the primary leaders of India's anti-colonial movement. Gandhi did not seek primarily to recruit the middle and upper classes, but rather the farmers, peasants, and city laborers who were most affected by discrimination and unjust taxes. For example, one British law established a colonial monopoly on salt, such that even people living on coasts were forbidden to harvest salt themselves, but had to purchase it from colonial markets. In 1930, Gandhi led his followers on the Dandi Salt March, which spanned close to 250 miles and lasted 24 days. Crowds of 50,000 or more were present at various stages of this journey, joining Gandhi in making salt by evaporation along the way in defiance of the British salt legislations. This show of power by the people of India, along with other protests that Gandhi helped lead, helped to convey to British authorities that India had the power and the will to resist their colonization (Homer, 1994).

21.3.2 The Mothers and Grandmothers of Plaza de Mayo

During Argentina's military dictatorship (1976–1983), military authorities used brutal force against political opponents, torturing, killing, and abducting thousands. Children were seen as particularly valuable targets. In 1977, a small network of mothers learned that the disappearances of their children were not isolated instances but were part of organized tactics by military authorities. A group of just over a dozen of these women began marching arm in arm in front of the presidential home in Buenos Aires each Thursday, despite the fact that the government banned gatherings of four people or more. Their movement grew to include hundreds of women, who often marched with white scarves on their heads, embroidered with their missing children's names and birthdays.

Alongside Las Madres de Plaza de Mayo, Las Abuelas de Plaza de Mayo demanded to know the whereabouts of another group of children: the approximately 500 babies who were born to mothers in detention. These mothers were then most likely executed and their children given up for illegal adoption. A few hundred now-adult children separated from their families in this manner have been identified through collaborations with genetic and legal experts.

Together, the Madres and Abuelas generated and sustained international attention on these disappearances through their weekly walks, continuing these protests despite the torture and murder of several founding members. In 1992, the Madres received the European Parliament's Sakharov Prize honoring their freedom of thought. Their search for other relatives who were abducted and killed continues into the present day.

21.3.3 South Africa's Soweto Uprising

During the long years of colonization and apartheid, educational inequities plagued South Africa along the lines of race, with most resources for schooling granted to White Afrikaaner students. In the mid-1970s, furthering this inequity, a national decree limited the use of African languages and English in schools in favor of Afrikaans. Many students and teachers alike saw this change as further eroding their autonomy and cultural sovereignty, hampering Black students' learning, and forcing the use of the colonizers' language. In June of 1976, students in Soweto began to walk out of their classrooms in protest of overarching inequities in education. Over the course of three days, these protests included around 20,000 students. After law enforcement set a police dog on the protesters, which the protesters killed, the police opened fire. Hundreds of students were killed. Meanwhile, uprisings erupted across South Africa, growing to include people far from Soweto, along with White South Africans who were horrified by the massacre of high school students and even younger children. It would be 14 years before Nelson Mandela was released from prison under mounting national and international pressure, and almost 16 years before a referendum vote abolished apartheid and ended rule by the minority White settler class. However, the Soweto uprising is credited as a pivotal moment in the fight to end apartheid, with sustained protest movements continuing across the country and international outrage resulting in universities, corporations, and other nations ending their relationships with those who financially supported the South African apartheid government.

21.4 Recent Protests for Children's Rights

As described in Chapter 17, the last few centuries have seen an evolving concept of childhood, with nearly unanimous agreement among the world's nations that it is the job of adults to provide a safe and nurturing environment in which children can develop. The world has seen the emergence of the principle of "the best interest of the child" and, with it, the establishment of protections for children in the home (e.g., from neglect and abuse), in schools (e.g., from corporal punishment), and in the broader community (e.g., from exploitative labor, educational neglect, and armed conflict). Language and international agreement about child rights has helped to fuel protests in recent years. For example, threats and violence against schoolchildren and teachers in English-speaking regions of Cameroon have resulted in two out of three schools closed and around 700,000 children deprived of an education. Teachers and parents have vocally protested this treatment and demanded that schools are once again kept safe from armed separatists (Davies, 2021). In 2014, members of majority-Black communities in Flint, Michigan began to complain of foul-smelling and mud-colored water from their pipes following a change in the city's water supply. The city's denial and inaction (a result of structural racism) resulted in countless residents being exposed for long periods of time to water-borne pathogens and, for over 100,000 residents, lead (Riley, 2024). Babies and children, whose rapidly developing brains are especially susceptible to damage from this toxin, were often centered in protest movements surrounding the crisis in Flint.

Embedded in the principle of acting in the best interest of the child is the premise that children ought to be listened to. Indeed, youth voices increasingly play a role in shaping community and planetary trajectories, especially in domains in which adults have routinely failed to act in children's best interest.

Climate change and environmental degradation present obvious examples. In 1980, U.S. President Jimmy Carter commissioned a group of scientists to study the impact of human activity on natural environments, and the impacts of these changes on society. This work, "Global 2000," identified some of the risks of pollution and resource depletion that would occur in the absence of policy changes, including desertification, deforestation, rising food costs, carbon accumulation in the atmosphere, and mounting inequities (Barney, 1980). Since that time, communities and countries around the globe have made incremental but insufficient changes to slow the rate of damage to environments and the global climate. Despite the fact that nearly 200 parties have signed on to the United Nations Framework Convention on Climate Change (UNFCCC), and despite several landmark agreements like the Kyoto Protocol (1997) and the Paris Agreement of 2015, inaction is the norm in the global fight against climate change—at least, among high-income and high-polluting parties. The 1.5°C threshold established as the maximum increase in global temperatures from preindustrial levels (that is, the threshold needed to reduce the risk of serious global catastrophe) was exceeded in 2024.

Chapter 23 describes some ways in which youth have taken up the burden of protesting for climate and environmental justice. A few additional stories are worth mentioning here. One is the example of Anna Lee Rain Yellowhammer, who, at 13 years old, helped launch a petition to stop the construction of the Dakota Access Pipeline through the Standing Rock Indian Reservation where she lived with her community and family, noting the damage it would cause to the ecosystem and the water supply (Revesz, 2016). It is also notable that many of the children affected by Flint, Michigan's contaminated water supply have gone on to research and participate in environmental justice causes (Webber, 2024).

Frequently, children protest to assert their own rights to survive and develop. Even before the 2023 Israel-Hamas War began, children in Gaza marched to protest Israeli blockades of their communities, releasing balloons to help the world see that they were asking for the right to be treated as children (Middle East Monitor, 2021). American youth have organized their own rallies to fight against structural racism in their communities, adding the urgency of young voices to the broader calls to protect and honor Black lives (Bryant, 2020). In the United States, the youth-led organization March for our Lives organizes rallies and lobbies for political change to end gun violence (March for our Lives, 2025).

Opportunities abound for adults to be involved in youth-led protests as supporters and allies. Most obviously, adults can advertise the causes that youth are advocating for, speak positively about youth's engagement to other adults, and offer scaffolding and practical supports to young protesters, like safety tips or transportation to events. There are also examples of people using their privilege as adults to protect youth from some of the risks associated with protesting. During the Soweto uprising, doctors treating child victims of police violence were told to report anyone with a gunshot wound to the authorities as a protester. Instead, they recorded the children's bullet wounds as "abscesses" to shield children from prosecution. Youth marching for climate justice in Australia recently received "doctors' notes" from climate scientists asking that they be excused from class "due to a major climate health concern" and the need for "a sick day to protest for a sick planet" (McIntyre, 2022).

Case Study: Mahsa Amini

In 2022, 22-year-old Jina Mahsa Amini was arrested in Iran by the religious morality police for failing to properly wear her hijab. She died shortly after this in police custody. While Iranian officials have denied a part in this death, eyewitness accounts state that she was beaten severely, and a UN fact-finding mission found that Ms. Amini's death resulted from violence she suffered during detention (Pelham, 2024). The resulting protests were among the largest in Iran's history, with the famous rallying cry—"Women, Life, Freedom"—demanding justice for Ms. Amini, freedom from gender-based violence, accountability for those who hurt women and girls, and equitable access to opportunities. Many organizers of these protests were youth, including young men, who worked on the local level to connect their communities' needs to the broader movement for gender equity. The UN has found that security forces committed human rights violations toward protesters, including sexual violence and "extrajudicial" killings, that disproportionately targeted people from minoritized ethnic and religious groups, as well as women and children. Amid these challenges, the Women, Life, Freedom movement has adapted to rely more on diffuse networks of leaders, including various members of opposition movements. It has been instrumental in keeping international attention on gender equity in Iran (Zeidan, n.d.). Ms. Amini was included in the *Forbes* list of the World's 100 Most Powerful Women in 2022.

21.5 Conclusion

Peaceful protest, which can take many forms, involves drawing on one's sources of power to bring about change. This right is protected by international law and has often proven effective at safeguarding the rights of children and other people who are vulnerable. The obligation to leverage one's power to protect children's rights should, of course, fall to adults, and yet it is increasingly a burden borne by children. Youth who speak up about their treatment deserve special attention and protection.

Reflection Questions

Question 1. Who are the youth in your community who are speaking out about child rights?
Question 2. When have you been invited to engage in protest? What were your reactions?
Question 3. What are your sources of power right now? How can they play a role in protecting child rights?

References

Barney, G. O. (1980). *The Global 2000 Report to the President--entering the Twenty-first Century: The technical report* (Vol. 2). US Government Printing Office.

Brantley, A. P. (2025). The power of boycotts. In Moore, M., Scherrer, C., & van der Lindent, M. (Eds.). *The Elgar companion to decent work and the sustainable development goals* (pp. 487–498). Edward Elgar Publishing.

Bryant, M. (2020). 'It was time to take charge': The Black youth leading the George Floyd protests. *The Guardian.* https://www.theguardian.com/world/2020/jun/15/black-youth-activism-george-floyd-protests

Davies, L. (2021). 'They punished me for having books': Schools in Cameroon terrorised by armed groups. *The Guardian.* https://www.theguardian.com/global-development/2021/dec/16/they-punished-me-for-having-books-schools-in-cameroon-terrorised-by-armed-groups

Homer, A. D. (Ed.). (1994). *The Gandhi reader: A source book of his life and writings.* Grove Press. ISBN 978-0-8021-3161-4.

March for Our Lives (2025). https://marchforourlives.org/

McIntyre, I. (2022). "When the bombs drop, school stops" – over 100 years of Australian school strikes and direct action. *The Commons Social Change Library.* https://commonslibrary.org/when-the-bombs-drop-school-stops-eight-decades-of-australian-school-strikes-and-direct-action/#Newcastle_2024

Middle East Monitor (2021). Gaza children unleash balloons into sky, demand end to Israeli blockade. *Middle East Monitor.* https://www.middleeastmonitor.com/20210824-gaza-children-unleash-balloons-into-sky-demand-end-to-israeli-blockade/

Pansardi, P., & Bindi, M. (2021). The new concepts of power? Power-over, power-to and power-with. In Giulio M. Gallarotti (Ed.). *Essays on Evolutions in the Study of Political Power* (pp. 51–71). Routledge.

Pelham, L. (2024). Mahsa Amini: Iran responsible for 'physical violence' leading to death, UN says. BBC. https://www.bbc.com/news/world-middle-east-68511112
Revesz, R. (2016). 13-year-old Native American's petition to stop oil pipeline reaches 80,000 signatures. *The Independent.* https://www.independent.co.uk/news/world/americas/13yearold-native-american-s-petition-to-stop-oil-pipeline-reaches-80-000-signatures-a7024426.html
Riley, S. (2024). The children of Flint, ten years later. *Harvard Public Health.* https://harvardpublichealth.org/environmental-health/the-children-of-the-flint-michigan-water-crisis-ten-years-later/
UDHR. Universal Declaration of Human Rights. 1948. https://www.un.org/en/about-us/universal-declaration-of-human-rights
Wall, I.rua. (2023). The right to protest. *The International Journal of Human Rights, 28*(8–9), 1378–1393. https://doi.org/10.1080/13642987.2023.2262395.
Webber, T. (2024). Children ofFlint water crisis make change as young environmental and health activists. *AP.* https://apnews.com/article/flint-water-crisis-youth-activists-10-year-anniversary-2e2c8605bf94631ba878d95a1b53bf5e
Zeidan, A. (n.d.). Women, life, freedom. *Britannica.* https://www.britannica.com/topic/Woman-Life-Freedom

22 Promoting Peace through Social Justice

22.1 Introduction: Resilience as a Path to Peace

Thus far, this text has discussed several ways in which environmental and climate events interact with sociopolitical events, such as armed conflict and social fractionalization, to shape the lives of children. In addition, it has proposed that these crises are worsening, with climate change exponentially multiplying these threats independently and strengthening their relationships to each other (for example, by magnifying existing inequities and vulnerabilities). Section IV has explored a number of solutions that can improve the lives of children faced with this impending storm. Thus far, many of these proposed strategies have fallen into the domains of the microsystem and exosystem. However, to improve the present and future well-being of children and youth, larger societal changes also need to occur. These final chapters will explore a number of changes in the macrosystem—in culture, collective values, and international resourcing, for example—that can support children through present and future challenges.

The best way to protect children from the risks of conflict, famine, and other harms to their development is to invest proactively in peace and justice. Peace is more than the absence of armed conflict and other existential challenges, and also refers to the health and resilience of individuals, families, communities, societies, and their relationships to one another. As climate crises intensify resource scarcity around the globe, the time is now to invest in the health of these individual systems and their relationships to one another (Masten, 2021; Oberg et al., 2021). It is impossible to predict the specific challenges that the next generations of children will predict, but fortunately, many of the tools that will protect them are present in societies already, and also are malleable—that is, they can be supported through interventions.

Multisystem resilience science increasingly plays a role in peacemaking efforts among humanitarian and international groups, reflecting the growing realization that peace depends on the functioning and adaptability of basic social systems like education, healthcare, economic opportunities, and governance (Masten, 2014). Scholars have also noted that there is a clear concordance of goals between those aiming to nurture child development at multiple

DOI: 10.4324/9781003488385-26

system levels and those working to prevent the onset or intensification of conflict (Panter-Brick, 2021). For example, reducing ethnic fractionalization in a society, promoting gender equity in education, boosting economic prosperity, and increasing access to sustainable sources of water and fuel can all help children and families stay healthy and also reduce the risk that future challenges escalate to conflict (Holleman et al., 2017; Ide et al., 2021). Similarly, the tools of building multisystem resilience overlap with those used to build peace and justice. These include supportive relationships, positive education and work opportunities, chances to be a leader, a sense of agency and hope, and problem-solving skills (Masten & Barnes, 2018). Readers may note that these factors can exist at the individual level and also at the collective level. Resilience is defined as a dynamic system's ability to adapt successfully to threats to its functioning (Masten & Hodges, 2025). As such, it is easy to see how building resilience at the level of individuals, families, communities, nations, and the planet is so critical to bringing about peace and justice. For example, when a community reliant on agriculture for livelihood faces a serious drought, this is less likely to result in food scarcity or armed conflict if members confidently solve problems together on a regular basis, share a strong sense of agency, and have positive reciprocal relationships with other communities and nations.

Case Study: Peacebuilding in Mozambique Through L-INGOs

After its 15-year civil war ended in 1992, Mozambique enjoyed several decades of relative peace. However, the process of ending this war is criticized for focusing on the cessation of violence but failing to sufficiently attend to the factors that support sustainable peace, such as political enfranchisement, economic prosperity, accountability of leaders, and gender equity (Saraiva, 2023). The risk of violence escalated in the 2010s and 2020s, exacerbated by growing inequities that accompanied the COVID-19 pandemic and mounting climate shocks (Manuel et al., 2020). Sociopolitical vulnerabilities made it possible for the Islamic State-linked group Mashababos (also called al-Shabab) to become entrenched in the north of the country.

In response, Mozambique has developed and implemented "localized international non-governmental organizations" (L-INGOs). L-INGOs are internationally connected, and therefore benefit from the resources and experiences of a large global community. However, all leadership, design, and implementation of programs occurs at the local level. Implementers are able to respond rapidly to changing situations in their local communities. These L-INGOs have launched successful initiatives like birth registration drives to reduce the risk of trafficking and other rights violations; education programs that focus on youth agency and peacebuilding; sustainable agriculture projects; and literacy initiatives

(Saraiva, 2023). These organizations are distinguished by their grounding in local contexts, their permanence in the community, and their responsiveness to the changing needs of those they serve. Notably, Mozambique's L-INGOs depend on collaborations with diverse religious groups. As such, they present a model for problem-solving across lines of difference.

22.2 Reforming and Reimagining International Law

As noted previously, child development and health professionals benefit from a general understanding of the international laws that concern human rights. A summary of key points from Chapters 11 and 17 is offered here.

The Charter of the United Nations opens by defining the primary purpose of the UN: "To maintain the international peace and security, and to that end: …bring about by peaceful means, and in conformity with the principles of justice and international law, adjustment, or settlement of international disputes" (UN Charter, 1945). This broad goal of maintaining peace and security was always grounded in a commitment to upholding human rights, and in fact, one of the first actions of the newly formed UN was to establish the Universal Declaration of Human Rights (UDHR, 1948).

Gaps existed, however, with regard to children's particular rights and needs. In 1959, member states reaffirmed their commitment to child rights by expanding the Geneva Declaration on the Rights of the Child that had been adopted by the League of Nations following WWI (Geneva Declaration, 1928). However, its role was aspirational and lacked any provisions for holding countries accountable. Then, in 1989, the UN General Assembly passed the UN Convention on the Rights of the Child (CRC), establishing the responsibility of member states and their citizens to act in the best interest of children, protect them from harm, and promote their wellbeing and optimal development, whether during peacetime or conflict (Goldhagen, et al. 2020; Oberg, 2021; UNICEF, 2009). Notably, however, enforcement of these articles is still somewhat limited: While signatory nations agree to uphold these principles, and submit regular summaries of their progress, it is dependent on these individual countries to ensure the CRC is upheld.

In parallel, the field of international humanitarian law (IHL) is concerned with parties' adherence to a set of conventions that safeguard military and civilian personnel alike during unrest and conflict. Among the most notable documents underpinning IHL are the Geneva Conventions, adopted over the decades following WWII, which include special protections for children and other civilians (Geneva Conventions, 1949; Miles, 2016). Enforcement bodies like the International Criminal Court (ICC) exist to prosecute war crimes, crimes of aggression, and crimes against humanity. However, the ICC can only prosecute crimes committed after July 1st, 2002, leaving gaps in its jurisdiction. IHL also lacks specificity with regard to violence that occurs between parties of the same nation, like civil war and insurrection, which is growing more common. Of note, bodies like the ICC often launch investigations only after accounts of crimes against humanity reach a certain threshold of severity or magnitude. By this point, countless children have often been killed, injured, or deprived of critical developmental resources (Alexander, 2015; Gegout, 2013). Child rights experts and advocates are likely to be essential voices in ensuring that the ICC responds with urgency to possible threats to development.

22.2.1 Proposed Structural Changes to the United Nations

Historically, those who work with the UN to promote peace and protect people from the effects of conflict and crimes against humanity have focused their efforts on changing international law. In many cases, they have succeeded. As arduous and complex it is to amend these treaties and conventions, the international community has worked to make deletions, additions, and clarifications where necessary. Much more difficult to implement, though, are suggestions to change the basic structure of the UN, in part because this was established many years ago, following WWII. However, a few structural reforms may help the world to prepare for the changing demands of the present century, particularly with regard to climate change.

There are six major bodies within the United Nations, including the UN Security Council and the UN General Assembly. It is the Security Council that is tasked with determining when political or military action is threatening to peace, to impose sanctions, and, if needed, authorize the use of force. The Security Council is made up of five permanent members (China, France, Russia, the United Kingdom, and the United States) and ten non-permanent member states, which are elected by the General Assembly for two-year terms.

As discussed throughout this text, many of the stakes of global geopolitical crises are felt most acutely in the Global South, especially as climate change accelerates. Some changes to the Security Council could ensure that nations that may have the highest vulnerability to climate shocks, environmental crises, and, therefore, armed conflict are also afforded adequate decision-making power. First, there is no guarantee that any nations from Africa, the Middle East, Latin America, or Oceania will be represented on the Council at a given time. It will be critical for the international community to formally honor the voices, priorities, and strategies of people from these regions as the world works to adapt to and mitigate the climate crisis. Guaranteeing diverse regional representation on the Security Council is one step toward this goal. Relatedly, it may be time to consider adding additional permanent members, such as Brazil, India, or other nations. At present, member nations that are permanently part of the Security Council have the power to veto and table resolutions and proposals brought by non-permanent members. While such a longstanding practice is likely difficult to change, it may be beneficial to reconsider the veto rule, or to instead require Council members to recuse themselves from votes when they have conflicts of interest or direct involvement in a crisis at hand; they could participate in deliberations and conversations but would not vote on the issue. Finally, it will be important for the UN to invest in greater transparency around Security Council discussions and decisions. Publicizing more of these conversations would help to build trust among UN members.

22.3 Economic and Trade Contributions to Injustice and Conflict

Poverty is a root cause of conflict. Among the root causes of poverty that persist today are the exploitative and harmful economic practices of wealthier nations—for example, through consumption of goods that are made by unpaid or low-paid workers, and by commitments to energy sources that accelerate damage to global climates. At times, economic exploitation has been addressed through combinations of rights-based campaigns, civil liability, consumer habit change, domestic regulation, and international regulation (Feasley, 2016).

One important way to protect children from conflict is to limit the production, sale, and use of weapons. The increasing ease of purchasing weapons, and their ever-growing sophistication and destructiveness, are partially responsible for the intensification of armed conflict around the world, as well as the mounting loss of civilian lives during these events (Oberg et al., 2022). Around a hundred billion U.S. dollars' worth of weapons are purchased worldwide each year, the vast majority of which are produced and exported by the United States (Stockholm International Peace Research Institute, 2025). At present, it is the job of arms manufacturers to monitor their sale, distribution, and use, and these bodies are generally unable or unwilling to ensure that IHL is upheld during the use of their products, though it is known that these weapons are predominantly used in the context of armed conflict (Amnesty International, 2025). The UN's 2013 adoption of the Arms Trade Treaty was a step toward reducing the illicit sale of weapons, promoting transparency in their distribution, and requiring states to ensure that weapons are not used for human rights abuses. This treaty has been minimally enforced and monitored to date.

22.4 Frameworks for Peacebuilding

As noted above, peacebuilding depends on preventing conflict and also on promoting resilience. One promising effort toward this goal is UNICEF's Learning for Peace program, which is designed to foster young people's multi-system resilience, including through social cohesion, conflict resolution skills, and access to developmental and cultural resources (UNICEF, 2016). Nations participating in Learning for Peace receive support in making sure that schools stay open during unrest, equipping educators and school systems to help communities cope with armed conflict, and infusing the goals of peacebuilding into curricula and school cultures. As shown in Figure 22.1, Learning for

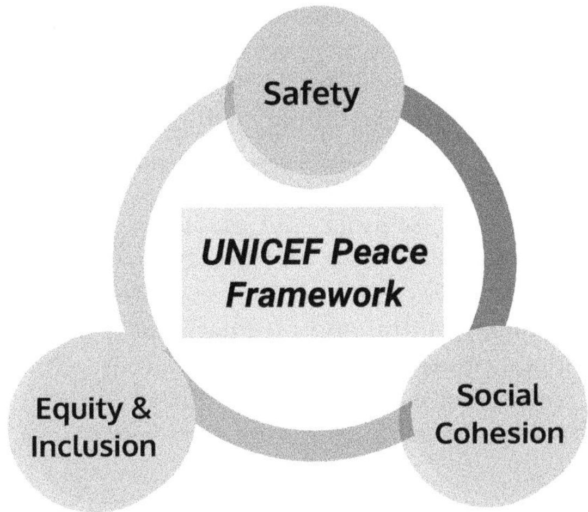

Figure 22.1 UNICEF's Learning for Peace framework.

Peace addresses three major themes: safety; social cohesion; and equity and inclusion. Safety is understood to occur when children, even the most vulnerable, are free from fear of violence. Social cohesion describes a state in which children feel that they matter, are protected, and are meaningful participants in their world. The principles of equity and inclusion refer to the safeguarding of all children's rights to healthy, fulfilled, engaged, and connected lives (UNICEF, 2023).

The Learning for Peace Framework was launched in 2012 and implemented in 14 countries across Africa, Asia, and the Middle East. As described above, many of its interventions target factors well upstream from a conflict. Its primary methods include curriculum development, guidance in educational policy, recruitment of teachers, and distribution of resources to educators and school systems that can support peacebuilding efforts in school communities. Community events, workshops, and discussions invite those in various spheres of children's ecosystems to see their own roles in raising the next generations of peacebuilders. All of this work is capacity-building, amplifying the confidence and skill of education agencies, religious communities, and other organizations and individuals to promote the multisystem resilience that yields sustained peace. Success stories from this UNICEF initiative include the education of Afghan refugee girls in a Pakistan community; increased community cohesion through school social events in Burundi; and the evolution of relationships between parents of differing ethnic backgrounds in Côte d'Ivoire, centered on engagement in women's adult education programs and early childhood development services (Affolter & Azaryeva Valente, 2019).

In 2020, the International Society of Social Pediatrics and Child Health adopted what is known as the Beirut Convention, which prohibits injury and harm to children affected by armed conflict (ISSOP, 2020). A few generalizable principles that can be derived from this document and the surrounding discussions may prove useful in the development of child-centered humanitarian response protocols (Oberg et al., 2023). First, conflict must be kept far from the places where children live, play, and learn, including from the resources that children most directly need for their development, such as homes, wells, hospitals, schools, and places of worship. Child-friendly zones in conflict-affected areas must be enforced by international law. Additionally, in accordance with the CDC, the best interests of children should be considered centrally in intra- and international dialogue about conflict, including states' decisions to levy sanctions. Relatedly, children deserve the enforcement of consequences for those who disregard their rights, whether these violators be policy makers, militaries, arms manufacturers, or financial interests.

Finally, there is a growing movement for behavioral health approaches to peacebuilding. Peace scholars and mental health practitioners alike note that individual and collective psychosocial wellbeing can play large roles in preventing the likelihood of armed conflict (Frasco et al., 2024). Behavioral health strategies of special relevance to peacebuilding include renewed investments in communities' mental health sovereignty (i.e., when communities design resources and supports that can bring about wellness as they conceptualize it together); delivering therapies that promote interpersonal skills (e.g., Papke et al., 2025); and addressing the structural inequities that shape mental health and conflict risks simultaneously. Additionally, some groups have formulated lists of socioemotional tools that individuals can use to promote peaceful discourse and reduce conflict in their own lives. For example, a group of psychologists from the Australian Psychological Society describes individual-level skills relevant to peacebuilding like cultural humility, empathy, seeking out role models, the capacity to critique the actions of one's in-groups, and the ability to maintain hope (APS, 2024).

22.5 Conclusion

Despite international efforts to safeguard child rights and hold violators accountable, children's risk of death and injury from armed conflict continues to grow (Adamkiewicz & Goldhagen, 2021). Peace efforts are most likely to succeed when they are multi-pronged, combining rapid solutions—such as the instantaneous activation of child-friendly zones during armed conflict, or the immediate imposition of sanctions toward child rights violators—with long-term solutions. Long-term solutions for peacebuilding are most likely to be effective and sustainable when they not only focus on preventing conflict, but also work to positively create "quality peace" for children, an environment in which community members engage with maximal respect toward one another (Frasco et al., 2024).

Reflection Questions

Question 1. How do you think international bodies like the UN are doing in fulfilling their obligations to children?

Question 2. Can you think of three ways that schools can be a part of reducing the risk of conflict? What about city- and state-level governments?

References

Adamkiewicz, T., & Goldhagen, J. (2021). Mitigating armed conflict casualties in children. *Pediatrics*, *147*(2), e2020027847.

Affolter, F. W., & Azaryeva Valente, A. (2019). Learning for peace: Lessons learned from UNICEF's peacebuilding, education, and advocacy in conflict-affected context programme. In Balvin, N. & Christie, D.J. (Eds.), *Children and peace: From research to action* (pp. 219–239). Springer International Publishing.

Alexander, A. (2015). A short history of international humanitarian law. *The European Journal of International Law*, *26*, 109–138.

Amnesty International (2025). Arms control. *Amnesty International.* https://www.amnesty.org/en/what-we-do/arms-control/

Australian Psychological Society (2024). https://psychology.org.au/for-the-public/psychology-topics/tragic-events-community-violence/community-safety/ten-ways-you-can-promote-peace

Feasley, A. (2016). Eliminating corporate exploitation: Examining accountability regimes as means to eradicate forced labor from supply chains. *Journal of Human Trafficking*, *2*(1), 15–31. https://doi.org/10.1080/23322705.2016.1137194

Frasco, E., Sherr, L., & Burgess, R. A. (2024). Reconstructing theory in mental health and psychosocial support and peacebuilding: Towards an integrated model for psychosocial peacebuilding. *Journal of Community & Applied Social Psychology*, *34*(4), e2848.

Gegout, G. (2013). The international criminal court: Limits, potential and conditions for the promotion of justice and peace, *Third World Quarterly*, *34*(5), 800–818. https://doi.org/10.1080/01436597.2013.800737

Geneva Convention (1949). *Summary of the Geneva conventions of 12 August 1949 and their additional protocols-in brief.* International Committee of the Red Cross.

Geneva Declaration (1928). Geneva declaration on the rights of the child. https://www.humanium.org/en/geneva-declaration/

Goldhagen, J. L., Shenoda, S., Oberg, C. N., Mercer, R., Kadir, A., Raman, S., Waterston, T., & Spencer, R. J. (2020). Rights, justice, and equity: A global agenda for child health and wellbeing. *Lancet Child/Adolescent*, *4*(1), 80–90. https://doi.org/10.1016/S2352-4642(19)30346-3

Holleman, C., Jackson, J., Sánchez, M. V., & Vos, R. (2017). Sowing the seeds of peace for food security. Disentangling the nexus between conflict, food security and peace.

Ide, T., Kristensen, A., & Bartusevičius, H. (2021). First comes the river, then comes the conflict? A qualitative comparative analysis of flood-related political unrest. *Journal of Peace Research*, *58*(1), 83–97.

International Society of Social Pediatrics and Child Health (2020). Beirut declaration-prohibition of harm to children in armed conflict. https://www.issop.org/2020/01/23/beirut-declaration-prohibition-of-harm-to-children-in-armed-conflict/

Manuel, L., Tostão, E., Vilanculos, O., Mandlhate, G., & Hartley, F. (2020). Economic implications of climate change in Mozambique. *SA-TIED Working Paper, 36.*

Masten, A. S. (2014). Promoting the capacity for peace in early childhood: Perspectives from research on resilience in children and families. In Leckman, J. F., Panterp Brick, C., & Salah, R. (Eds.), *Pathways to peace: The transformative power of children and families.* MIT Press. ProQuest Ebook Central, https://ebookcentral.proquest.com/lib/umn/detail.action?docID=3339906

Masten, A. S. (2021). Resilience of children in disasters: A multisystem perspective. *International Journal of Psychology*, *56*(1), 1–11. https://doi.org/10.1002/ijop.12737

Masten, A. S., & Barnes, A. J. (2018). Resilience in children: Developmental perspectives. *Children*, *5*(7), 98.

Masten, A. S., & Hodges, H. R. (2025). Children and war: Perspectives from developmental resilience theory and research. *Psychiatry: Interpersonal and Biological Perspectives, 88*(3), 293–299. https://doi.org/10.1080/00332747.2025.2530347

Miles N. (2016). International humanitarian law-a comprehensive introduction, international committee of the red cross, August.

Oberg, C., Goldhagen, J., & Spencer, N. (2023). Renewing our commitment to protect children experiencing armed conflict. *Journal of Paediatrics and Child Health*, *59*, 427–430. https://doi.org/10.1111/jpc.16367

Oberg, C. N., Hodges, H. R., & Masten, A. S. (2022). Conflict, war, and famine in childhood: Risks and resilience for social development. In Smith, P.K. & Hart, C.H. (Eds.), *The Wiley-Blackwell handbook of childhood social development* (pp. 189–205). Wiley-Blackwell.

Oberg, C. N., Hodges, H. R., & Masten, A. S. (2021). Risk and resilience of Somali children in the context of climate change, famine, and conflict. *Journal of Applied Research on Children: Informing Policy for Children at Risk*, *12*(1), Article 10. https://digitalcommons.library.tmc.edu/childrenatrisk/vol12/iss1/10

Oberg, C. N., Nathawad, R., Raman, S., & Goldhagen, J. (2021). Violence against children recognition, rights, responses. *Pediatric Clinics of North America*, *68*(2), 357–369.

Panter-Brick, C. (2021). Resilience humanitarianism and peacebuilding. In Michael Ungar (Ed.), *Multisystemic resilience: Adaptation and transformation in contexts of change* (pp. 361–374). Oxford University Press.

Papke, V., Hayee, S., Hodges, H., Simenec, T., Reigstad, K., Gunlicks-Stoessel, M., & Klimes-Dougan, B. (2025). Considerations for cross-cultural adaptations and implementation of interpersonal psychotherapy: A review. *American Journal of Psychotherapy*, appi-psychotherapy.

Saraiva, R. (2023). Adaptive peacebuilding in Mozambique: Examples of localized international non-governmental organization (L-INGOs) in complex and uncertain environments. In C. de Coning, R. Saraiva, A. Muto (Eds.), *Adaptive Peacebuilding, Twenty-first Century Perspectives on War, Peace, and Human Conflict.* https://doi.org/10.1007/978-3-031-18219-8_5

Stockholm International Peace Research Institute (2025). Ukraine the world's biggest arms importer; United States' dominance of global arms exports grows as Russian exports continue to fall. *SIPRI.* https://www.sipri.org/media/press-release/2025/

ukraine-worlds-biggest-arms-importer-united-states-dominance-global-arms-exports-grows-russian
UN Charter (1945). Charter of the United Nations and statute of the International Court of Justice. San Francisco. https://treaties.un.org/doc/publication/ctc/uncharter.pdf
UDHR (1948). The universal declaration of human rights. https://www.un.org/en/about-us/universal-declaration-of-human-rights
UNICEF (2009). *The state of the world's children special edition. Celebrating 20 years of the convention on the rights of the child.* UNICEF, November.
UNICEF (2016). Peacebuilding, education, and advocacy in conflict-affected contexts programme (PBEA): 2012–2016 programme report. Retrieved August 8, 2022, at https://www.unicef.org/media/96556/file/UNICEF-PBEA-Final-Report.pdf
UNICEF (2023). *UNICEF peacebuilding programing framework.* UNICEF, New York. ISBN: 978–92–806–5543–8.

23 Climate Solutions and Champions

23.1 Climate Adaptation and Mitigation

It is common for adults and youth alike to feel daunted and hopeless in the face of our climate crises. Some readers may react this way to reading this book, in fact. Sections I, II, and III described in detail some of the ways in which sustained injury to global climates can harm children, including through direct exposure to worsening natural disasters, damage to caregiving and community systems, reduced availability of food and water, and forced displacement. Climate change has been framed here as an ***exponential modifier*** of the effects of any challenge on children's health and wellbeing. It is therefore appropriate to end with attention to climate, and with the potential that our beautiful planet has to support children's survival and thriving well into the future.

There are two major strategies for responding to climate change: climate adaptation and mitigation (VijayaVenkataRaman et al., 2012). As shown in Figure 23.1, these are not mutually exclusive and can be thought of as companion approaches.

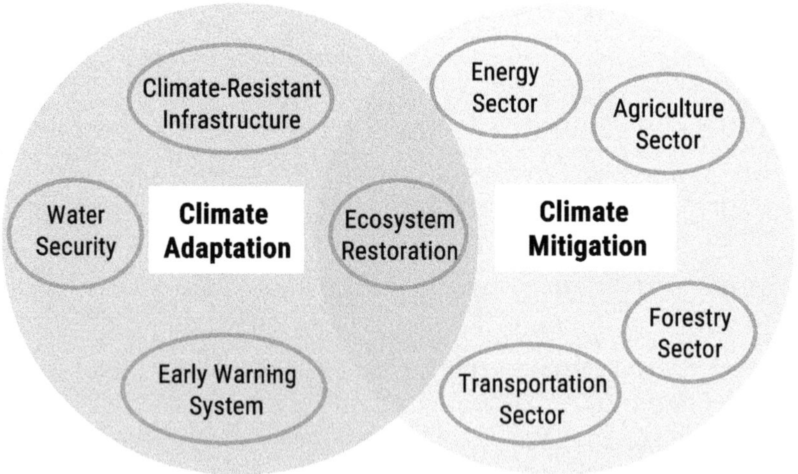

Figure 23.1 Climate adaptation and mitigation strategies.

DOI: 10.4324/9781003488385-27

Climate adaptation entails adjusting human activities to minimize adverse events related to climate change. It examines what capacity individuals and communities have to moderate the impact of potential damages and explores strategies for coping with the effects of climate change right now. In contrast, climate mitigation involves social, economic and technological activities intended to end or reverse the dangers of climate change, such as cutting down drastically on use of fossil fuels.

23.2 Successful Climate Adaptation Approaches

The United Nations Environment Programme recently identified five ways countries can adapt to climate change. They included:

23.2.1 Climate-Resistant Infrastructure

Climate-resistant infrastructure includes roads, bridges, tunnels, and powerlines that can withstand shocks from extreme weather events. The World Bank estimated that each dollar invested in climate-resilient infrastructure can have a return on investment of four dollars (UNEP, 2022). For example, Malaysia has seen recent floods that caused considerable damage. In Kuala Lumpur, a Stormwater Management and Road Tunnel (SMART Tunnel) was built with three levels. It serves a dual purpose of traffic dispersal to reduce congestion and a flood-mitigation initiative to reduce the occurrence of flash floods in the city (Mohammad, 2014). Normally, the top two levels carry road traffic. However, they can be temporarily used as storm drains during major weather related events. It is estimated that the SMART Tunnel will prevent more than $1.5 million in flood damage over the coming decades. It is also expected to reduce the cost of traffic congestion by more than $1 billion (ITS International, 2012).

23.2.2 Early Warning Systems

Early warning systems are extremely cost-effective in providing timely warnings so people can take action prior to weather events, like sandbagging buildings, evacuating, or stockpiling resources. In 2022, the UN Secretary-General unveiled the "Early Warning for All" Initiative by the World Meteorological Organization that will work to develop early warning systems covering the whole world's population by 2027 (UMO, 2022).

23.2.3 Ecosystem Restoration

The UN Decade on Ecosystem Restoration is an effort of the UN Environment Program (UNEP) launched in 2021. Ecosystem restoration is both a climate adaptation approach and also a mitigation strategy: The global repair of the world's ecosystems will increase carbon absorption while also decreasing the impact of climate events. In Laos, for example, UNEP and partners are engaged in a five-year effort to restore wetlands and streams in and around four cities with the expectation of reducing flooding for 700,000 people (UNEP, 2020).

23.2.4 *Water Supplies and Security*

It is expected that by 2030, 50% of the world's population will face severe water shortage (UNEP, 2022). Governments are in the process of creating holistic Integrated Water Resource Management plans to improve the health and resilience of local water systems. In Bagamoyo, Tanzania, for example, the government partnered with the community to install rooftop gutters and storage tanks that help retain rainwater and improve access to potable water.

23.2.5 *Long-Term Planning*

The development of National Adaptation Plans (NAPs) for long range planning and implementation purposes is a difficult but very impactful approach to climate adaptation. This approach involves examining climate scenarios decades into the future to try to identify vulnerabilities in distinct sectors. Seventy nations have developed such plans (UNEP, 2024).

23.3 Climate Mitigation

Climate mitigation approaches often involve coordinated global efforts implemented at the local level. The purpose of these efforts is to decrease the global carbon footprint so as to keep the global temperature below the 1.5°C target set by the Paris Accord. The world faces a significant challenge in reaching such a goal, and each year reflects the global inaction from the previous years and decades. In fact, 2024 was the warmest year in 10,000 years, just as 2023 was the year before. In addition, 2024 was the first year the world surpassed the 1.5°C threshold.

So, what can be done for the world's children? The task is daunting, but the goal, by necessity, is reachable. Four major societal and economic sectors can play key roles in this effort.

23.3.1 *Energy Sector*

Unsurprisingly, this sector has the potential to be a substantial driver of global progress toward reducing carbon emissions and adopting cleaner technologies. First, the energy sector can drive the continued *transition to renewable energy sources*, like solar, wind, geothermal, hydropower, and nuclear, both fission and fusion. Fossil fuels are the largest contributor to global climate change, accounting for 75% of global greenhouse gas emissions and nearly

90% of all carbon dioxide emissions. Unfortunately, fossil fuels still account for 80% of global energy production (UN, 2024). It is imperative to halve emissions by 2030 and reach net-zero by 2050. Second, this sector can help protect the climate by ***developing improved carbon capture and storage (CCS)*** technologies. Though carbon capture is in its early stages of development, it is promising. As of 2024, there are fifteen CCS facilities operating in the United States with an additional 121 under construction or in development. Third, engineers, architects, and urban planners can collaborate to improve energy-efficient ***buildings and appliances.***

23.3.2 *Transportation Sector*

Globally, transportation remains largely dependent on fossil fuels. Coordinated industry-spanning efforts and policy can continue incentivizing and driving improvements in fuel efficiency and electrification across air, water, and land travel. These efforts can also involve the promotion of walking, cycling and use of public transportation, including through urban planning approaches like walkable cities initiatives (Southworth, 2005).

23.3.3 *Agriculture Sector*

The agriculture sector can reduce global methane and carbon dioxide emissions by supporting efforts to reduce the world's dependence on animal consumption and engaging in climate-sensitive industry reforms. Sustainable land management practices and regenerative approaches to farming and harvesting can reduce carbon emissions while promoting the sustainability of supplies and yielding social and economic benefits for local communities (e.g., Branca et al., 2013).

23.3.4 *Forestry Sector*

One of the most powerful adaptive systems built into our climate is the capture of carbon by the world's trees and other plants. These incredible organisms remove carbon dioxide from the atmosphere while increasing oxygen availability. Sustainably reforesting lands that were previously cleared marks a key investment in planetary health, though preservation of old-growth forests is much more efficient, of course. Afforestation—the deliberate introduction of trees to areas that have never or not recently had trees—can also help with the re-treeing of the world.

23.4 Major International Climate Treaties

There have been numerous climate treaties over the course of the last 30 years, since concerns about the impacts of the climate crisis began gaining global attention in the early 1990s. This section does not discuss all such

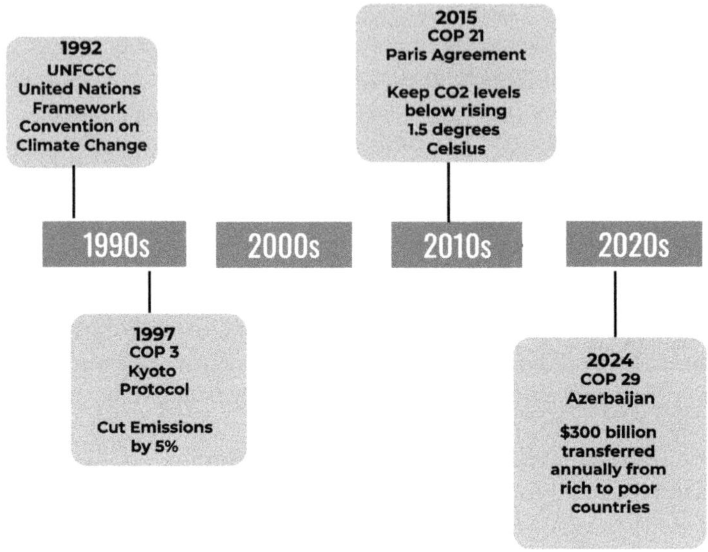

Figure 23.2 A timeline of major climate agreements.

agreements, but rather focuses on several of the major international accords. Despite widespread agreement across nations about the basic science of climate change, there is disagreement about who should be held morally and financially accountable for past, present, and future damages.

23.4.1 UN Framework Convention on Climate Change (UNFCCC)

The UNFCCC was introduced in 1992 and ratified by 197 countries, including the United States. It was the first global agreement to explicitly address climate change, and it set up the Conference of Parties (COP) that establishes the international gatherings that have occurred regularly since its ratification (CFR, 2023).

23.4.2 Kyoto Protocol

Though established in 1997, the Kyoto Protocol did not go into force until 2005. The first legally binding international agreement, Kyoto established a system to track countries' progress toward climate goals. In addition, Kyoto mandated that 37 industrialized nations, plus the European community, cut their greenhouse gas emissions by an average of 5% below 1990 levels (UN, 2022). The protocol only binds high-income countries, as these nations are largely responsible for the present state of climate change and greenhouse gases in the atmosphere.

Kyoto also established two market-based mechanisms to help achieve the 5% goal. First, emission trading allows countries that emit less greenhouse gasses to sell this credit to other industrialized countries that exceed the 5% target. Second, the clean development mechanism with joint implementation allows countries to invest and gain credit in emission-reducing projects.

23.4.3 Paris Agreement

The Paris Agreement was approved in 2015 and required all countries to set emission-reduction pledges. A system known as national determined contributions (NDCs) was established that set goals of preventing the global average temperature from rising 2°C/3.6°F and keeping global levels to below a 1.5°C/2.7°F elevation. It also set a standard of climate or carbon neutrality, where the amount of greenhouse gases emitted does not exceed the amount removed from the atmosphere (Savaresi, 2016). The United States, the world's second largest emitter, has been the only country to withdraw from the accord.

23.4.4 COP29 Azerbaijan

The 29th Conference of Parties (COP29) was held in Baku, Azerbaijan in 2024. At the conclusion of the conference, countries agreed to drastically reduce greenhouse gas emissions by 2035 and protect the world from the worsening impacts of climate change. Rich nations pledged to contribute at least $300 billion annually to the global fight against climate change. However, this was seen as insufficient and insulting by developing nations who bear the worst impacts of climate change. These nations had sought over $1 trillion in assistance (COP29). There was also conflict over who would finance these efforts.

23.5 Youth Voices from Around the World

Youth have increasingly demanded that adults take aggressive steps to safeguard the global climate, often calling out the international community for their inaction. One obvious example is that of Greta Thunberg of Sweden, who has helped mobilize youth to take immediate action on climate change. She first took individual action in her early teens by encouraging her family to reduce their carbon footprint. At the age of 15, she took her voice beyond the family and encouraged peers to skip school every Friday until Sweden was in compliance with the Paris Agreement. She went on to address the 2018 United Nations Climate Change conference. Her visibility on social media and her commitment has led her to become an ad hoc leader in the climate justice movement. The BBC and others have discussed the "Greta Effect," the profound impact of this young woman's ability to raise public awareness of climate change, especially among children, adolescents, and young adults (CBBC, 2020).

Case Study: Maguette Ba

Young people's climate activism is frequently marked by persistence and passion. It is also creative and multi-sector. Maguette Ba, a young Senegalese woman, uses her skills at storytelling to tell the world about the harsh realities of living with extreme weather events, with a special emphasis on women's and children's experiences. She also works to encourage education efforts that help communities care for and benefit from their resources in sustainable ways, while simultaneously working to improve corporations' responsibility to their surrounding communities (Kuwonu, 2024).

At 15, Ms. Ba took a class on climate change and its impacts that served as a turning point for her. She joined an environmental club at her high school and became involved in an ecological management project. This initiative, supported by partners such as the European Union, inspired other schools to adopt similar practices. The next step was to find ways to extend the effort beyond schools. She became a Youth Advocate for Senegal and the founder of Kèw Gi Agency, which is working to disseminate African models of environmental protection. Ms. Ba's mission is to protect natural resources, empower youth, and build solutions rooted in the needs and strengths of African communities.

Like Ms. Ba, many young activists are known for grounding their climate activism and engagement in the values and identities of their cultural communities. For example, the young crop scientist Aung Sing works directly with farmers in Bangladesh to help them improve the yield and sustainability of their farming. His status and insights as a member of the Indigenous Marma community help him to leverage shared spiritual beliefs in these conversations, and the messages that he shares are also sensitive to his community's experiences of marginalization within their broader nation (UN Global Climate Promise, 2023). Young climate activists are often using their voices globally, while keeping their feet planted in their own communities, allowing them to keep their strategies culturally and contextually specific to the lived realities of those around them.

A growing movement of young people use legal avenues to address climate change. A group of activists, including Ms. Thunberg, brought a landmark case before the European Court of Human Rights (ECHR), which agreed that Switzerland had violated the rights of older Swiss women for the lack of action in reducing carbon dioxide and other greenhouse gases. Another group of U.S. youth in Montana joined with Our Children's Trust, a nonprofit firm in the state, to bring a climate lawsuit setting a precedent that the state's citizens had the right to a clean and healthy environment. The lawsuit was begun in 2020 with a positive judgment in 2024. In 2018, children, youth, and adult partners sued the Colombian government for allowing deforestation of the Amazon rainforest. The court partially agreed and ordered the government to create and implement plans to reduce deforestation.

Several similar cases are pending. In Portugal, as of 2023, a small group of youth pleaded before the European Court of Human Rights that 32 European countries failed to act on climate change. In 2020, South Korean youth sued the government for failing to provide a specific plan to reduce greenhouse gases, violating their right to live and thrive in a clean environment. In December of 2024, 27 law students from Fiji brought a case before the International Court of Justice (ICJ) at the Hague, Netherlands, which was established in 1948 by the United Nations to, among other things, issue non-binding advisory opinions that clarify international law. These students, whose island is sinking as sea levels rise, are leading the largest climate case in history, and the largest case ever brought before the IJC, with 98 countries and 12 international NGOs participating (AP, 2024).

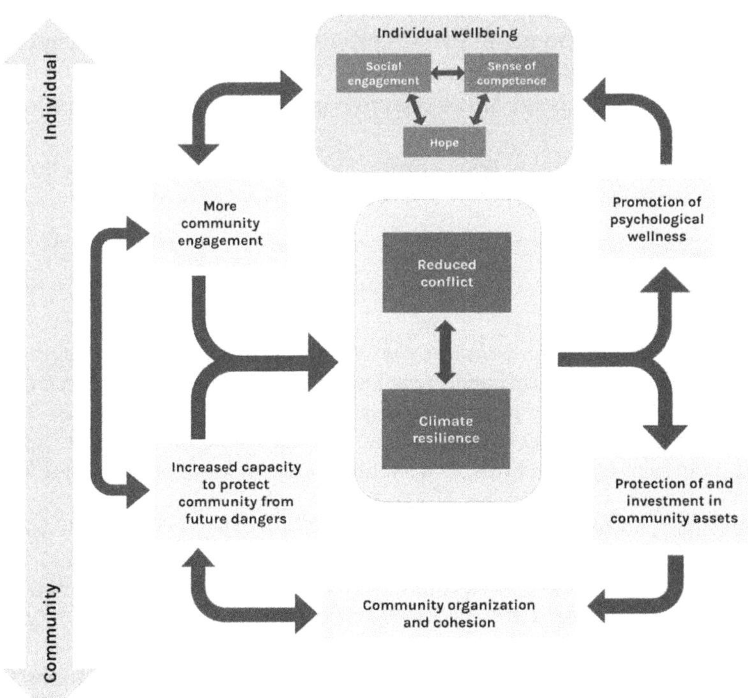

Figure 23.3 Climate resilience at the collective and individual levels.

23.6 Climate Resilience

As discussed, damage to environments and to the global climate relates bidirectionally to social adversities like armed conflict and interpersonal violence. Conversely, though, efforts to restore climate health have the potential to initiate cascades of wellbeing—not only for ecosystems and global weather patterns, but also for individuals and communities, as shown in Figure 23.3.

25.7 Conclusion

Due to adults' current and historic failure to prioritize the needs of children, the young people of today disproportionately bear the burden of climate injustice. Many are speaking out about this, using insights from their communities' lived experience to effect awareness and action around the globe. Meanwhile, several promising efforts in national politics, international collaboration, science, and industry have the potential to support climate adaptation and mitigation.

Reflection Questions

Question 1. Can you name two examples of climate adaptation and two examples of climate mitigation?
Question 2. What is the most effective messaging you have seen about climate justice?
Question 3. What helps your community take steps for climate justice? What makes it harder?

References

AP News (2024). *A landmark climate change case opens at the top UN court as island nations fear rising seas.* Associated Press, December 2. https://apnews.com/article/eu-world-court-icj-climate-global-warming-e954301f0258509f67e66ae2762da6f6

BBC (2020) Greta effect' sees young people making voices heard online says Ofcom report. February 4, 2020. https://www.bbc.co.uk/newsround/51358462

Branca, G., Lipper, L., McCarthy, N., & Jolejole, M. C. (2013). Food security, climate change, and sustainable land management. A review. *Agronomy for Sustainable Development*, *33*, 635–650. https://doi.org/10.1007/s13593-013-0133-1

CBBC (2020). "Greta Effect" sees young people making a voice heard online, according to an Ofcom report. *CBBC nNewsround*, February 4, 2020. https://www.bbc.co.uk/newsround/51358462

COP29 (2024). CoP29 concludes with climate fiancé deal. United Nations Climate Action. https://www.un.org/en/climatechange/cop29?gad_source=1&gbraid=0AAAAAD9kiAfXUgiUnBzXv-CyqnE0bQb4E&gclid=CjwKCAiA0rW

6BhAcEiwAQH28InYDrcQ8H7bHGyy3R6EP_wqEcf9Q05H97VYo48Cw2aKdf-h3vG1mdSBoCkf8QAvD_BwE

Council of Foreign Relations (CFR) (2023). *Global climate agreements: Successes and failures.* Council of Foreign Relations Backgrounder, December 5. https://www.cfr.org/backgrounder/paris-global-climate-change-agreements

ITS International (2012). *Success of Kuala Lumpur's dual purpose tunnel.* ITS International, September 12.

Kuwonu, F. (2024). Climate youth advocate making a difference. United Nations: Africa Renewal. https://africarenewal.un.org/en/magazine/climate-youth-advocate-making-difference

Mohammad, S. (2014). Malaysia country report. In F. Zen & M. Regan (Eds.), *Financing ASEAN connectivity* (pp.167–220). ERIA Research Project Report FY2013, No.15. ERIA.

Savaresi, A. (2016). The Paris agreement: A new beginning? *Journal of Energy & Natural Resources Law, 34*(1), 16–26. https://doi.org/10.1080/02646811.2016.1133983

Southworth, M. (2005). Designing the walkable city. *Journal of Urban Planning and Development, 131*(4), 246–257. https://doi.org/10.1061/(ASCE)0733-9488(2005)131:4(246)

(WNO, 2022). The world meteorological organization. WMO and the Early Warnings for All Initiative. 2022. WMO and the Early Warnings for All Initiative

UN (2022). Marking the Kyoto Protocol's 25th anniversary. United Nations Climate Action, December 11. https://www.un.org/en/climatechange/marking-kyoto-protocol's-25th-anniversary

UN (2024). *Renewable energy powering a safer future.* United Nations Climate Action. https://www.un.org/en/climatechange/raising-ambition/renewable-energy

UNEP (2020). Ecosystem-based Adaptation in Lao PDR. https://www.unep.org/ecosystem-based-adaptation-lao-pdr

UNEP (2022). 5 ways countries can adapt to the climate crisis. UN Environment Program. October 12. https://www.unep.org/news-and-stories/story/5-ways-countries-can-adapt-climate-crisis

UNEP (2024). What is Integrated Water Resource Management (IWRM). UN Environment Programme. https://www.unep.org/explore-topics/disasters-conflicts/where-we-work/sudan/what-integrated-water-resources-management

UN Global Climate Promise (2023). *These 4 young leaders from Asia and the Pacific region are at the forefront of climate action.* UNDP. https://climatepromise.undp.org/news-and-stories/these-4-young-leaders-asia-and-pacific-region-are-forefront-climate-action

VijayaVenkataRaman, S., Iniyan, S., & Goic, R. (2012). A review of climate change, mitigation and adaptation. *Renewable and Sustainable Energy Reviews, 16*, 879–897. ISSN 1364-0321, https://doi.org/10.1016/j.rser.2011.09.009

Epilogue

A Clarion Call for Hope, Hospitality, and Resilience

Congratulations! You have made it to the end of the book. Whether you have read the text from cover to cover, skimmed, or selected portions at random, we have a few thoughts to leave you with.

First, we appreciate that this book is a difficult read in many ways, for those who have directly experienced complex risks to development like those described in this text, as well as those just learning about some of these challenges. Part I is about the scope and scale of our century's complex, converging crises, which likely have already caused sadness, anxiety, and anger for many readers. Parts II and III describe some of the ways in which these crises of armed conflict, environmental disasters, and climate change can harm children as they develop.

The emotional, cognitive, and moral burden of these insights can lead us to despair and inaction. This state is an understandable response to overwhelming challenges. However, simply put, despair and inaction are not what children need. Therefore, woven throughout this book—and especially in its final part—is a subtle intervention with which we wanted to reach you. The intervention is *hope*. Each chapter concretely references the children who depend on adults for their daily needs, since hope needs humans at its center. In each corner of the text, you will find, too, opportunities to become unstuck from despair and inaction. For example, we have shared strategies known to protect children; evidence that simple interventions can make a difference for them; and stories of what is possible when adults collectively decide that children matter and are worth sacrificing for. We have also pointed out "doors" that readers from all walks of life, disciplines, and developmental stages may walk through in their search to improve children's lives, such as policy design, direct service, advocacy, caregiving, research, storytelling, and art. This book's resilience lens has hopefully made it clear, too, that children's wellbeing is bound up in the adaptive functioning of surrounding systems (Masten, 2020). In other words, the movement to protect children in the 21st century needs everyone, in every sector. It certainly needs you.

We have attempted throughout this book to positively articulate our visions for children's lives—in other words, that children are not simply protected from developmental damages, but reach levels of freedom, relatedness,

DOI: 10.4324/9781003488385-28

creativity, and joy we ourselves cannot currently imagine; that they get to build and participate in equitable, just communities that celebrate them for who they are. We, as authors, have promised each other to do something each day to maintain our hope that a better world is possible for children. This practice has helped us to stay both motivated and creative in our work. Perhaps you will consider doing the same with a friend.

Finally, allow us to articulate the ethical value at the core of this book: *hospitality*. This is the manner of a host who receives a guest with welcome and goodwill, the *virtue of a great soul that cares for the whole universe through the ties of humanity* (de Jaucourt, 1765). In an expanded definition, hospitality is the absolute fruit of good, an action—individual or collective—that magnifies the felt dignity of body and soul, while minimizing or reversing the power differential between giver and receiver (Hallie, 1981). It can be understood as the greatest virtue, an antidote to cruelty. What children need in the 21st century, we argue, is our hospitality, our eagerness to give the best of what we have—to give *better* than what we have—for the love of the small guests at the door.

References

de Jaucourt, chevalier Louis (1765). Hospitality. In Sophie Bourgault (trans.), *Encyclopédie ou Dictionnaire raisonné des sciences, des arts et des métiers* (vol. 8). The Encyclopedia of Diderot & d'Alembert Collaborative Translation Project, hdl:2027/spo.did2222.0002.761.

Hallie, P. (1981). From cruelty to goodness. *Hastings Center Report* (pp. 23–28).

Masten, A. S. (2021). Resilience of children in disasters: A multisystem perspective. *International Journal of Psychology*. https://onlinelibrary.wiley.com/doi/full/10.1002/ijop.12737

Index

Note: **Bold** page numbers refer to tables and *italic* page numbers refer to figures.

For Product Safety Concerns and Information please contact our EU
representative GPSR@taylorandfrancis.com
Taylor & Francis Verlag GmbH, Kaufingerstraße 24, 80331 München, Germany

www.ingramcontent.com/pod-product-compliance
Ingram Content Group UK Ltd.
Pitfield, Milton Keynes, MK11 3LW, UK
UKHW020152200926
475702UK00016B/2676

* 9 7 8 1 0 3 2 7 7 4 8 7 9 *